DR. HARRIOT
KEZIA HUNT

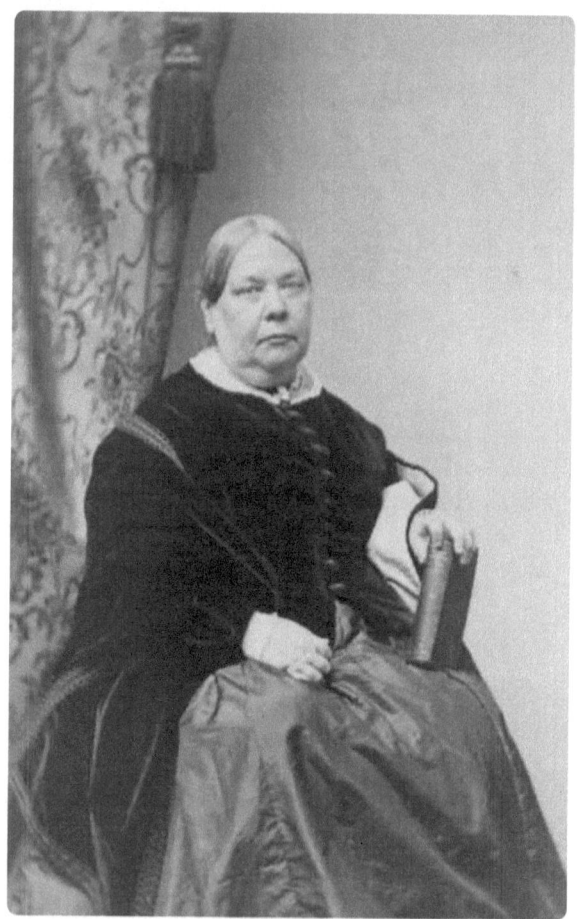

Undated Portrait of Harriot Kezia Hunt.
—*Schlesinger Library, Radcliffe Institute, Harvard University.*

DR. HARRIOT KEZIA HUNT

NINETEENTH-CENTURY PHYSICIAN AND WOMAN'S RIGHTS ADVOCATE

MYRA C. GLENN

UNIVERSITY OF MASSACHUSETTS PRESS
Amherst and Boston

Copyright © 2018 by University of Massachusetts Press
All rights reserved
Printed in the United States of America

ISBN 978-1-62534-376-5 (paper); 375-8 (hardcover)

Designed by Sally Nichols
Set in Minion Pro and Open Sans
Printed and bound by Maple Press, Inc.

Cover design by Milenda Nan Ok Lee
Cover art: *Hygieia, goddess of health, holding a pentangle and a staff encircled by a snake.*
Engraving by Théodore Galle, c. 1600.
CC BY, courtesy Wellcome Collection.

Library of Congress Cataloging-in-Publication Data
Names: Glenn, Myra C., author.
Title: Dr. Harriot Kezia Hunt : nineteenth-century physician and woman's rights advocate / Myra C. Glenn.
Description: Amherst : University of Massachusetts Press, [2018] | Includes bibliographical references and index. |
Identifiers: LCCN 2018019144 (print) | LCCN 2018047287 (ebook) | ISBN 9781613766224 (e-book) | ISBN 9781613766231 (e-book) | ISBN 9781625343765 | ISBN 9781625343765?(pbk.) | ISBN 9781625343758?(hardcover)
Subjects: LCSH: Hunt, Harriot Kezia, 1805–1875. | Women physicians—Massachusetts—Boston—19th century—Biography. | Women's rights—United States—History—19th century.
Classification: LCC R154.H8 (ebook) | LCC R154.H8 A28 2018 (print) | DDC 305.43/61092 [B] —dc23
LC record available at https://lccn.loc.gov/2018019144

British Library Cataloguing-in-Publication Data
A catalog record for this book is available from the British Library.

Portions of chapters 2, 3, and 4 were previously published in
"Women's Struggles to Practice Medicine in Antebellum America: The Troubled Career of Boston Physician Harriot Kezia Hunt," *New England Quarterly* 90, no. 2 (June 2017): 223–251.

For David, steadfast friend,
incisive critic,
and beloved husband.

Contents

Author's Note on the Text ix

Preface xi

Acknowledgments xiii

Introduction 1

CHAPTER 1
The Making of a Maverick
Harriot Hunt's Early Years 7

CHAPTER 2
Establishing a Medical Career 25

CHAPTER 3
Coping with Family Tragedy and Professional Rejection
during the 1840s 45

CHAPTER 4
Battling Harvard Medical School,
Becoming a Woman's Rights Activist 69

CHAPTER 5
Seeking Political Power, Gender Equality,
and Female Friendship 90

CHAPTER 6
Forging New Connections in the Mid-1850s
*Hunt's Involvement with Abolitionists,
Western Feminists, and Female Doctors* 113

CHAPTER 7
Glances and Glimpses—Harriot Hunt's "Heart History,"
Jeremiad, and Reform Manifesto 136

CHAPTER 8
Confronting War, Old Age, and Other Challenges 165

Note on Digitized Nineteenth-Century
Newspapers and Journals 189

Notes 191

Index 219

Author's Note on Text

When I cite Harriot Kezia Hunt's autobiography, *Glances and Glimpses; Or Fifty Years Social, Including Twenty Years Professional Life* (Boston: John P. Jewett and Company, 1856), I will use the abbreviated title *Glances and Glimpses*. When I quote from this book I will cite the pages parenthetically.

Preface

Years ago, while investigating the autobiographical narratives of antebellum women, I was struck by how few of these existed in comparison with the numerous works by men. Most female memoirs were brief and episodic. But then I stumbled on *Glances and Glimpses*, Harriot Kezia Hunt's richly detailed 1856 autobiography. At the time I had no idea who Hunt was. Although little remembered now, even by professional historians, Hunt was a prominent woman in nineteenth-century America. She was a pioneering female physician, well established in her medical practice in Boston by the time Elizabeth Blackwell, the first licensed female physician in the United States, graduated from Geneva Medical College in 1849. By the 1850s Hunt enjoyed a national reputation as a health reformer and woman's rights advocate. She was especially noted for her annual protests demanding woman's right to the suffrage and for her speeches at national woman's rights conventions.

As I began researching different sources, including institutional records and newspaper accounts about Hunt's activities, I realized that she merited a full-length biography. *Glances and Glimpses* also deserved extensive analysis not only as the major historical document describing Hunt's life but also as a multivalent literary and political text. So I had several purposes in writing this book. It is the first biography of a prominent professional woman and reformer in nineteenth-century America, one whose life illuminated how seemingly disparate issues, especially the transformation of American medicine, the impetus for health reform, and the struggle for woman's rights, intersected. My book is also an analysis of how Hunt used the genre of autobiography to promote her reformist agenda in medicine and woman's rights and to craft a public persona for herself, one that burnished her reputation, lambasted her critics, and challenged prescribed gender roles in mid-nineteenth-century America.

Acknowledgments

Four historians offered me invaluable help. Tamara Thornton and Lisa Francavilla read drafts of several chapters that explored Hunt's life. Patricia Cline Cohen perused my initial discussion of Hunt's autobiography, *Glances and Glimpses*. Beth Salerno gamely read the first six chapters of this book in their earliest form. These scholars' incisive comments encouraged me to think more critically about my work and to dig deeper in the archives. Their friendship and support nurtured me during the years I spent investigating Hunt's life and work.

Numerous archivists, librarians, and their supporting staff have helped me with my research, especially when they sent me copies of various documents from their repositories. Particular thanks to Robin Carlaw at the Harvard University Archives; Jack Eckert at the Francis A. Countway Library of Medicine, Harvard Medical School; Christian Goodwillie at the Daniel Burke Library, Hamilton College; Ann K. Sindelar at the Cleveland History Center of the Western Reserve Historical Society; Jeanne Solensky at the Winterthur Museum; Karen V. Kukil at the William Allan Neilson Library, Smith College; Crosby Diana Enright at the Library of Congress; Sabina Beauchard at the Massachusetts Historical Society; Charles Daniello and Mary Soom at the Lockwood Library, State University of New York at Buffalo; and Kathleen Gale at the Gannett Tripp Library, Elmira College. Thanks also to the staffs of the William L. Clements Library, University of Michigan; the Arthur and Elizabeth Schlesinger Library on the History of Women in America, Radcliffe Institute for Advanced Study, Harvard University; the Boston Public Library, especially the Microtext Department; the Ohio Historical Society; and the College of Medicine, Archives & Special Collections, Drexel University.

The anonymous readers and staff of the University of Massachusetts Press offered constructive criticism and encouragement. I also thank Jennifer Spanier for her work on the index. Thanks go as well to the *New England Quarterly* for publishing my article, "Women's Struggles to Practice Medicine in Antebellum America: The Troubled Career of Boston Physician Harriot Kezia Hunt," in its June 2017 issue.

I am also grateful to Justin Frank DeFreitas, a descendant of the Hunt family, for sending me excerpts from the unpublished journal of Harriot Hunt's nephew Edmund Wentworth Wright that discuss his "Aunty." Historian Susan Porter conversed with me about her research on Elizabeth Mott and provided me with several references on her. Friends and colleagues listened patiently while I talked at length about Harriot Hunt. Particular thanks to Beth Mattingly, Cynthia Smith, and Mary Jo Mahoney. As always, I have relied on the support and love of my husband, David.

DR. HARRIOT KEZIA HUNT

Introduction

When Harriot Kezia Hunt of Boston, Massachusetts, died in early January 1875 at the age of sixty-nine, area newspapers remembered her as a noted female physician and woman's rights advocate. The *Boston Daily Advertiser*, for example, praised her as "one of the pioneers in female medical practice" who established "an excellent reputation" among her female patients. It also stressed that Hunt achieved national renown for her annual protests against forcing women to pay taxes when they could not vote.[1] Leading nineteenth-century feminists also paid tribute to Hunt. At an 1875 woman's rights convention Elizabeth Cady Stanton mourned Hunt's death and portrayed her as the first woman doctor and also one of the "most steadfast advocates of woman suffrage."[2] When the first volume of the now classic work *History of Woman Suffrage* appeared in 1881, Stanton and the other authors honored Hunt by including her in the list of women activists to whom they dedicated their book. Hunt's name appeared with those of Mary Wollstonecraft, Lucretia Mott, Margaret Fuller, and other founding mothers of modern feminism.[3]

Hunt merited such tribute for many reasons. She was the first woman to establish a successful medical practice in the United States.[4] Although denied the opportunity to earn a medical degree, Hunt had begun treating patients, women and children, in Boston in 1835. By the time Elizabeth Blackwell, the first female licensed doctor in the United States, earned her degree at Geneva Medical College in 1849, Hunt already had a flourishing medical practice. Convinced that many of her patients' physical maladies were rooted in their spiritual and mental anguish, Hunt became renowned for listening to women's troubles, or "heart histories," and counseling them.[5]

Hunt was also the first woman to formally demand admission into Harvard's medical school. Her first petition to attend lectures at the school occurred in 1847 and met with a quick refusal. Yet in 1850 Harvard did accede to Hunt's second application. But various issues, including the request of three male students of color to attend medical lectures and the remonstrations of Harvard medical students, all of whom were white men, caused the faculty to regret its initial acceptance of Hunt and to privately urge her not to attend their institution.[6]

In the early 1850s Hunt emerged as a leading woman's rights advocate. She became the first woman in Massachusetts to publicly protest the injustice of taxing propertied women like herself while denying them the right to vote. Her annual petitions declaring "no taxation without representation" were widely reprinted in newspapers throughout the Northeast and Midwest.[7] Hunt was also prominent in the annual woman's rights conventions of the 1850s where she championed health reform, female doctors, higher education for women, and their enfranchisement.[8]

Hunt played a pivotal role in forging institutions that educated women and mobilized them on behalf of various reform causes. In 1843, for example, she helped establish the Ladies' Physiological Institute, an organization that instructed women about the human body and how to keep it healthy. Hunt spoke repeatedly at the institute and served as its president during the years 1856 and 1857.[9] In 1868 she was one of the founders of the New England Women's Club, soon renowned for numerous civic projects and reforms, including demands for female suffrage.[10]

Hunt also gained funding for impecunious women to study medicine, nurtured their careers, and helped create hospitals that trained female doctors and ministered to women patients. One of the students Hunt aided was the German immigrant Marie Zakrzewska, a leading American female physician in the latter part of the nineteenth century. Hunt enabled Zakrzewska to finance her studies at the Cleveland Medical College. She also advocated for Zakrzewska and Elizabeth Blackwell when they began planning the New York Infirmary for Women and Children. Established in 1857, this hospital was the first in the United States to be completely staffed by women. Finally, Hunt supported the pioneering New England Hospital for Women and Children, founded by Zakrzewska in 1862.[11]

Another one of Hunt's major achievements was her 1856 autobiography entitled *Glances and Glimpses*. At a time when few women wrote life narratives

Hunt offered a richly detailed and revealing work. Her text was the first autobiography published by a leading antebellum feminist and also by a female physician. Analysis of *Glances and Glimpses* elucidates the public personas or identities that Hunt constructed for herself. These included that of the loving, dutiful daughter and sister, the dedicated and innovative doctor and health reformer, the committed political activist and defender of woman's rights, and the lonely spinster who sacrificed herself for the cause of humanity.

Harriot Hunt was a remarkable woman who forged multiple careers for herself. Leading nineteenth-century feminists predicted that she would be "long remembered" for her pioneering efforts in medicine and woman's rights.[12] Yet Hunt is mostly forgotten today. Part of the reason for this is that few of her letters have survived. Hunt also ordered the destruction of her patients' records. But her fate is sadly that of many women and minorities who have been marginalized and at times even erased from the historical record.

Scholars exploring the development of antebellum medicine and health reform have discussed Hunt's medical career in the context of examining the role of women physicians in nineteenth-century medicine.[13] In recent years the way that Hunt wrote about medicine, especially in her autobiography, has snagged the interest of those studying nineteenth-century literature and rhetoric.[14] Although these writers have contributed to our understanding of Hunt, they have folded her story into a larger one about either the study of medical literature or the emergence of female physicians in nineteenth-century America. Many have also accepted *Glances and Glimpses* at face value and not mined other sources to explore Hunt's life.

Dr. Harriot Kezia Hunt is the first biography of this exceptional individual and utilizes a wide range of documents to investigate her life and work. These sources include Hunt's last will and testament, her annual protests against "taxation without representation," her speeches at national woman's rights conventions, newspaper editorials and articles about Hunt's myriad activities, and various institutional records, especially those of the Harvard Medical School, the Ladies' Physiological Institute, and the Shaker settlements that Hunt regularly visited. Letters written to and from Hunt, including the numerous ones that Hunt's dear friend, the noted abolitionist and pioneering feminist Sarah Grimké, wrote to her, as well as the unpublished journal of her nephew Edmund Wentworth Wright offer insight into Hunt's private life.

Harriot Hunt offers a rare, fascinating case study of how a single woman from a working-class Boston home became a successful professional and renowned reformer in nineteenth-century America. Recent excellent biographies of Lucy

Stone, Dr. Mary Putnam Jacobi, and Dr. Marie Zakrzewska highlight the importance of investigating noted nineteenth-century feminists and female physicians.[15] *Dr. Harriot Kezia Hunt* examines a person who was both a pioneering woman doctor *and* prominent feminist in antebellum America. Hunt's activism in various endeavors, especially her establishment of an innovative medical practice and campaigns on behalf of health reform, female suffrage, and education, illuminates how these multiple issues resonated with one another and often intersected in the nineteenth century. Hunt's life also illustrates how personal crises served as a springboard to professional advancement and reform activism for nineteenth-century women. Finally, Hunt's experiences with Harvard elucidate how the politics of gender and race as well as concerns about professionalism and student retention shaped antebellum efforts to admit women to medical schools.

The first six chapters of this book examine Hunt's life until 1856, the year *Glances and Glimpses* appeared. Chapter 1 discusses Hunt's childhood and youth in the dynamic but unstable maritime world of Boston's North End during the early nineteenth century. It also considers how the Hunt family's allegiance to Universalism and the Masons nurtured their commitment to female education and reform activism. Chapter 2 explores how Harriot and her younger sister, Sarah, navigated the vibrant, fractious world of medicine in Boston during the latter 1830s to establish their medical practice. It also investigates how Harriot's focus on her patients' "heart histories" heightened her sensitivity to Boston's gender and class divisions. Chapter 3 examines various familial, religious, and professional challenges Harriot Hunt faced during the 1840s. These included Sarah's marriage and her decision to leave the Hunt medical practice, the deaths of Harriot's beloved niece and mother, Harvard Medical School's rejection of her first petition to attend lectures there, and her temporary breakdown in 1849. Discussion of how Hunt responded to each crisis shows her resiliency and commitment to both medicine and reform. Chapter 3 also explores how Hunt's involvement with the Shakers and her conversion to the ideas of the Swedish philosopher and mystic Emanuel Swedenborg helped anchor her life after professional setbacks and family deaths. Analysis of Hunt's emotionally intense friendships with other women, particularly Sarah Grimké, shows the complexity of female relationships in nineteenth-century America.

Chapters 4, 5, and 6 focus on an especially rich and busy decade in Hunt's life, the 1850s. During this time Hunt became a nationally renowned figure in health reform and the woman's rights struggle. She also participated in the temperance and abolitionist movements. Analysis of her involvement in these disparate reforms highlights how they resonated with each other. Hunt also created a wide reform network that nurtured her both professionally and personally.

These three chapters discuss specific incidents in Hunt's life as a way to elucidate different issues in antebellum America. Study of Hunt's second failed attempt to attend lectures at the Harvard Medical School in November 1850, for example, illuminates how entwined racial and gender discrimination were at this institution. Discussions of Hunt's annual public protests against "taxation without representation" highlight how contested were notions of citizenship and voting during the antebellum era. These chapters also explore paradoxes in Hunt's life. Chapter six, for example, investigates how the growing professionalization of medicine and Hunt's persistent commitment to a "mind-cure" approach to healing at times distanced her from the younger generation of licensed female physicians she nurtured.

Chapter 7 analyzes Hunt's autobiography primarily as a literary and political text. *Glances and Glimpses* was in the vanguard of life narratives produced by pioneering woman's rights advocates. The few antebellum feminists who published their autobiographies generally did not do so until years after the Civil War. *Dr. Harriot Kezia Hunt* discusses why Hunt chose to produce her book while she was still at the height of her activism. It also considers another unusual feature of her text—its repeated and pointed expressions of anger against patriarchal power. While examining this theme *Dr. Harriot Kezia Hunt* explores how antebellum debates over gender, citizenship, medicine, and politics shaped Hunt's autobiography. As noted earlier, this book also discusses the various public personas that Hunt constructed for herself to gain her readers' respect and sympathy. In addressing these issues, chapter 7 contextualizes *Glances and Glimpses* by exploring how its ideas and language built on earlier texts produced by leading antebellum feminists and other women.

Chapter 8 examines the last quarter of Hunt's life with respect to numerous topics, including the elaborate celebration of her twenty-five years in medicine, Hunt's ambivalence about the Civil War and Reconstruction, her continued involvement in the woman's rights movement, and her efforts to shape her legacy through her detailed will. Chapter 8 also explores how Hunt forged closer relationships with female reformers who came of age during the latter part of the nineteenth century, especially Ednah Dow Cheney, Caroline Severance, and Caroline Dall.

Dr. Harriot Kezia Hunt contributes to different historiographies, particularly those of antebellum medicine, health reform, woman's rights, and liberal

Protestantism. It also enriches and complicates our understanding of women's life narratives during the nineteenth century by viewing *Glances and Glimpses* as a multivalent text. But, ultimately, the major purpose of *Dr. Harriot Kezia Hunt* is to tell the story of a fascinating, complicated woman who despite her many contributions remains little known in contemporary America.

Chapter 1

The Making of a Maverick

Harriot Hunt's Early Years

On November 9, 1805, thirty-five-year-old Kezia Wentworth Hunt achieved a long-desired goal—motherhood. After fourteen years of marriage to thirty-six-year-old Joab Hunt, a Boston shipwright and joiner, Kezia gave birth to her first daughter. The family named her Harriot Kezia Hunt (1).[1] The difficult birth had both Kezia's family and neighbors worried. When Harriot was born after three days of labor, she seemed to be a stillborn. Fortunately, Kezia's oldest sister massaged Harriot until she let out a yelp (6). Three years later on December 25, 1808, the Hunts welcomed their second and last child, another daughter named Sarah (9).[2]

What kind of family were the Hunts? What was their world like in early nineteenth-century Boston? To what extent did they nurture Harriot's careers in medicine and reform? How did she remember her childhood? Exploration of these questions illuminates how Harriot Hunt came of age in a rapidly changing society, one where life was precarious for working-class families like hers.

Hunt offered an idyllic portrait of her childhood home in *Glances and Glimpses*. She gushed that it "might truly have been called 'The Great Joy'" because there was so much love and "oneness in spirit" in her "happy elevated home." Her parents, she stressed, were wise, gentle, and nurturing. Kezia was allegedly a paragon of Christian virtue, domesticity, and love; Joab was a "bright, glad, witty man" who practiced a "genial benevolence" toward others; and Sarah was a beloved sister (40, v, 2, 9).

Although the Hunt family was probably not as ideal as Harriot depicted in her autobiography, her recollections highlighted several key facts about them. First, Harriot stressed that her father was "entirely 'a North-Ender'" (2). In early nineteenth-century Boston, this meant that he lived in a maritime community.[3] Harriot noted that in his youth her father had wanted to be a sailor but gave up this goal owing to his family's opposition. Yet many of his friends were sea captains (2–3). Of course Joab's occupations as shipwright and joiner meant that his living depended on Boston's seafaring trade.

After Sarah's birth the family moved from Lynn Street, an area increasingly dominated by commercial establishments, to Fleet Street, which had more individual residences (11).[4] By the early nineteenth century, however, the North End had begun to decline as a neighborhood. It increasingly became a place from which residents, especially those with families, moved to more fashionable parts of the city. In the 1840s the North End would be noted for its dance halls, brothels, gaming dens, taverns, and cheap boardinghouses. It would also have the dubious distinction of having the city's highest crime rate, an area where burglaries and assaults were common. Some of Boston's earliest tenements, domiciles that unfortunately promoted the spread of deadly epidemics such as tuberculosis and smallpox, were also in the North End.[5]

But Harriot Hunt remembered the neighborhood in which she grew up as a wonderful place, whose homes had "nice little gardens in the rear" and "verdant grass plots in the front." The North End also featured "a pleasant neighborhood of children" with whom she played and went to school. As a child Hunt also saw the mansions where "opulent" North End merchants and political leaders, such as Governor Thomas Hutchinson, used to live. These homes were still "elegant" if "old-fashioned" (11–12).

Early morning walks with her father deepened Hunt's appreciation for the North End (14). Joab used these occasions to educate as well as entertain his daughter. His stories about the overseas adventures of his seafaring friends as well as Harriot's own reading of "ship-news" in area papers made her realize that there was a large, diverse world outside of Boston, one that merited study and understanding (3).

Joab Hunt loved Boston's North End neighborhood and its maritime world. Although at times he scrambled to earn a living, his skills as a repairer and builder of ships often enabled him to prosper. In 1802, for example, he earned the handsome sum of $178.94 for helping repair the French corvette *Le Berceau*,[6] presumably one of the eighty-two privateers the United States Navy captured during its Quasi-War with France from 1798 to 1801.[7] By his midthirties Hunt was a man of property, owning a place of business on Merry's Wharf as well as his own home.[8] In 1803 Hunt advertised to sell or rent a house having eight acres of land in a nearby township.[9]

A dutiful citizen, Joab Hunt participated from an early age in different civic and charitable activities. At the age of twenty he was "Captain of Engine No. II," and in the spring of 1816 he was chosen to be a vote distributor from ward number two.[10] In 1822 he was one of the organizers of the Associated Housewrights in Boston, designed to assist impoverished mechanics and their families.[11] Hunt also served as one of the trustees of the Massachusetts Charitable Mechanic Association, an organization that sponsored various educational and civic activities and nurtured the development of a "middling-class consciousness" among its members, many of whom were artisans like Hunt.[12]

But Joab's most important public activity was belonging to the Freemasons, an international secret fraternity first established in early eighteenth-century Europe. The Masons, especially in the United States, saw themselves as a band of brothers committed to nonsectarian Christian values, science, and philanthropy. Loyalty to fellow members and a pledge on pain of death never to reveal the secret rituals and ceremonies of their organization also characterized the Masons. The fact that many of the nation's founding fathers, including George Washington and Benjamin Franklin, were Masons, as were many of the political and economic elites of various urban areas, heightened the fraternity's prestige and influence.[13]

Yet a man did not have to be part of the elite to be accepted into the Masons. Boston's St. Andrew's Lodge, which initiated Joab Hunt in 1795 and where he remained for the rest of his life, was comprised primarily of artisans and small retailers from the North End rather than "gentlemen."[14] Neither rich nor destitute, the St. Andrew Masons belonged to a "middling" group. Many of these men were ambitious, upwardly mobile, skilled laborers committed to bettering themselves as well as their city and nation. The most famous member of St. Andrews Lodge was not a wealthy, college-educated gentleman but Paul Revere, the artisan and Revolutionary hero.[15]

Like all Masons, the members of St. Andrew's Lodge sought to promote a "school of moral virtue" throughout their society.[16] But the modest socioeconomic status of these men must also have made them especially responsive to one of Masonry's key tenets: a pledge to promote the advancement of their members and to provide them financial and other assistance in hard times.

Ultimately the Masonic fraternity offered its members a way to forge bonds of community in a world increasingly characterized by an expansive, volatile market economy. It promised not only to promote its members' welfare but also to offer them a buffer or haven from the onslaught of class divisions and fierce competition that was rapidly eroding the traditional order of New England.[17]

Joab Hunt and his fellow Masons in St. Andrew's Lodge would need all the help they could get to weather numerous developments that roiled their city and nation during the early nineteenth century. The titanic struggle between Great Britain and France which began in the late eighteenth century and continued until Napoleon's defeat in 1815 caught maritime workers such as Hunt in the maw of global war, economic depression, and partisan politics. The Embargo Act of 1807, designed to prevent war with Great Britain by prohibiting American vessels from sailing to a foreign port, devastated New England's maritime economy. When war did come in 1812, it hammered New England's economy, especially when the British Navy blockaded Boston and other ports. American seafaring trade and shipbuilding ground almost to a halt. Exports plummeted from $61 million in 1811 to $7 million in 1814; imports declined during the same period from $53 million to $13 million.[18] As ships rotted in port and destitution increased, the political mood in New England soured. Late in 1814 at their Hartford Convention, the Federalists even flirted with the idea of secession. The disgruntled remarks of one Massachusetts Federalist perhaps best captured the bitterness of his region when he groused: "We are in a deplorable situation, our commerce dead; our revenue gone; our ships rotting at the wharves . . . Our treasury drained—we are bankrupts [sic]."[19]

New Englanders were understandably jubilant when the War of 1812 ended. The Hunt family shared in this joy. Harriot recounted that her family was awakened by "the ringing of bells and the firing of guns" when "the joyful news of peace" reached Boston in early January 1815. Like so many of their fellow Americans, the Hunts took to the streets that evening to celebrate with fireworks their nation's victory over John Bull (22–23).

If Bostonians living in the North End hoped for good economic times in the postwar period they were soon disappointed. According to historian Samuel Eliot Morison, "the first few years of peace were the severest test that maritime Massachusetts had ever met" for several reasons, including Britain's initial refusal to allow American vessels into its colonial ports.[20] Even when Boston's maritime economy began to rebound after several years, it faced new challenges. First, this economy lost ground as the port of New York increasingly dominated the major routes of international shipping and also trade with the southern states. The completion of the Erie Canal in 1825 cemented New York's preeminence by making it the entrepôt for the lucrative trade with the western interior.[21] This latter development highlighted another major challenge for Boston's mercantile community in the early Republic—the development of a market revolution shifted the nation's economic center to the West and the South and also to the early manufacturing hubs found in New England and New York. Various developments promoted this change, including improvements in transportation and mass communications, a more commercialized agriculture, the manufacturing of shoes, textiles, and other commodities, the cotton boom, and westward expansion.[22] The rise of manufacturing with its de-skilling of labor hurt both the status and the income of artisans in such cities as Boston.[23] It also exacerbated class divisions as many artisans became struggling wage earners while the mercantile elite grew richer as it invested in manufacturing. The shift in Massachusetts's economy "from wharf to waterfall," therefore, often came at the expense of workers who lived in Boston's North End.[24]

The Panic of 1819, which lasted for years, also hurt many Bostonians. By 1820 thousands of banks and businesses throughout the United States had failed, creating widespread unemployment, especially in urban areas such as Boston.[25] Countless destitute Americans, unable to pay their debts, suffered imprisonment. In 1820, for example, over 1,440 debtors were jailed in Boston alone.[26]

Many working-class Bostonians mobilized politically to demand relief. In 1820 printer Joseph T. Buckingham organized a protest movement called the "Middling Interest" that attracted many fellow artisans and other working-class people. They demanded a new kind of politics, one responsive to the mass of voters, many of whom felt oppressed by an entrenched political elite catering to the interests of wealthier residents. To achieve their goals, Buckingham and his supporters demanded an end to imprisonment for debt, compulsory militia service, and property qualifications for voting. They also urged the disestablishment of the Congregational Church. Their popularity in the early 1820s highlighted how hard times challenged the established political order in Boston.[27] The politics of earlier decades, based on people deferring to their alleged "betters," gave way to a more populist and democratic politics where voters mobilized to address their class interests.[28]

The erosion of deferential politics also reflected Boston's rapid growth in the first few decades of the nineteenth century. A city that had a little over 18,000 people in 1790 had grown to over 61,000 by 1830.[29] Boston's incorporation as a city in 1822 reflected not only its rapid growth but also the fact that it was becoming a more diverse society fractured by all sorts of divisions.[30] One of these was ethnic divisions caused by the influx of immigrants from different parts of Europe, but particularly from Ireland. Although the potato famine, precipitating a huge exodus from Ireland, did not occur until 1845, growing numbers of Irish began arriving to America during the 1820s. One of the cities to which they immigrated was Boston. There were approximately 2,000 Irish in Boston in 1820, 5,000 in 1825, and 7,000 in 1830.[31] Willing to work for low wages, these immigrants often offered competition to Anglo-American workers already facing a tight job market.

The hard times many working-class families faced in 1820s Boston offer another vantage point from which to view the charitable activities of Joab Hunt. Committed to helping his fellow artisans, especially if they were Masons, he sought to alleviate their plight during the economic downturn. Although there is no proof that Joab Hunt belonged to the Middling Interest movement, he may well have. Like Hunt, Buckingham was an artisan committed to defending what he saw as the imperiled interests of this group in a rapidly changing society. Like Hunt, he was also a Mason and in fact in 1817 began publishing the *New England Galaxy and Freemason's Weekly*.[32] Finally, like Hunt, Buckingham was a leading member of the Massachusetts Charitable Mechanic Association, the organization for which Hunt had served as a trustee.[33] So it is likely that the two men crossed paths in Boston and that Buckingham's political message resonated with Hunt.

But irrespective of Joab Hunt's political affiliation, the fact remains that as major changes roiled his community, he valued the fellowship offered by St. Andrew's Lodge with its preponderance of North End skilled workmen like himself. What seems to have particularly attracted Hunt about the Masons was not its penchant for elaborate, secret ceremonies and initiations but rather its good works. One of Hunt's Masonic brethren recalled that he was not a man who "took any active part" in their lodge's rituals, but Joab Hunt readily volunteered for civic or charitable projects designed to help those buffeted by hard times.[34]

Part of Hunt's commitment to helping others stemmed from his religion. Although he was raised a Congregationalist and Kezia was initially an Episcopalian, they were committed Universalists by the time Harriot was born in 1805 (4–5). Asserting that salvation was possible for all, even unbelievers, Universalists challenged the use of public taxes to support established churches, including the Congregational Church in Massachusetts. Even before the first American Universalist society appeared in Gloucester, Massachusetts, in 1781, polemicists, pamphleteers, newspaper editors, and leading orthodox clergymen excoriated Universalism as heretical, atheistic, and immoral. Yet despite these denunciations, this faith spread throughout America. By 1820 Universalists had approximately two hundred churches and societies. New England, especially Boston, was the area where Universalism attracted its widest support.[35]

Much of the credit for Universalism's success goes to John Murray, an Englishman who introduced this faith to America and became the friend of as well as pastor to the Hunt family during his long ministry of Boston's Universalist Church from 1793 until his death in 1815.[36] Joab Hunt "zealously" embraced Universalism after listening to Murray's dynamic sermons (4). Yet Kezia Hunt initially resisted Murray's ideas and even refused to enter the Universalist church that her husband attended. But Murray was a persistent as well as effective minister. He repeatedly visited the Hunt home and patiently answered Kezia's many scriptural objections to Universalism; he debated theological issues with her. Finally, after a number of meetings with Murray, Kezia Hunt converted to Universalism. Her eldest daughter noted that her mother then became even more devout than her father in her new faith (5).

The conversion of Kezia and Joab Hunt to Universalism liberated them from the Calvinist orthodoxy that still permeated much of New England in the early Republic. It led them to embrace a liberal Protestantism that stressed aiding one's fellow human beings as the essence of genuine Christianity. This belief fueled Universalists' involvement in various reforms, including the temperance, peace, and anti–capital punishment movements.[37] Most Universalists also opposed slavery, although they generally did not support abolitionists owing to their vitriolic denunciations of slaveholders as sinners facing eternal damnation. The fact that many evangelical abolitionists condemned Universalists as "near infidels" also antagonized members of this church.[38]

Universalists, however, were active in the antebellum labor movement. Their ministers in the working-class neighborhood of Southwark, Philadelphia, for example, allowed labor activists to conduct meetings in their churches.[39] Many Universalists were also Masons. In fact their clergy were often high-ranking Masons. One of these was the Reverend Hosea Ballou, the leading Universalist theologian who served as pastor of the Second Universalist Church in Boston from December 1817 until his death in June 1852.[40] Among the parishioners he befriended was the Hunt family (61). The prominence of Universalists in the Masonic movement reflected the resonance between these two organizations. Both Universalists and Masons believed in a benevolent God who offered salvation to all; they also rejected sectarian, evangelical churches and stressed the improvement of the human race through good works.

Another common thread that united Masons and Universalists was their commitment to educating all people, including women. In the early Republic this remained a controversial idea. Many Americans feared that educating women would "unsex" them and make them more masculine. The belief that most women were not as rational or analytic as men convinced many that schooling females was a waste of money and effort. Others argued that education hindered women from fulfilling their "natural" roles as mothers and homemakers.[41]

Yet postrevolutionary America saw a sea change in attitudes about female education. The idea of "republican motherhood" urged the education of women so that they could better cultivate civic virtue in their children, especially their sons, and thereby ensure the success of the newly created Republic.[42] This ideology promoted the establishment of numerous female academies starting in the 1790s and gaining momentum throughout the first half of the nineteenth century. Although many of these schools focused on teaching their female pupils social graces and ornamental arts, some, such as Emma Willard's Troy Female Seminary and Mary Lyon's Mount Holyoke Seminary, offered a rigorous academic curriculum.[43]

One of the nation's strongest proponents for female education in the early Republic was Murray's second wife, whom he married in 1788 after his first wife and only child had died. Judith Sargent Murray was the widow of a Gloucester merchant and already a Universalist before she met Murray. She defied the conventions of her day not only by embracing a controversial faith and marrying its founder but also by becoming a published author. Judith Sargent Murray's texts, especially her popular "Gleaner" essays and "On the Equality of the Sexes," published in the 1790s, demanded a more egalitarian society, one that granted basic rights to women. Unlike postrevolutionary male leaders who saw female education as a way to improve domestic life and nurture patriotism in children, Judith Murray argued that it was the innate, natural right of all human beings, including women, to develop their intellect. A rigorous education, comparable with what privileged men received, she boldly proclaimed, was essential for women's emancipation and self-reliance.[44]

John Murray supported his wife's views and encouraged her to publish her work. His actions highlighted how Universalism encouraged its female followers to assume a more public and forceful role in their society. As Judith Murray's biographer has noted, Universalism gave her the "religious legitimacy" she needed to challenge traditional patriarchy and seek greater freedom and rights for women.[45]

The feminist ideas espoused by Judith and John Murray resonated throughout their church. Universalists were in the vanguard of campaigning for woman's rights, including the right to vote.[46] They also pioneered in the ordination of women into the ministry, allowing women preachers in their churches by the 1850s. In the 1860s Olympia Brown, Augusta Chapin, and Phebe Hanaford were ordained Universalist ministers, and other women soon followed their path. Many of these ministers became active in the woman's rights movement during the latter part of the nineteenth century. In fact Brown and Hanaford achieved national prominence as they filled leadership positions in various female suffrage associations.[47]

Not surprisingly, Universalists challenged patriarchal authority in the home, encouraging women to assume a more prominent role in the training of their children, especially their daughters. This was evident in a December 6, 1806, letter that John Murray wrote to Kezia Hunt. Although he praised Joab's love for his baby daughter Harriot, Murray contended that it was Kezia who should train her child's mind and shape her character: "A mother is the best tutor for a daughter" (27).

Universalism's commitment to empowering and educating women resonated with Kezia Hunt. Although ostensibly a conventional homemaker, she was a woman who diligently educated herself and sought to transcend the confines of domesticity by cultivating an interest in civic affairs, including politics. Harriot stressed that her mother was an avid reader. Fourteen years of married life without children afforded Kezia the opportunity to read widely on diverse subjects (3). This reading not only enriched her intellectually but also nurtured in her a public identity. Kezia Hunt illustrated what historian Mary Kelley has stressed about educated women in the early Republic: reading enabled women, most of whom remained within the female sphere of domesticity, to forge a civic identity for themselves. They learned to "stand and speak" about public issues in their society.[48]

According to Harriot Hunt, her mother also participated in reform and had "a strong love for politics," even more than her father did (4). Kezia helped establish the first Industrial School for impoverished girls in Boston (12). She also nurtured an interest in politics in her daughters. Kezia required them to read and discuss the annual messages of presidents and Massachusetts governors, a task which Harriot recalled dreading when she was young but which she later appreciated (4). As this remembrance suggests, Kezia Hunt helped instill in her eldest daughter an awareness of the importance of politics.

Both Kezia and Joab were committed to educating their daughters, to nurturing in them an appreciation for the world outside the prescribed female sphere of home. Kezia, of course, did this when she required her children to read and report about current political events. Joab did this when he told Harriot stories about sailors' overseas journeys and encouraged her to read the "ship-news."

Although the Hunt family did not have the money to send their daughters to expensive boarding schools, they were committed to providing them with the best education possible. Joab and Kezia refused to enroll their children in the public schools, thinking them inadequate. Instead, Harriot and Sarah attended several private schools, which the former praised for their excellent teachers. Kezia Hunt saved the bills for their schooling so that years later she could show her daughters how the family had sacrificed for their education. Kezia also made it a point to know her children's teachers. She regularly invited them to her home where they not only had tea but also discussed the progress of the Hunt children (16–17).

Her mother, stressed Harriot, was determined that her daughters excel in school. Harriot did not disappoint. She recalled with obvious pride that she won prizes for her excellent spelling and writing (39). One major advantage that both Harriot and Sarah had was that their mother fostered in them a love of reading. Kezia carefully chose books for her daughters designed to cultivate their character as well as intellect. She had her children read aloud regularly and also discuss numerous topics at home (14, 41–42). Through such practices Kezia developed her daughters' self-confidence as well as intellect.

Committed to educating, not merely schooling, her daughters, Kezia taught them the importance of practicing Christian charity by helping those less fortunate than themselves. She also wanted them to experience firsthand the grueling and poorly paid labor that countless people, especially women, did in order to scrounge a living. Kezia drove home these lessons by requiring Harriot and Sarah to help a shirtmaker with poor eyesight stitch, make button holes, and "ruffled bosoms" (13). She also had her daughters help distant relatives who were "book-folders" so as to alleviate their heavy labor (40).

Growing up in the Hunt household was a nurturing experience for Harriot. She was the long-awaited, much-beloved child of parents who gave her a stable home and a good education and instilled in her an obligation to help those in need. The Reverend John Murray and the Universalist Church also had a major impact on Harriot Hunt. He "dedicated" her to the church shortly after her birth (8). When Hunt was a young child, Murray gave her a Bible, a gift she regarded with "reverence" and carried with her on her many adult travels (24). Hunt credited Murray with saving her from the straitjacket of dogmatic, sectarian religion. Murray, as well as her parents' "bold, earnest reception of the liberal doctrines of this wonderful man," she asserted, enabled her to embrace truths even when they challenged entrenched orthodoxies. Hunt pointedly added: "New truths never seem strange to me." Murray's benign, loving approach to religion enabled her to appreciate the crucial distinction between professing religion as opposed to actually possessing "its life-giving principles." His deeply felt piety and rejection of conventional religion also caused Hunt to recognize the "hollowness" of most churches (23). As Hunt's remarks suggest, Murray nurtured in her a spirit of rebellion and a willingness to challenge orthodoxy and to strike out on her own in the search for truth. Eventually this search led Hunt to question her society's most basic institutions and strictures.

But in the mid-1820s, Harriot Hunt and her family faced more immediate challenges. In her autobiography Harriot recalled that a "depression of business" hurt her family financially (55). Although she did not state what caused this "depression," action by the Massachusetts State Legislature did harm Boston's seafaring trade. In 1824 this legislature, in its quest for additional revenue, levied a "tax of one per cent on all sales of merchandise at auction," including cargoes from Canton. This action badly hurt Boston's maritime economy because it drove the lucrative Canton trade to New York, where no tax was levied.[49] Newspaper articles proclaiming that the "TAX ON SALES BY AUCTION" was "*impolitic* as well as *unjust*" and particularly damaged the "seaports" articulated the anger felt by many in the maritime community.[50] On October 11, 1827, merchants and traders gathered at Boston's Exchange Coffee House. They denounced the tax on sales by auction as "injurious to the trade of [their] city" and demanded its repeal.[51] Despite such protests, the Massachusetts State Legislature did not rescind the tax until 1852.[52]

Although the downturn in Boston's maritime economy hurt families like the Hunts, Harriot stressed that it was not the only reason why her father was in financial straits by the latter 1820s. His "hospitable nature" and commitment to helping the needy, as well as his increasingly ill health, also contributed to his financial problems. Her family's economic difficulties, recalled Harriot, made it a "duty" for her to become a wage earner. In early April 1827 when she was twenty-two years old, Hunt did what many young, literate women her age did when they needed to earn money—she became a teacher (55).

Historian Thomas Woody has aptly described antebellum school teaching as a "most lowly, lonely, and unattractive means to a living."[53] The paucity of "respectable" occupations for young, single women as well as the widely held belief that school teaching was an extension of mothering and so best designated "woman's work" fostered the feminization of this profession during the antebellum era. By 1840 women held 61 percent of all teaching positions in Massachusetts.[54] But school officials also hired female teachers because they could pay them significantly less than their male counterparts. During the 1830s and 1840s it was not unusual for women teachers to earn anywhere from one-half to as much as three-quarters less than their male colleagues.[55]

Given the problems young female teachers faced, it is not surprising that many became dispirited. This was the case with Gail Hamilton, who gave up teaching after four years. She confessed to a friend that she was "wearing out my life, and soul, and brain, and lungs, in teaching" and barely keeping "body and soul together."[56] Fortunately, teaching was not as dispiriting for Hunt as it was for Hamilton. No doubt the fact that she could run her school in her family home and did not have to board with strangers made her job more palatable. So too did the fact that her students came from her neighborhood and that she knew their families were of "the highest respectability" (54).

Hunt also saw school teaching as an opportunity not only to help her financially strapped family but also to achieve some independence, to come into her own. She remembered 1827 as a "momentous period" in her life, the "first year, strictly speaking, of individual responsibility—of a going out alone" (47). With obvious pride Hunt noted how quickly her school grew—from eight pupils in April 1827 to twenty-three by October (55). The success of her school brought in badly needed income. It also fostered Hunt's view of herself as a productive, independent young woman. "I had earned my first money—had tasted the joy of exerting myself for a useful purpose," she emphatically declared (56).

Hunt was innovative in her approach to school discipline. At a time when most schools relied on corporal punishment, she appealed to students' sense of honor and guilt. She also utilized the practice of public confession to shame disobedient students. Once, when she had to be absent from her school, Hunt put her father's "large old-fashioned slate" on her chair and wrote the names of all her pupils with instructions for them to state if they had misbehaved. She told her class that the next day they would assemble, their remarks would be read out loud, and their fellow students would then vouch for their accuracy. "I *trust* in you," she told her pupils. When she returned to her school the following day Hunt confirmed to her satisfaction that all students, with one exception, had behaved. One "open, bright, brave" girl, she remembered, did admit laughing several times at the idea that *"a slate was keeping school!"* Hunt readily conceded that this humorous anecdote merely recounted a minor incident, a "trifle," but added that "trifles are of great importance. We test very mighty principles by small experiments" (96).

By the time Hunt published these comments in 1856, a broad, disparate movement had emerged, one designed to discipline human beings by reforming their minds rather than merely repressing or punishing their bodies. Fundamental shifts in attitudes about punishment and discipline fueled various reform endeavors, including the campaign against capital punishment, the establishment of penitentiaries, and movements to end corporal punishment in schools, prisons, and the military.[57]

Like leading antebellum reformers who spearheaded the above campaigns, Hunt often seemed oblivious to how her disciplinary techniques could be oppressive, especially if children were publicly shamed by classmates who exposed their misbehavior in public.[58] As with so many of her adult recollections of her early years, Hunt saw her experience as a young teacher mostly in a positive light. She recalled that she "loved" teaching and that keeping a schoolroom in her home did not detract from the "joys" of domestic life (81, 57). If anything, she claimed, her school heightened her family's enjoyment of home. It allegedly broadened the already wide circle of friends she and her parents had since now they deepened their relationships with the families of the children they taught (57).

Yet Hunt did admit that her new career as a teacher soured her friendships with some of her former schoolmates. The fact that she now worked for a living caused her to lose "some caste" with young women who were not wage earners: "A chasm had yawned between our friendships—for I was at work—they were at play." This development rankled Hunt. In her autobiography she condemned those who slighted her. Her former classmates, she bristled, were "like parasites," living off their parents and leading unproductive lives as they waited to be married off to the highest bidder. In the meantime, "too many" of these idle women, she added, "sank down into a monotonous half-life," indulging in a "selfish, contemptible indolence" (57–58).

Hunt predictably counterposed her former schoolmates' allegedly wasted lives with her busy and useful one. But teaching was ultimately a rite of passage for Hunt, just as it was for so many other young women.[59] She taught for only several years. In *Glances and Glimpses* Hunt recounted that even when she most enjoyed her school and it was flourishing, she knew that it was merely a stepping-stone to another profession. She "never felt" that teaching was her "true vocation" but instead was preparing her "for something higher and more permanent,—it was but transitional" (81).

In the end what forced Hunt to forge a new career path for herself were several family tragedies. The first was the sudden death of her father on November 15, 1827, while he was attending the annual meeting to elect next year's officers at his Masonic lodge.[60] Although he was in ill health and still recovering from a serious injury incurred when shingles fell on his head (59), Hunt had insisted on attending the meeting.[61] Numerous accounts reported that while he was conversing with a fellow Mason, Joab Hunt abruptly "falter[ed] and fell" and "expired without a groan."[62] Most newspapers wrongly reported his age as being sixty-two. But as Harriot sadly recalled, he had turned fifty-eight only the preceding week (60). Both newspapers and fellow Masons eulogized Joab Hunt as a "highly respected man," a "gentleman of upright conduct, and cheerful and happy disposition."[63]

Kezia Hunt and her two daughters were devastated by Joab's death. Despite his health problems, the family was shocked as well as deeply saddened by his abrupt departure. Recounting this tragedy in her family's life almost two decades later in her autobiography, Harriot Hunt conveyed the anguish she, her mother, and her sister suffered after her father's death. Only Kezia's strength and her "folding her motherly arms" around her daughters, declared Harriot, enabled them to endure the pain of bereavement (65).

The Hunt family's shock and sorrow turned to anger when Joab's death was used to discredit the Masons. By late 1827 this fraternity had become a lightning rod for controversy throughout the United States. Mobs attacked Masonic lodges, pamphlets and newspapers denounced the Masons, state legislators conducted hearings on the threat these men allegedly posed to the nation, and an Antimasonic Party emerged. What precipitated this powerful backlash against the Masons was the kidnapping and probable murder of an apostate Mason named William Morgan in September 1826. Rumors circulated that Morgan was about to publish an exposé of the Masons' secret rituals. When Masons derailed investigation of Morgan's disappearance and subsequent death, public opprobrium against them mounted.

But other factors besides the Morgan case fueled the Antimasonic crusade. The fact that many Masons were well-to-do and politically powerful leaders of their communities, with a well-deserved reputation for helping their fraternity brothers, exacerbated class resentment and fears of a conspiratorial elite. The Masons' secret rituals attracted widespread suspicion, while their embrace of liberal Protestantism and rejection of sectarian, evangelical churches aroused public ire. By the late 1820s, therefore, the Masons were out of step with mainstream Americans. The public increasingly viewed the Masonic fraternity as an elitist, secretive, and non-Christian society that threatened the Republic and its commitment to democracy, transparency, equality, and evangelical Protestantism.[64]

Joab Hunt's death occurred as the Antimasonic movement crested. Accusations that Masons committed heinous crimes, such as the torture and murder of lodge brothers suspected of exposing them, gained credibility. Given the public hysteria against the Masons, it is not surprising that soon after Joab's death rumors began to circulate that he had been murdered by his fellow Masons. Posters appeared in the streets of Boston and even New York City claiming this as fact.[65] A number of newspaper editorials reiterated this view. They often reprinted articles from Boston's Antimasonic press that accused Joab Hunt's lodge brothers of killing him because he condemned the murder of William Morgan. These accounts contended that Hunt was a man in good health and unlikely to die so suddenly. They also asserted that the Masons were suspiciously able to quickly produce a coffin that fit Hunt's corpse, which suggested that they had planned his death. Newspapers also asserted that the "blush of guilt" appeared on Masons' faces whenever the subject of Hunt's death was raised and that Hunt's body had suspicious marks indicative of foul play. There was allegedly "a black indentation all around" his neck, and his eyeballs looked "blood shot and as if started from their sockets." Newspapers also stressed that Masons were secretive, uncommunicative, and "under the most terrible oaths not to tell the truth if it will injure a brother mason." In short, these were men who would kill or at the very least lie to protect Masons who committed murder. Their fraternities were "Blood Knights of the Skull Bone," and they needed to face *"hard questions"* about Joab Hunt's abrupt and suspicious death.[66]

These accusations dismayed the Hunt family. Harriot denounced the "wicked and slanderous accusations" made against the Masons (74). She stressed that her father "loved his masonic brethren" and valued his participation in their various charitable activities (61). She also indignantly recalled that some "antimasons" even visited the Hunt home hoping to dredge up evidence to support their accusations of foul play. They received "the rebuke they deserved," curtly noted Harriot (74).

To quell the rumors about Hunt's death, several of his Masonic brethren gave depositions testifying in detail about his abrupt collapse and failed efforts to revive him (74). But the belief that Hunt was murdered persisted. As one member of St. Andrew's Lodge bitterly recalled over forty years later, people continued to misrepresent Joab Hunt's death as a way to spread "wicked and slanderous accusations" against the Masons.[67] Ironically, therefore, the death of a man who loved Masonry put his lodge brothers in the crosshairs of a powerful national movement against their organization.

Meanwhile, Joab Hunt's death as well as economic hard times in the North End whipsawed his family's finances. On the face of it, the inventory of Hunt's estate made it seem as if he was well off, particularly for a maritime worker in 1820s Boston. The total value of his estate came to $7,882.50. Most of this was in properties—the Hunt family home on Fleet Street was appraised at $5,000, and another house on a nearby wharf, presumably Joab's place of business, was worth $1,600. But both properties were mortgaged at $800 each. Joab Hunt also owned shares of three schooners. His "undivided" fourth, eighth, and sixteenth shares of these schooners totaled $825. He also owned a tomb worth $100. The remaining part of his estate, valued at only $357.50, consisted mostly of household furnishings.[68]

Unfortunately, Joab Hunt was heavily in debt by the time he died. Probate records document that he owed $3,360.34. His personal estate, after the sale of his stake in the three schooners, amounted to only $1,182.50. Hunt's creditors received most of this money. But still left was a debt of $2,291.77.[69] This was a daunting sum for a middle-aged homemaker like Kezia Hunt and her two young daughters to pay.

The Hunt women scrambled to survive. They rented out part of their home (70–71); Sarah started teaching an "infant school" (78); and Harriot continued in her position. Since the family was now taking in boarders and space was at a premium, Harriot's class now met in a small room constructed in their garden (75). Kezia also publicly announced that as administrator of Joab's estate, she took it on herself to give "bonds as the law directs" in order to eventually pay off her husband's creditors.[70]

But health and financial problems dogged the family. Harriot seems to have suffered a temporary breakdown. After her father's death, she remembered, a "morbid dreaminess" overtook her. "I pined for my father," she admitted, and suffered "a kind of home-sickness" for the happy family life that had been so abruptly shattered (77). Hunt also developed a severe cough that required her to suspend her teaching and recuperate in the country at a friend's house. She conceded that her illness was exacerbated if not caused by her anguish over her father's death: "My physical powers sympathized too much with my mental states" (77).

Fortunately Hunt recovered enough of her health to resume teaching. But her family's finances remained precarious. Of course the sluggish maritime market in Boston hurt the Hunts' efforts to sell Joab's property. When recalling this troubled time, Harriot stressed that the "general mercantile depression" made it "the very worst period for profitable settlement" of her father's estate (70).

But according to Harriot, the economic downturn was the "least" of her family's problems. What most hurt them was being swindled by men they had trusted. Hunt did not identify who these men were or what they did, but her anger was still evident years later when she declared in her autobiography, "To be defrauded by persons we had considered honorable and truthful, was very hard" (79). Hunt was also bitter when even relatives refused to aid her family. A "distant relation" whom her father had repeatedly helped, she angrily noted, did not offer the Hunts any assistance but only "vented his pique and ill-nature" (79).

The year 1828 was very difficult for Hunt and her family. Yet, at the very end of that year, she heard a sermon from a remarkable young clergyman whose ideas would impact not only her life but those of countless others—Ralph Waldo Emerson. In 1828 he was just starting his career as a Unitarian minister and preaching periodically in one of the oldest and most distinguished churches in Boston, the Second Church located in the North End. In January 1829 Emerson would be ordained minister of that church and would remain there until he resigned in 1832 to travel and pursue a career as a public lecturer and author. Although he would not start to publish many of his famous essays, especially "Self-Reliance," until 1841, Emerson was already urging individuals to rely on themselves and defy convention and custom. He stressed that the things of this world were ephemeral and transitory and that what was important was the spiritual, eternal realm. Emerson also urged his congregation to view Christ as a spiritual guide and teacher but not as divine.[71]

His sermons had a deep impact on Harriot Hunt. She recalled that she "often" heard him preach in the Second Church and "enjoyed it deeply." Perhaps more important, Hunt thought Emerson's sermons were "very searching" (78). The fact that her pastor, the Reverend Hosea Ballou, encouraged Universalists to espouse Unitarian views undoubtedly made Emerson's theology more compelling to Hunt.[72]

Emerson's emphasis on self-reliance and the need to defy convention touched a particularly resonant chord with Hunt. Repeatedly her life narrative echoed Emerson's ideas to justify her embrace of nonconventional career paths. When she recounted her decision to study medicine, for example, Hunt declared that one must seize life's opportunities, even if it meant rejecting the advice of one's friends: "It becomes us to do our own thinking, and not send it out to our neighbor to have him do it for us" (114). When she started her medical practice in Boston, Hunt significantly quoted the famous lines from *Hamlet* that Emerson's later lectures echoed:

> To thine own self be true,
> And it must follow as the night the day,
> Thou canst not then be false to any man. (126)

As further chapters will document, one of the driving themes in Hunt's multifaceted career as a woman's rights activist was to nurture women's self-reliance. She worked to give women the opportunities and freedom that would enable them to forge independent lives, ones where they would not have to rely on men for either their security or their rights. Ultimately, Hunt took to heart Emerson's injunction to "trust thyself: every heart vibrates to that iron string."[73]

In the late 1820s and early 1830s, Hunt was still groping for ways to create a meaningful life for herself, one that not only nurtured her but also helped her impoverished family. During this trying period, the Hunt women soldiered on, desperately trying to keep up with mortgage payments and repay outstanding debts. The year 1830 began auspiciously as Harriot's school grew and attracted "a very interesting group of children" (81). But, unfortunately, Sarah soon became so sick that she was incapacitated. Her sister's illness, emphasized Harriot Hunt, was "the great turning-point of my life" (81). It caused her to give up teaching and to begin a new career for herself as a doctor and a health reformer.

Chapter 2

Establishing a Medical Career

By the spring of 1833, Sarah Hunt had been gravely ill for three years. Her doctors diagnosed a heart ailment. Harriot's anguish was evident as she recounted how the treatments prescribed by the family physician, such as the use of blisters, mercury, and leeches, failed to cure Sarah. Indeed her condition worsened, forcing her to abandon teaching and confining her to bed. Sarah also began experiencing "terrible spasms," attacks that were harrowing to witness as well as endure. They "agonized our very souls" to watch, Harriot remembered (82).

But anger as well as sorrow characterized Harriot's response to her sister's condition. Even several decades after Sarah's illness and recovery, Harriot's indignation was still palpable when she described how her sister became an invalid, subject to her doctor's "harsh and severe measures," which at times bordered on the "truly barbarous" (81, 83). As these treatments continued, Harriot began voicing her concerns to Sarah's physician. "I could hardly conceal my horror," she recalled, when the doctor prescribed a seton, a knotted thread of cotton inserted below the skin to facilitate the draining of fluid. She also remonstrated against his administering a large dose of prussic acid (83).

Harriot Hunt also had vivid, bitter memories of the harsh medicine this same doctor administered when she became ill with flu-like symptoms. On his orders she took calomel to alleviate her bad cold and aching limbs. *Glances and Glimpses* conveys her disillusionment with the conventional medical treatment she received: "I remember those pains as though they were yesterday! I remember also my wonder that so simple a malady required such severe treatment"

(84). When the doctor prescribed leeches to treat eye troubles, Harriot finally "revolted." Her eyesight improved when she applied a mild lotion (92).

Sarah also rebelled against conventional doctors and their prescribed treatment. Her "own *health-instinct* revolted," recalled Harriot, when the Hunt family physician told Sarah that she must remain cloistered in her room for the entire winter (83). Fortunately, Sarah's health improved decidedly in June 1833 when two recent émigrés from England, Dr. Richard Mott and his wife, Elizabeth, began treating her. By then, Harriot added with obvious resentment, "the best physicians had given up an only sister!" (113). She credited the Motts with Sarah's full recovery and counterposed their allegedly helpful therapy with the useless and harmful ones prescribed by conventional doctors.

Sarah's recovery led to another significant development for the Hunt family. In March 1834 they rented out their home on Fleet Street and boarded with the Motts. Kezia helped run the Mott household, while her daughters studied medicine with the English couple and assisted them with patients (113). In October 1835 Harriot and Sarah began their own medical practice, one that the former continued until shortly before her death in 1875 (123).

The medical practices of the Motts and Hunts were part of a populist revolt that contested the authority of the male medical profession. They belonged to a vibrant and eclectic alternative health care movement that trumpeted women's traditional roles as healers. Discussion of these developments provides a necessary context for understanding how Harriot Hunt created a pioneering medical career in antebellum Boston.

American medicine was a diverse, contentious, and gendered activity during the antebellum era. This was especially evident in large urban areas such as Boston, where different kinds of medical practitioners competed for patients and often criticized one another. During the first two decades of the nineteenth century, medical schools, many of them fledgling institutions, tried to establish a monopoly over the practice of medicine. They sought to discredit traditional healers, including herbalists and other practitioners of folkloric remedies. They also successfully pressured state legislatures to restrict the practice of medicine only to licensed doctors and to penalize those without proper medical credentials. In 1806, for example, the Massachusetts State Legislature prohibited doctors from consulting with "unlicensed practitioners," and in 1827 the New York State Legislature declared that no person could receive a medical degree unless he gave proof that he had studied for three years under a "regular physician."[1]

Committed to establishing their professional status, doctors in the early Republic continued to prescribe therapies popularized in the late eighteenth century—bloodletting, blistering, purging, and harsh, often addictive medicines such as mercury, calomel, arsenic, and opium. Although growing numbers of physicians in Boston and other cities began to decrease their use of these "heroic therapies," they were still widely employed. Fortunately, countless Americans rebelled against such practices and the physicians who relied on them. A growing chorus of people argued that many doctors used dangerous and overly harsh medicines that made patients sicker or even killed them.[2]

The 1830s and 1840s were the heyday of popular alternative therapies. Various patent medicines and do-it-yourself manuals, promising to cure ills without consulting doctors, became widespread. *Gunn's Domestic Medicine: The Poor Man's Friend*, for example, quickly became a bestseller when it appeared in 1830 and by 1871 was in its hundredth edition. Samuel Thomson's *New Guide to Health*, first published in the early 1820s, enjoyed enormous popularity and spawned an entire health reform movement that promised to cure all sorts of ills relying on plant remedies. Homeopathic practitioners who advocated using only a tiny dose of the drugs prescribed by physicians gained a large following in antebellum America, as did advocates of hydropathy, who argued that immersing oneself in baths was a panacea for all sorts of maladies.[3]

This populist revolt against licensed physicians reflected the democratization of antebellum America, one committed to empowering the individual and challenging the privilege of elites. Numerous developments illustrated this theme—religious revivals urged people to take charge of their spiritual lives and challenged established churches; abolitionists denounced slavery as a "relic of barbarism" that violated an individual's human rights and civil liberties; Jacksonian Democrats condemned the National Bank as a bastion of moneyed privilege and an insult to the "common man"; and Emerson's popular lectures and writings glorified self-reliance and rebellion against conformity to traditional customs.[4]

Many leading health reformers portrayed themselves as rebels who empowered people by challenging a privileged minority. Thomson, for example, proclaimed that "every man [should] be his own physician" and denounced medical schools as elitist monopolies. Another influential health practitioner, Joseph Buchanan, stressed that he waged war against "old school" medicine. Buchanan also boasted that although lacking formal medical training, he instead relied on common sense and "natural" remedies, readily available to all people.[5] Such claims were, of course, an insult to those who insisted on the need to study medicine formally.

Predictably, the medical establishment denounced alternative health care practitioners as quacks and charlatans. The American Medical Society, established in 1847, condemned hydropathists and other nonconventional healers, but the latter's popularity only grew. State legislatures responded to public pressure to rescind their earlier prohibitions against unlicensed medical practitioners. Beginning in the 1830s, one state after another stopped penalizing nonlicensed physicians.[6]

This development illustrated that licensed doctors were fighting a losing battle to monopolize the practice of medicine. They were also facing another challenge in antebellum America: the growing movement to allow women to practice medicine. In sharp contrast to conventional medical colleges, hydropathic schools and water-cure establishments welcomed female students. In fact, these organizations were gateway institutions that allowed women to practice medicine. Popular water cures, such as the one run by Silas and Rachel Gleason in Elmira, New York, as well as the Water Cure College, founded in 1851 in New York City by Thomas and Mary Gove Nichols, gave women needed medical training, credentials, and experience.[7] Eclectic medical schools, so named because they espoused a wide variety of alternative health therapies, graduated many of the earliest female doctors in the United States. Doctors Lydia Folger Fowler, Sarah Adamson Dolley, and Rachel Gleason, the second, third, and fourth women to earn medical degrees in antebellum America, respectively, graduated during the years 1850 and 1851 from the Central Medical College, an early eclectic school located initially in Syracuse, New York.[8]

During the 1840s and 1850s, women intent on earning a medical degree from a "regular" medical school faced staunch opposition. Most of these schools summarily rejected their admission. The few who initially did allow female students quickly rescinded this policy. This occurred, for example, at Geneva Medical College. Shortly after Elizabeth Blackwell graduated, the dean declared that no more female applicants would be admitted. Similarly, the Western Reserve College in Cleveland graduated six female doctors, including Elizabeth Blackwell's younger sister Emily, between 1852 and 1856 but then barred women students.[9]

The reluctance of medical schools to accept women led to the establishment of two all-female medical colleges in the late 1840s and early 1850s. The Boston (later New England) Female Medical College, founded in late 1848, was notably substandard, trained women mostly to be nurses and midwives, and was led by an eccentric lecturer and reformer named Samuel Gregory who lacked any medical training and marginalized female staff.[10] The Female (later, the Woman's) Medical College of Pennsylvania, established in Philadelphia in 1850, enjoyed a better reputation, and many of its graduates established successful careers during the last third of the nineteenth century.[11]

In 1861 there were over 280 female doctors in the United States, over twenty of whom practiced primarily in Boston. Most of these women were graduates of eclectic schools or separate women's colleges.[12] These women faced widespread public opprobrium, especially from licensed male doctors. As numerous historians have documented, gender discrimination went hand in hand with the professionalization of medicine in antebellum America. Medical schools and most of their male graduates sought to monopolize the lucrative practices of obstetrics and gynecology and denigrated traditional female healers as incompetent, even dangerous. Male physicians repeatedly argued that women's brains were too small, their emotions too volatile, and their bodies too delicate to practice medicine. They predicted that female physicians would soon prove incompetent and undermine the professionalism and status of medicine. Ironically, even as they made these assertions, many male doctors feared that women physicians would succeed and take female and child patients from them.[13]

Underlying these comments was the belief that women were invading, violating, traditional masculine spheres as well as stripping themselves of their allegedly natural, "feminine" virtues.[14] Such views promoted various hostile actions against women who dared to study medicine in nineteenth-century America. In December 1851, for example, over five hundred male medical students from different schools in Philadelphia trooped to the first graduation ceremonies of the Woman's Medical College, where their boisterous behavior threatened to disrupt the proceedings. Only the presence of fifty police officers allowed the eight women graduates to receive their diplomas.[15]

Yet the male medical establishment was not uniformly against women joining their profession. By the mid-nineteenth century, a small number of licensed male physicians, some affiliated with accredited medical schools, supported female doctors. These men often had religious and reform convictions that led them to question established gender norms. Often they championed abolition, woman's rights, pacifism, and various other activist causes. The Female Medical College, for example, relied on the support of noted Quaker reformers and physicians, including Drs. Joseph Longshore, Bartholomew Fussell, and Hiram Corson, committed to the innate equality of all human beings.[16] Dr. Henry Ingersoll Bowditch, noted supporter of radical causes, especially abolition, and professor of clinical medicine at Harvard from 1859 to 1867, was another champion of female physicians. He befriended pioneering women doctors, including Hunt and Marie Zakrzewska, and supported the latter when she established the New England Hospital for Women and Children in 1862.[17]

Although a minority of licensed male physicians advocated on behalf of women in medicine, they were outliers in the medical profession. These men braved public criticism, even ostracism, from their colleagues when they agreed to teach at women's colleges or consulted with female physicians. The nation's leading medical societies remained closed to women throughout the antebellum era and forbade their male members to have any professional contact with female physicians, including the few licensed ones. In November 1858, for example, the Philadelphia County Medical Society prohibited its members to "consult or hold professional medical intercourse" with the "professors or alumnae" of the Female Medical College.[18]

Such strictures underscore how daring as well as challenging Harriot Hunt's medical career was in antebellum Boston. Long before women were able to study medicine formally, let alone establish themselves professionally, Hunt had forged a successful medical practice. How did she do this? What kind of medicine did she practice? How did she deal with those who questioned her right to be a doctor? Discussion of the Motts' medical career in Boston and their training of the Hunt sisters helps answer these questions.

Shortly after their arrival in Boston in 1833, the Motts established a medical practice where Richard treated men and Elizabeth ministered to women and children.[19] Despite Richard calling himself a doctor, there is no evidence that he was a certified physician. Instead, he and his wife peddled all sorts of vegetable compounds, shampoo baths, and medicated lotions that they concocted and patented. Newspaper advertisements trumpeted their remedies. The Motts claimed that their "champoo baths" and "vegetable medicine" could cure cancers, "contagious diseases," and all other sorts of "internal or external" maladies.[20] Elizabeth Mott's book *The Ladies Medical Oracle*, published in 1834, made similar boasts. Elizabeth claimed that she and her husband used only natural ingredients, such as herbs, roots, and various flowers and vegetables, in their medicines.[21] Mott assured her readers that such remedies, especially one concoction she dubbed her "Life Elixir," could cure a wide range of illnesses, including cancer, cardiovascular disease, cholera, and typhus.[22]

Predictably, such claims soon attracted the derision of Boston's licensed doctors. Mott noted at the beginning of her book that she and her husband were condemned as quacks by the medical establishment. She also asserted that this establishment had particularly singled her out for criticism, spreading "foolish and slanderous reports" about her, such as the charge that she was "an *impostor*" and an "ignorant" woman who "relieved no one . . . [and] killed many"[23]

But Mott gave as good as she got. Her counterattacks articulated criticisms that other nonconventional health therapists leveled against licensed doctors. Such physicians, she contended, were "useless" and kept their patients in the dark about the medicines they prescribed: "The doctor mystifies himself" and needlessly complicates what should be simple, transparent treatments. Like other health reformers, Elizabeth Mott also accused male doctors of sexually exploiting their women patients. She looked forward to the day when women's "morality, modesty, virtue" would be protected by female doctors and "male intruders" would no longer have access to the bodies or "secrets" of female patients. At times Mott's anger against Boston physicians veered into rage. This was apparent when she asserted that their false accusations against her could only be made by "a venomous designing reptile who lives on slander and exuberates on the unwholesome air of evil."[24]

Harriot Hunt was well aware of the controversy surrounding the Motts. In *Glances and Glimpses* she conceded that friends had warned her family against consorting with "quacks" like the Motts (112). She also admitted that the Motts' claim to cure all diseases was extravagant, full of "bombast" (110–11). Yet Harriot and her sister still decided to live and study with the Motts for various reasons. First and foremost, of course, was the fact that the Hunts credited the Motts with curing Sarah of a debilitating illness. The "joy that pervaded our souls at sister's recovery," remembered Harriot, "overbalanced every other consideration," including moving to a new home (113). Boarding with the Motts must also have alleviated financial constraints on the Hunt family, especially since they could now rent their house on Fleet Street.

Last and perhaps most important, Harriot suggested that she and her family viewed the association with the Motts as a way for them to begin anew, to put behind them the sorrows they had experienced after their father's death. When the Hunt women began boarding with the Motts, they stopped wearing the mourning clothes they had worn for six and a half years in remembrance of Joab. Harriot recalled how this development revived her family's spirits: "To have been shrouded in black all that time! A change came over us, my sister and myself put on colors again. This action had much to do with our cheerfulness" (115). Harriot, Sarah, and their mother eagerly embarked on a new life.

This change was a particularly welcome opportunity for Harriot Hunt. She was at loose ends when she met the Motts. Her frequent headaches, perhaps rooted in the stress she experienced due to her family's problems, made her eager to stop teaching. The fact that she was in her late twenties and so unsettled in her life also seemed to bother her. One wonders if Hunt's unmarried state heightened her dissatisfaction. Most women her age in antebellum America were wives and mothers. Hunt stressed that when she met the Motts she was "twenty-eight years old," adding that her mother was twenty-one when she made a major life change by marrying (112). But irrespective of whether she regretted her single state, Hunt was eager to change her life. When the Motts invited the Hunt family to live and study under their roof, Harriot snapped up their proposal: "I left my school, and adventured on a new life" (112).

She credited Elizabeth Mott with offering her a needed role model. As Mott ministered to Sarah, Harriot began to entertain the idea that she too might become a physician (111). Not surprisingly, she dismissed those who warned the Hunt family against associating with the Motts. "We were not of the metal to mind such nonsense," she curtly stated (112). Hunt remembered her family's move from Fleet Street to the Mott home on March 19, 1834, as "epochal" for her. It was a time of "joy" and "satisfaction" when she risked all to forge a new life for herself and her family (113).

But boarding with the Motts lasted only until July 1835 (120). Afterward the Hunts leased a house in Boston's West End, a working-class neighborhood filled with artisans, and continued renting out their home on Fleet Street. In October the family moved to another rented house, and the Hunt sisters launched their own medical practice (123). What had happened to the relationship between the Motts and Hunts? What kind of practice did the Hunt sisters establish? Who were their patients? What kinds of treatments did they offer? How did they deal with the hostility of Boston's all-male medical establishment? How did the sisters' personal lives shape their professional one? Exploration of these questions shows how Harriot Hunt matured both as a woman and a physician.

All began well when the Hunts moved in with the Motts. Harriot remembered that she spent her days working with Elizabeth Mott, not only doing daily correspondence but also seeing patients, some of whom urged her to become a physician (116). But in June 1835 Elizabeth Mott abruptly left for Europe (119).[25] The reason for her departure remains unknown. Although Kezia Hunt and her daughters set up their own household on the West End shortly after Mott's departure, their involvement with the Motts had not ended. The Hunt sisters nursed Richard Mott when he became gravely ill (123). After his death in September 1835, Mott was buried in the Hunt family tomb.[26]

When the Hunt sisters started their own medical practice in October they used the techniques and medicines they learned from the Motts. Like Elizabeth Mott they limited their practice to women and children. Their newspaper advertisements appeared with particular regularity in the *Boston Traveler* and illustrate how Harriot and Sarah marketed their medical practice. The "Misses Hunt" trumpeted the fact that they had been the "only" students of Elizabeth Mott and had the patent rights for the Motts' many medicines. Like their English teachers, the Hunt sisters made extravagant claims for their "medicated champoo baths" and "vegetable medicines." They asserted that such remedies could cure or relieve a broad range of ills, including asthma, scrofula, rheumatism, spinal and nervous maladies, and "female weaknesses."[27]

Harriot and Sarah Hunt soon had to share their practice with another woman—Elizabeth Mott. Starting in November 1836 newspaper advertisements announced that Mott had returned to the city and was resuming her profession by working with the Hunt sisters. As before, Elizabeth Mott tried to drum up business by making extravagant claims about her medical remedies and skills. She declared that the "herbs, roots, and essential oils" she brought from Europe, allegedly unavailable in America, enabled her to combat diseases "in their most formidable appearances." She also stressed that her well-known "medicated champoo baths" could be administered to female patients "at any hour of the day." These baths, claimed Mott, were "not only a cure but also a preventive against chronic and contagious diseases."[28] Many newspaper advertisements also noted that Mott and the Hunt sisters treated children as well as women.[29]

The shared medical practice between Elizabeth Mott and the Hunt sisters did not last. In her autobiography Harriot Hunt is vague about when this association ended, other than to note that after practicing with her and Sarah for "some time," Elizabeth Mott left for New York (136). Newspaper advertisements suggest that by the end of the 1830s the Hunt sisters and Mott had each gone their own way. In regular notices in the *Boston Traveler*, for example, Harriot and Sarah thanked patients for their "extensive patronage" and declared that they would "still continue to attend to their profession." They made it a point of adding that they would persist in administering their medicated shampoos to "ladies as usual" and also treat children's diseases.[30] By then Harriot had also begun to travel to nearby towns and cities, thereby expanding her patient pool. Numerous newspaper advertisements in the late 1830s and early 1840s noted that she regularly traveled to Gloucester and surrounding towns, such as Newburyport and Rockport, to treat her numerous patients there.[31]

As for Elizabeth Mott, she did practice in New York City for a while but returned to Boston in 1842. There she expanded her practice to include men. She also traveled to nearby towns and cities, hawking her patented medicines and treating patients.[32] Throughout the 1840s her advertisements appeared in various newspapers, touting her various remedies and medicated baths. But now she pointedly added that she had "no connexion with the Misses Hunt of Boston, whatever."[33]

Glances and Glimpses offers a brief but suggestive account of why the relationship between Harriot Hunt and Elizabeth Mott ended. Despite claiming that her feelings for Mott had not altered, Hunt admitted in her narrative that Mott's approach to medicine increasingly worried her. Apparently Hunt had begun reevaluating Mott's methods even while the latter was in Europe: "A great change had passed over my mind in her [Mott's] absence, both as regards diseases and remedies." Hunt then drily added that "it was well for us all when she removed to New York" (136).

The brevity of Hunt's comments and the lack of archival evidence make it impossible to answer with certainty why there was a break in the Hunt-Mott relationship. But Mott's reliance on various vegetable concoctions and medicated lotions, her claims that she could cure all diseases, especially by prescribing her "Life Elixir" with its secret ingredients, and her reputation in the medical community as a charlatan likely made Hunt realize that continued association with Mott would hurt her professionally. She brusquely ended her discussion of Mott by stressing that there were times in a person's life when "connections which are injurious to us must be surrendered" (136).

Although the Hunt sisters initially used "medicated champoo baths" (129), their approach to medicine increasingly diverged from that of the Motts. Hunt stressed that she and Sarah soon found themselves "differing from our teachers" and learned "not to trust too much to medication" (127). Reflecting the influence of hydropathy, the Hunt sisters touted the benefits of bathing in plain water. In her autobiography Hunt was effusive in proclaiming water to be a panacea for bodily ills. Quoting Methodist leader John Wesley's aphorism, "cleanliness is next to godliness," she even asserted that water "tends to induce godliness" (130).

The Hunt sisters were in the thick of a populist revolt that challenged the authority, competency, and morality of conventional physicians. When Harriot and Sarah began their medical practice in the mid-1830s, they were in the vanguard of a pioneering group of female physicians who sought entrance into a profession that excluded and denigrated women. *Glances and Glimpses* conveys the excitement and happiness Harriot Hunt felt at the beginning of her medical career: "I remember vividly the earnestness—the enthusiasm—with which we received our first patients . . . every case . . . was a new revelation—a new wonder—a new study *in* itself, and *by* itself." She also relished the opportunity to study the marvels of the human body: "Anatomy had partially opened its treasures to me; and the wonderful deposits from the blood to develop, perfect, and sustain the system, even the bony structure, filled my soul with reverent awe" (127).

Glances and Glimpses details the challenges and vexations as well as joys that Hunt encountered at the start of her medical career. This author addressed how she tackled a number of practical but crucial issues: Should she and Sarah remain in Boston or start their practice in a new area? What therapies should they use? Should they offer gynecological and obstetric services? How could they continue to educate themselves about medicine? How should they handle those who ostracized them, especially the all-male medical establishment?

Hunt quickly dispatched the first question. "Boston was my birthright," she proudly asserted. So the Hunt sisters resolved to remain in their hometown, hopeful that their "parentage" and "character" would smooth their way and mitigate the "slights" some neighbors and even "old friends and schoolmates" gave them on learning of the sisters' plans (126, 125). Recognizing that it would initially be difficult for two young women without credentials or experience to attract patients, the Hunt sisters charged considerably less than did licensed physicians (152).[34] Aware that she and Sarah were under public scrutiny, Hunt recalled how careful they were to avoid the appearance of impropriety. Limiting their practice to women and children was one way to enhance their respectability.

They also did not practice midwifery. Such a decision undoubtedly reflected the recognition that many would object to two unmarried young women practicing obstetrics. Hunt also stressed how the hostility of Boston area physicians shaped this decision. No licensed doctor, she bitterly remembered, spoke "one encouraging word" to her or Sarah (135). The sisters' pariah status in their city's medical community meant that if they ran into complications with a birth, they could not turn to a licensed medical doctor for consultation.

Despite the Hunt sisters' enthusiasm and dedication, the first several years of their medical practice grew "very slowly" (127). Yet the crucial point is that it grew. Because Hunt ordered in her will that her patients' records be destroyed, one cannot identify these people, what treatments they received, or how much they paid. But in *Glances and Glimpses* Hunt stressed that initially most of her patients were working-class women, including "many dress-makers and seamstresses" (134). These women often lived on very tight budgets—Hunt noted that she treated patients who had "no superfluity of wages" and managed to survive only by living lives of "painful self-denial" (150).

With cases like these, Hunt may well have waived any doctor's fee. She recalled doing this, for example, when one woman informed her that she was bankrupt and unable to pay. Hunt promptly told her "forget my bill" (396). Her generosity toward her financially strapped patients was also evident in her will when she directed that no bills be sent to any of her patients but to leave it to "their discretion" to pay whatever amount for which "they may feel indebted."[35]

Fortunately for the Hunt family's finances, women who came from "homes filled with every luxury" started consulting Harriot and Sarah as their reputation grew (151). In a remark that revealed her own class prejudices and yearning for respectability, Harriot proudly declared that by the late 1830s the Hunt practice included "patients from the highly cultivated, the delicate, and the sensible portion of the community" (135).

But the Hunt sisters became increasingly frustrated by their lack of medical knowledge. They quickly recognized that the much-touted water cure was not a panacea for illness any more than were the Motts' vegetable concoctions or medicated shampoos. Harriot and Sarah therefore embarked on a rigorous course of study to better treat their patients. They studied late into the night, quizzing each other about what they learned with "unwearying zeal" (128). Such actions suggest a certain defensiveness on Harriot's part about her lack of formal medical training and credentials.

This defensiveness was also apparent when Hunt remembered how a writer in a medical journal derided the sisters after seeing one of their advertisements depicting themselves as physicians. The author, stated Harriot, sarcastically asked if the Hunts even knew the difference between the "sternum and the spinal column." Although she dismissed such remarks as "a thin jest," Hunt also admitted that the author's quip was "a palpable hit" (127, 128).

As she recalled her early medical practice, Hunt emphasized how the lack of university training and professional colleagues as well as the public's hostility to female doctors disadvantaged her and Sarah. "Being entirely shut out from the medical world," she declared, prevented them from consulting physicians who could have helped them understand what they read and, more important, "cheered and encouraged" the sisters (142). Hunt also stressed how the public's opprobrium against female physicians made it counterproductive for her and Sarah to make house calls, as male doctors regularly did. "There was so much opposition to the attendance of a woman as physician among the friends of the invalids," she remarked dryly, "that the good of our visits was neutralized" (136).

To read this portion of *Glances and Glimpses* is to recognize how disheartened Harriot and Sarah must have felt at the outset of their medical career. Their lack of either formal training or degrees, their ostracism from the larger medical community, the snubs and consternation they faced from neighbors, friends, and some patients' families—these developments undermined the Hunt sisters' confidence and made them feel acutely alone, isolated.

Hunt's narrative is particularly revealing and plaintive when she declared: "In looking back to this period of my life, I am forcibly struck with the fewness of those who understood us—with the scarcity of those who even caught a glimpse of our states. Had it not been for our mother, how sad would this have been!" (128–29). Such remarks underscored not only how discouraged the Hunt sisters felt at times but also how pivotal Kezia remained in their lives. She anchored and comforted her daughters as they worked hard to build up their practice and faced hostility from Boston's medical establishment.

Hunt's autobiography makes clear her sadness and also resentment as she and Sarah faced an uphill battle to educate themselves about medicine and establish a "respectable" practice in Boston. Fortunately, Hunt recalled, she experienced at this dispiriting time a sort of epiphany. In October of 1838 she attended the lectures of George Combe, the renowned Scottish phrenologist popular on both sides of the Atlantic during the Victorian era. Touted as a science when it crested in influence during the 1830s and 1840s, phrenology purported to reveal a person's character by studying the shape and protuberances of their skulls.

As David Stack, Combe's biographer, has shown, this Scotsman was primarily an educator and a reformer, steeped in Enlightenment values. He rejected sectarian religion and instead urged the development of a secular "science of man." Combe sought to discover the allegedly natural laws of the universe that governed the human body as well as the mind. If human beings followed these organic laws, he asserted, they could banish disease and prolong life indefinitely. More important, Combe believed that adherence to such laws would enable humans to institute a thoroughgoing reformation of the world, one characterized by peace, tolerance, reason, and civic virtue.[36]

He popularized these ideas through a series of well-attended lectures and popular books. The most celebrated and influential of his works was *Constitution of Man*, first published in 1828. Combe stressed that this text should be read as "an essay on education," one that enlightened human beings about natural laws and offered them a guide for following them.[37]

Combe's tenets dovetailed with the alternative health care movement of which the Hunt sisters were a part. Like health reformers, Combe rejected the harsh medicines used by conventional physicians and advocated reliance on diet, cleanliness, and exercise. Such a regimen, he stressed, accorded with natural laws and cured or prevented disease.[38] Combe's beliefs, especially his commitment to improving the world through rational, scientific means, also resonated with liberal Protestants, such as Universalists and Unitarians.

His two-year lecture tour of the United States in 1838–41 was a triumph for Combe. By then *Constitution of Man* had become a best-selling work, audiences flocked to hear him, and newspapers praised his presentations. Harriot Hunt was one of Combe's most enthusiastic listeners. She gushed in admiration when she described him and his lectures. The latter were "revelations—bread for a hungry spirit and water for a thirsty soul" (142). She credited Combe with offering a rational, scientific basis for comprehending human beings and the world: "He opened to us the labyrinth of life; he lighted up its mysterious chambers, and bade us enter and explore; he gave us the golden clue of connection between cause and effect and end. . . . I needed a more earnest consciousness of laws,-I needed to realize that they govern every department of life; and these lectures supplied my need. . . . They snapped the fetters that had manacled thought" (142–43).

Combe's ideas liberated Hunt. They infused her with confidence in her own abilities and reinforced her rejection of conventional medicine. According to Hunt, Combe enabled her "to see the inexpediency of the ideas cherished by time-servers" and "to scan the accumulated rubbish of the past with discrimination." Hunt's newfound assurance rested on her belief that Combe had provided her with a "key" for how to treat illness, how to make sense of the disparate and bewildering number of diseases that afflicted human beings. Because of him, she stressed, her practice grew "constantly and successfully" as patients regained or preserved their health by following nature's "physical laws" (143, 151).

Yet even as she praised Combe, Hunt increasingly embraced what Robert Fuller has called the "spiritualizing of alternative medicine."[39] Numerous unorthodox healers in antebellum America invoked spiritual forces to cure or prevent disease. Mesmerists put patients into a trance and sought to direct the allegedly life-giving magnetic forces permeating the universe to the diseased parts of the body. Prominent spiritualists, such as Andrew Jackson Davis, treated the sick while in a clairvoyant state. Although lacking any medical training, Davis soon became renowned for his seemingly miraculous healing powers. Phineas Quimby pioneered in the "mind-cure" approach to medicine. Attributing physical illness to spiritual and mental malaise, Quimby counseled patients to banish negative or evil thoughts, to tap into the spiritual force within them, to regain health. One of his patients, Mary Patterson (later known as Mary Baker Eddy) built on Quimby's ideas to create one of the nation's most popular and influential religious movements in the late nineteenth and early twentieth centuries, the Christian Science Church.[40]

The widespread belief that the body was an ephemeral vessel for the eternal spirit led many nineteenth-century Americans, including Hunt, to view illness merely as a manifestation of spiritual disease or disharmony. *Glances and Glimpses* highlighted how this conviction shaped Hunt's approach to medicine. She stressed that doctors must be first and foremost "physicians of the soul," who recognized that bodies were often "worn with pain," so that "spirits may be purified" (157). This conviction led Hunt to urge a return to earlier times when "the offices of priest and physician" had been allegedly "united." These offices, she asserted, should "never have been divorced" because "the functions of the pastor and of the doctor are so blended—they are so intimately connected— that they should be made one" (185).

Hunt's medical practice reinforced her belief that "physical maladies" were often caused by "concealed sorrows." She and Sarah were repeatedly exposed to "harrowing scenes" of anguish as they became privy to "the heart-histories of women" (139). Since Sarah specialized in treating children, women unburdened themselves more to Harriot. Not surprisingly, her working-class patients detailed their desperate struggles to eke out a living for themselves and their families. Hunt sympathetically recalled these women's tales in her autobiography. She recounted, for example, the story of an impoverished widow who had to "part with two of [her] children" since the wages she earned were "so small." Another woman told Hunt that because her "sick-headaches" often prevented her from working, she did "not have one cent laid up" (133). There were "many women among my patients," Hunt noted, "whose poverty denied them a home" (151). When "ill-health" added to these women's already deep troubles, their situation became desperate (133).

Hunt's working-class patients were not the only ones troubled. Hunt stressed that her affluent patients were also unhappy. She described women who led bored, empty lives in the midst of luxury and who seemingly suffered from a "drought . . . felt in the *soul*" (408). According to Hunt, such women became ill because they could not develop either their intellect or interests outside the home, their "mind[s] had been uncultivated—intelligence smothered—aspirations quenched. The result was physical suffering" (393). Hunt recalled that many of these women patients made comments that highlighted their frustration and anger with the circumscribed lives they led. One such patient, for example, asked Hunt not to "laugh" at her "over-dress," adding ruefully that she had "nothing else to do with my time" (412). Another wistfully stated that "had I been a man, I should have had some occupation," while a third patient complained, "I am a woman; my want of education forbade me to select the employment that would have been congenial to my taste" (393).

Hunt's well-to-do patients at times idealized the condition of those who suffered great injustice in antebellum America, such as Native Americans and the poor. But their comments reflected a yearning to escape the entrapment they felt in their gilded cage of affluence. This was evident when one of Hunt's patients told her: "I wish I had been an Indian, then I should have enjoyed freedom. Why is it that we are so feeble when rich, so strong when poor?" (393).

The stories Hunt recounted about her female patients, whether poor or rich, underscored the anguish many of them felt. They highlighted that such women felt imprisoned either by poverty or by affluent domesticity. Many of Hunt's female patients recognized how lack of educational and economic opportunity trapped them into unhappy, at times desperate, lives.

Their "heart histories" also revealed another theme—women's pain and anger about their relationships with men. A number of Hunt's patients had been hurt, at times swindled, by men who handled their business affairs. One woman who was pregnant and widowed, for example, had trusted in the administrator of her husband's estate to provide for her and her baby. But the man mishandled the estate, sold "stocks and lands" at a loss, causing the widow to lose her house and face poverty (72). Another initially affluent widow was impoverished by her brother-in-law who was a stockbroker and convinced her to invest in stock, which "ruined" her. A third woman, a dressmaker, was swindled of her meager savings by a "non-paying railroad" (396). No doubt such accounts touched a resonant chord with Hunt, given that her own widowed mother apparently had been "defrauded" by men who she wrongly thought were "honorable and truthful" (79).

But the most heartbreaking stories Hunt heard from her patients were those imprisoned in unhappy marriages. Patients told her of how they had nothing in common with their husbands, how often these men ignored or belittled them.

One woman, for example, related that her husband was a successful but very busy businessman who had no time for her or their home life. He ate breakfast alone, dined at a hotel with business associates, and came home late at night too "weary to talk at all." When their only child, a daughter, died, the wife experienced "utter desolation," recalled Hunt, and her "health failed" (391–92).

Other patients confessed how their husbands betrayed them by committing adultery and the pain they suffered because of this. One case Hunt recounted was especially sad. The young wife had traveled to California with her baby to reunite with her husband only to find that he had played her "false" and "deserted" her. The devastated wife almost died but "clung to life" so as to care for her young daughter (386). At times, Hunt noted, wives seemed resigned to their spouses' philandering. "Oh, he is a man," said one such woman, "you cannot expect purity" (393).

Hunt helped many of the women who came to her by doing something very important for them. She *listened* to these women; she offered them a haven or sanctuary where they could speak about their personal problems and obtain a sympathetic hearing. Hunt had a gift for asking probing questions about a woman's personal life in ways that enabled her patients to finally articulate long-suppressed memories and grievances. She offered a particularly poignant example when she described how one patient, "a suffering dyspeptic," revealingly confessed to her that "I have no language in which to utter myself." Only after Hunt got this woman to talk about her unhappy childhood, one where "petty tyranny ... nearly rendered her a mute," did this patient improve (397, 398).

She also used her patients' "heart histories" to forge a sense of community among them. Hunt recollected doing so when she introduced the widow impoverished by her brother-in-law to the dressmaker swindled by railroad officials. Despite their vastly different backgrounds, both women allegedly came together on "common ground" as they discussed their respective exploitation (396–97). Hunt did not claim that these women recovered their lost money. But she argued that at least they found a kinship with other women similarly exploited. Perhaps most important, these two women found a place where they could vent their anger, protest injustice, and receive sympathy and encouragement.

Her patients' "heart histories" convinced Hunt that the truly effective physician had to be a counselor, a confessor, who helped women uncover "the cancerous sores and corruption of *private* life" that sickened them (200). But before this healing process could occur, stressed Hunt, the patient and doctor had to forge a very close emotional bond. According to her, the sharing of confidences bound the patient and doctor together. They formed a "oneness," a partnership, and only this kind of relationship made recovery from illness possible. Hunt pointedly rejected the popular belief that doctors could cure their patients. "The doctor and the patient *together*," she emphatically declared, are "to cure or mitigate the disease. They must be coworkers" (156).

Hunt's views bring to mind how many contemporary psychotherapists and other mental health workers treat their patients. Living in a pre-Freudian world, Hunt groped toward what would today be labeled the "talking cure" to help people in emotional turmoil. Throughout her autobiography Hunt showcased how she increasingly focused on treating the mental or psychological problems of her patients, which she hoped would alleviate not only their anguish but also many of the physical maladies that plagued them.

Harriot Hunt was in the vanguard of a new approach to medicine, one that became popular among women practicing alternative health therapies during the first half of the nineteenth century. Some of these women, such as Rachel Gleason, used the term "heart histories" to describe how they ministered to ailing women by getting them to talk about personal, even intimate aspects of their lives. As Susan Wells has noted, medicine was a "heavily discursive practice" in the antebellum era, one where female healers encouraged their patients to confide in them, to voice their sorrows and anxieties in order to regain their health.[41] In the 1840s and 1850s, the first generation of women physicians to graduate from an accredited medical school continued to invoke the merits of "heart histories." Elizabeth Blackwell, for example, declared that a female doctor was like a "moral mother" who enabled her patients to regain their health by empathizing with them when they confided in her.[42]

The widespread belief that women were innately more emotional, intuitive, and empathetic than men fostered a commitment to "heart histories" among female healers. Conversely, these healers asserted that most male doctors lacked the ability to listen to and empathize with women. When these men did try to be the confidants of their women patients, many female medical practitioners accused them of ulterior motives. They argued that male doctors often sought to ensnare their women patients into sharing confidences so that they could seduce or manipulate them. The language these women used was revealing—male physicians were allegedly "intrusive" or "invasive" when they tried to worm confidences out of female patients. When they used such practices, male doctors were predatory; they engaged in a kind of psychological rape of unsuspecting women that was often the prelude to a literal rape or seduction.[43] Elizabeth Mott's description of physicians as lecherous "male intruders" who pried "secrets" from their women patients occurred in this context.

So too did the comments of Harriot Hunt. In *Glances and Glimpses* she dismissed the efforts of most male physicians to become their female patients' confidants. The preference of most "women of refinement and purity" to "reserve their confidence for those of their own sex," argued Hunt, meant that a male doctor should never demand "as his right" that "a woman shall make him her father-confessor" (156).

Hunt's injunction revealed her commitment to a gendered approach to medicine, in which it was primarily female doctors who had the understanding and empathy to hear their patients' woes. Although she conceded that it was possible for a male physician to possess these requisite attributes and forge a close, nonsexual bond with a female patient, Hunt stressed that such cases were extremely rare. Therefore, she emphatically asserted, "the female physician is *the* physician for the female patient" (157).

But who was to be her physician? Who was to hear her troubles and counsel her? For Harriot Hunt the people in whom she confided and who comforted and loved her were her sister and especially her mother. Sarah and Harriot made a good medical team. The latter remembered that it was a "great privilege" to work with Sarah, especially because she was so talented in treating sick children. "We enjoyed even our differences of opinion," claimed Hunt (162).

As for her relationship with her mother, Harriot readily conceded that even as an adult she remained emotionally dependent on Kezia, almost as if she were still a child. She recalled that her thirty-second birthday in November 1837 found her "childlike, resting on a mother." Sheepishly, Hunt admitted that this "childish feeling" was "very strong" in her and at times "conflicted" with her "dignity." Yet it fulfilled a deep need in Hunt. She was willing, she said, to assume all sorts of "responsibilities" as long as she could return home to her mother's nurturance and "be a child again" (137).

For a while in the late 1830s, Harriot Hunt seems to have achieved a good life. Her medical practice with Sarah was growing. She at times traveled to nearby towns, thereby gaining more patients. What made life particularly satisfying for Harriot Hunt, however, was that her family finally achieved a long-desired goal—paying off the mortgage on their house in Fleet Street. With obvious satisfaction she noted: "In ten years after my father's decease, our homestead was unfettered and free. . . . By our own efforts we had cancelled the mortgage on our homestead" (138). Understandably, Hunt felt a "thrill of joy" on reentering her childhood home (136).

Yet, in the end, her family did not move back to Fleet Street. In September 1839 they purchased a home on Green Street, where Harriot Hunt lived for many years. She gave no reason for her family not returning to their Fleet Street home other than to note that the site of their new house was "favorable" (160). No doubt the deteriorating neighborhood of the North End made it preferable to live in another part of Boston. Their new domicile may also have had better accommodations for the Hunts' medical practice. Perhaps the house on Fleet Street had too many painful memories. But what was crucial was that the days of scrambling to find cheap lodgings while they rented out their mortgaged house were over for Kezia Hunt and her two daughters. "There is a necessity from the very nature of woman for a *home*, a centre," asserted Hunt, and now she, her sister, and her aged mother, whose vision had been deteriorating, finally had a home again (160).

But in the 1840s the comfortable world Harriot Hunt had fashioned for herself shattered. Sarah married and left the medical practice. Kezia died. To cope with these events, Harriot created a new life, one in which she became a public lecturer in health reform, established an institute catering to women's physiological needs, and challenged the exclusion of women from Harvard's Medical College.

Chapter 3

Coping with Family Tragedy and Professional Rejection during the 1840s

October 4, 1840, was a bittersweet day for Harriot Kezia Hunt. Her sister married an attorney named Edmund Wright.[1] The match proved to be a good one for Sarah, who married several months before her thirty-second birthday. Her husband was the only son and namesake of the man who had helped the Hunt women after Joab's death. The senior Wright served as Kezia's bondsman and thereby risked his own money if she defaulted on any family debts. Like the Hunts, Wright Senior was a devout Universalist who had been friends with the Reverend John Murray. In her autobiography Harriot gratefully recalled Wright as a "valued friend," a "single-hearted man" who did her family a great service: "He trusted us!" Wright Senior did this when many others refused to help Joab Hunt's indebted widow and two daughters. Not surprisingly, the Hunt family mourned Wright's death in December 1837 at the age of seventy four (84, 138).[2]

When Sarah married Wright's son, the Hunt family, including Harriot, seemed to rejoice. In *Glances and Glimpses* Hunt offered almost fulsome praise for her brother-in-law: Wright showed "unselfish devotion" to family and quickly became a "son and a brother" to his mother- and sister-in-law. Hunt also stressed that Sarah's marriage did not immediately end her involvement in their medical practice. At first Sarah continued to treat her patients and to consult with Harriot on her cases. Initially, Sarah and presumably her bridegroom also lived with the Hunts (164–65).

But none of this could assuage Harriot's regret at her sister's marriage. Despite claiming that she had "not lost a sister, but gained a brother," Hunt conceded that she felt "a great loss" when Sarah wed. Her sister's marriage "loosened" the professional partnership and perhaps also the close personal ties the sisters had enjoyed. Harriot admitted that she felt abandoned, bereft after Sarah's wedding: "There was a widowed feeling about me, which passed away somewhat in time; but it has never wholly left me" (165–66).

Such reactions were not atypical in mid-nineteenth-century middle-class families. Various developments, including the erosion of patriarchy and the growing differentiation of siblings by age and gender, promoted the "reign of the elder sister" in these families. The oldest sister increasingly functioned as a surrogate or "deputy" mother, nurturing and guiding her younger female siblings. Sisters became especially close and often remained so throughout their lives. Yet the marriage of a young woman often caused anguish, a sense of abandonment, and at times jealousy in the unmarried sister, even if she recognized the merits of her sibling's husband.[3]

Although Harriot's pain over her sister's betrothal might not have been atypical for her time, it did not make it any easier to bear. Yet in some respects Sarah's marriage and withdrawal from the Hunt medical practice liberated Harriot. It forced her to rely on herself; it freed her to experiment with new ways to treat patients; it deepened her commitment to her profession. Harriot's recollection of this period in her life warrants extensive discussion because it underscores the exhilaration and creativity she experienced as she forged a life for herself without Sarah as her partner. Sarah's marriage, she remembered, "opened new channels of life and freedom. . . . It threw me back on my own individualism. My medical life received a new illumination: my patients gave me a new inspiration: new elements of thought came to me, which after experience was to shape and confirm. I had thought myself individual before, but it had only been at times. I had been in love with my profession: this change deepened the feeling very much. . . . My life had now assumed more distinctness—more identity. I knew I must now, in a great measure, act alone" (165–66).

Such comments highlight a crucial fact: Harriot faced a fundamental decision after Sarah married and became a full-time homemaker and mother in 1843. Harriot could abandon the medical practice she and her sister had worked so hard to establish and find another and perhaps more conventional means to make money, or she could forge ahead on her own as "Doctor Hunt." Harriot

Kezia Hunt chose the latter course, even though flying solo promised not only a life of greater "freedom" and "individualism" but also entailed serious risks. There would be no more reliance on others to share the responsibilities of running a pioneering medical practice. Hunt would have to cope on her own with myriad challenges, including the seriously ill patients, many of whom could not pay much, if at all; the continued hostility from Boston's male physicians; and the competition offered by other alternative health practitioners. As she juggled these challenges, she also had to deal with her mother, who at age seventy endured failing eyesight and other ailments.

Despite claiming that she became more adventurous in her medical practice after Sarah left it, Harriot Hunt initially proceeded cautiously. She admitted that after her sister's marriage she "relinquished travelling as a general thing, and quietly sat myself down to my home practice" (169). This decision likely reflected Hunt's desire to reassure her mother that her eldest daughter would remain at home to look after her. Perhaps Hunt also faced a heavy workload as Sarah withdrew from the practice and the latter's patients now relied on Harriot. Hunt may also have needed to stay close to the home that anchored and nourished her, especially when Sarah embarked on her new life.

Whatever the reason, Harriot Hunt hunkered down in Boston and focused on her patients. There is no evidence that she made radical changes in how she treated them. She continued to counsel patients to stop using the varied "heroic therapies" prescribed by conventional physicians, therapies that she derided as "quack medicines." She also urged patients to follow a regimen allegedly prescribed by the physiological laws of nature by eating healthy, exercising, and bathing regularly. The latter was especially important, asserted Hunt, since water was the "great remedial health-restoring agent" that most people ignored at their peril (173).

Such advice was no different from that offered by numerous other alternative health care practitioners in antebellum America. What distinguished Hunt from many of these people, however, was when she urged patients to keep a diary in which they could "faithfully" record their life's troubles (401). Such documents were grist for Hunt's mill and served as the basis for the "heart histories" patients confided to her. Hunt described herself as a kind of priest confessor, one who "sat in the confessional" and heard patients' troubles (171). Given the widespread anti-Catholicism in 1850s America, Hunt's analogy risked alienating her readers. But it was a risk she took since portraying herself as a priestly confessor dramatized a key point: she could help patients only if they revealed their deepest sorrows. Only through such therapy, she believed, could the soul and body reestablish a harmonious equilibrium, one that healed the sick and strengthened the healthy.

This belief led Hunt to participate in the establishment of an organization that incorporated many of her ideas about medicine and created a new professional opportunity for herself. The Ladies' Physiological Institute, formally incorporated in 1850, began in 1843 with a series of meetings held in the homes of middle- to upper-class Boston area women, including Hunt. The stated purpose of the institute was to educate women about human anatomy and the physiological laws that supposedly prevented disease and promoted good health. Members engaged in different activities. They had "conversational meetings" once a month, visited gymnasiums, established a library, and in the 1850s supported the medical training of women doctors and hospitals that focused on female health care.[4] An especially important activity for the institute was to sponsor weekly lectures about a wide variety of issues, including the need for dietary and dress reform, the merits of hydropathy and homeopathy, and the importance of good hygiene for women.[5] As historian Martha Verbrugge has shown, the Ladies' Physiological Institute reflected beliefs common among urban, educated, affluent Americans in the 1840s and 1850s: God had intended for human beings to live a long, healthy life; disease was therefore an abnormality; it represented a transgression of the divine plan; it must be cured or prevented altogether by adhering to basic natural laws that promoted good health.[6]

In *Glances and Glimpses* Hunt called the formation of the Ladies' Physiological Institute one of the major events in her life because it gave her "the first hint as to the possibility of lecturing to my own sex on physical laws" (170). The institute also affirmed Hunt's belief that a doctor's major duty was to prevent disease. With obvious satisfaction Hunt noted that some institute members stressed that now their physicians' bills were "one half reduced in consequence of their obedience to physical laws" (179); no doubt at least some of these women became her patients. Hunt was both wistful and effusive when she remembered her participation in the establishment of the Ladies' Physiological Institute: "Those afternoon meetings will never be forgotten by me. The earnest looks—the friendly greetings and farewells—the religious element that kindled there—gave them life. . . . There I learned more deeply the need of light for the people on medical subjects; there was *born* the thought of public speaking which I afterward realized. . . . Peace be unto every one who composed that Circle! . . . I loved my Charlestown meetings, and regretted when my duties forbade regular attendance" (180).

As Hunt's comments suggest, the Ladies' Physiological Institute nurtured her in personal as well as professional ways. Its members provided Hunt with needed companionship, sociability, and emotional support. She recalled with deep gratitude how the women who attended the organization's first meetings in Charlestown gave her not only "great satisfaction and encouragement" but also showed her "charity" and "tenderness" when she was "in affliction" (179).

By the mid-1840s Hunt would need all the support and nurturance that she could get as she suffered the tragic loss of loved ones. The first death was that of her niece, Sarah and Edmund Wright's oldest child and Harriot's namesake. Born in early 1843, Harriot Augusta weighed less than five pounds and was very frail (181). Her Aunt Harriot was quickly smitten with this child, admitting that she loved her almost to the point of "idolatry" (189). This child, gushed Hunt, was an "angelic little girl" who possessed an incomparable "baby beauty" (181–82).

Becoming an aunt was a wonderful experience for Harriot Hunt. Love for her niece created "a well-spring of pleasure" in her, it "opened new avenues of love for others," it forged "a link between the spiritual and material" (182). Although Sarah soon bore several other children, Harriot's favorite remained her niece, whom she appropriately nicknamed "Sunbeam" (187). That this little girl looked like Joab heightened her aunt's love for her (189).

But Harriot Augusta's frail health worried the family, especially her aunt and mother. Both worked diligently to make the child strong through diet, bathing, exercise in the fresh air, and other regimens. Years later Harriot claimed that she had a presentiment that her niece might succumb to illness and die (189). Certainly Harriot as a doctor knew firsthand the sadness of families who lost young children to illness. Her own aunt, her mother's eldest sister, had buried nine children and was survived by only one daughter by the time she died as an elderly woman (145).

But the tragic propensity of children to die young did not lessen the anguish Harriot and her family experienced when her niece died on October 10, 1845, approximately three months shy of her third birthday.[7] As Hunt grimly recalled, "the bereavement was severe: it ploughed up the ground" (196). Hunt seems to have experienced an emotional withdrawal or breakdown after her niece's death similar to the one she suffered after her father's demise. Just as she felt enveloped by a "sort of morbid dreaminess" after Joab died (77), she now felt "subdued" (190): "A sort of dreaminess, mistiness, and dampness of spirit rested upon me; I feared indifference and apathy" (196).

Kezia Hunt was able to bear the loss of her first grandchild because of her deep religious faith, but in the fall of 1845, Harriot admitted that she lacked her mother's comforting piety: "My religion was then more exterior, a response to my mother's. A sort of satisfied religious conventionality clothed me" (196). One cannot know why Harriot's commitment to the Universalist faith waned, but perhaps it is significant that the Hunts' longtime minister, Hosea Ballou, had become "infirm" and unable to continue his full-time clerical duties as the family mourned the loss of Harriot Augusta. Although Hunt recalled that the various ministers who preached "on trial" kept her mind "wide awake," they did not seem to evoke a deep emotional response in her (196).

Seeking a way to cope with her niece's death and to experience a heartfelt piety once again, Hunt became a Swedenborgian. The son of a prominent Lutheran theologian and minister, Emanuel Swedenborg (1688–1772) was one of Sweden's leading scientists. In the mid-1740s, however, he proclaimed that he experienced religious visions where he conversed with God, angels, and renowned early church leaders such as Saint Paul. Through a mysterious process he termed "intromission," Swedenborg stated that he was transported to the spiritual world and there discerned a central truth: the material, physical world was merely a manifestation of the eternal, spiritual one. He also articulated his theory of correspondence, or the belief that every physical object in the world corresponded to a spiritual, divine one.[8]

Swedenborg's ideas found numerous followers in America as well as Europe during the first half of the nineteenth century.[9] He was particularly popular in Boston, especially among liberal Protestants, such as Unitarians and Universalists, who sought respite from the pessimistic determinism of Calvinist orthodoxy. By the mid-1840s the Swedenborg church in Boston, the Church of New Jerusalem, better known as the New Church, had an imposing new building which seated one thousand and attracted many congregants.[10]

One of these was Harriot Hunt. During the winter of 1845–46 she attended a series of lectures at the New Church that changed her life. The speaker she heard was George Bush. He had been a professor of Hebrew and a philologist as well as Presbyterian minister. By the time Hunt encountered him, Bush rejected conventional religion. His disavowal of Presbyterian theology and church governance led to his expulsion from the clergy. But this did not deter Bush from pursuing his search for truth. In the mid-1840s he embraced the ideas of Swedenborg and proselytized them on the lecture circuit.[11]

Hunt credited Bush with converting her to Swedenborgianism. She was effusive in her praise of this former minister: "George Bush was the first New Church preacher I ever heard *interiorly*." Cherishing "the privilege of being awakened" by Bush, Hunt claimed that his "broad, comprehensive mind" enabled her to feel "a childlike confidence and trust" (197). Her comments are revealing for several reasons. First, they highlight Hunt's recurrent desire to be a child again, to reenter the idealized world of her childhood where her parents, especially her mother, cherished, comforted, and protected her. Hunt's comments about Bush also underscore the fact that she was in a difficult and sad time in her life when she met this man. She was in deep mourning for her beloved niece and sought reassurance that God existed and was benign.

Bush's lectures and more particularly Swedenborg's tenets provided Hunt with the solace she craved. Swedenborg offered a richly detailed view of a divine cosmos; he insisted that death served as a gateway to eternal life. His assertion that after children died they immediately came under the protection of angels and soon became angels themselves must have been especially consoling to Hunt.[12] But Swedenborg did not just comfort a grieving Hunt; he also deepened her commitment to a "mind-cure" approach to medicine. Convinced that the body became sick when it violated spiritual laws, Swedenborg proclaimed that the physician must be "a doctor of the soul as much as of the body." In a world before the advent of modern medicine, his belief influenced numerous health practitioners, including mesmerists, homeopaths, spiritualists, and "mind healers."[13]

Swedenborg's *Animal Kingdom* had a particular impact on Hunt. She fulsomely praised this text for allegedly revealing to her the key tenets of life and how to approach medicine: "My profession assumed a magical power over me, just in proportion as I recognized the material body as a *type* only of the spiritual. This great and powerful truth I found fully elaborated in Swedenborg's Animal Kingdom. . . . Light emanated from that work, which invested anatomy and physiology with golden robes. Clouds of mist vanished, and a flood of light dazzled me at first, but my mental vision became stronger by use. . . . Heaps of facts, gathered during my medical life, assumed form; . . . and order was evolved from chaos. Many truths were found to be centered in one. . . . I had found the philosopher's stone, the elixir of life" (197–98).

It is easy to dismiss Hunt's gushing admiration for Swedenborg as the prattle of someone caught in the throes of a powerful religious conversion, but Swedenborg offered Hunt a kind of psychological life raft—she had been in anguish since the death of her niece. Like other antebellum physicians, Hunt also had to watch helplessly as patients, many of them young, sickened and died. Swedenborg was a godsend to his followers because he provided them with a guide for allegedly curing and even preventing disease. He also reassured the bereaved that death ushered in immortal life.

Hunt's remarks about Swedenborg echo those she made about George Combe. Ignoring the significant differences between these men, Hunt often conflated their ideas. She credited both thinkers with enabling her to move beyond the confusing morass of facts about the human anatomy and to recognize spiritual and mental anguish as the cause of physical illness. But ultimately such an approach to medicine reflected Swedenborg's ideas more than Combe's. The former man's philosophy and view of medicine encouraged Hunt to reject mainstream doctors and their medical training. She recalled, for example, how reading Swedenborg's *Animal Kingdom* and attending the New Church revealed to her the "soulless character of medical works" and enabled her to perceive that "all truth was from the Lord alone." Hunt added that she viewed herself as "a medium" of God; she experienced "a delightful consciousness of *power through Him*" and "gloried in an utter *lack* of *self*-confidence" (198).

But Hunt's actions belied her words. By the time she published the above remarks in her 1856 autobiography, Harvard Medical School had twice rebuffed her efforts to attend lectures. Even as she embraced the religious mysticism of Swedenborg, Hunt still sought to acquire scientific medical training by studying at Harvard. In the end, Hunt straddled two conflicting approaches to medicine in nineteenth-century America: one that promised to banish illness and possibly even death through "mind cures," and one that focused on scientific study of the human body. Like the majority of antebellum alternative health practitioners, Hunt gravitated toward the former approach even as she tried to study medicine as a scientific discipline. Hunt was not opposed to science. Instead, she took an eclectic approach to healing.

Personal as well as professional factors motivated Hunt to study the causes of disease scientifically. The deaths of her father and niece seared her life and brought home the tragedy caused by illness. In the spring of 1847, Hunt saw her beloved mother deteriorating in health. It came at a particularly bad time because Sarah and her family, which now included three boys, moved to a new home. Harriot ruefully conceded that she "experienced a terrible heart-sickness" when her sister moved, especially since her mother was "not well" (209).

As her health deteriorated, Kezia Hunt had no fear of death and at one point asked hopefully if she was soon "going home" to heaven. But if she faced death with equanimity, her eldest daughter dreaded it: "I could not sympathize in [my mother's] gladness. My orphanage dawned upon me, a feeling of desolation seized me" (210). Yet Hunt's conversion to Swedenborgianism did offer her needed comfort. The "truths of the New Church," she gratefully recalled, enabled her to realize that she must not be "selfish" but accept the fact that her mother would soon enter a glorious eternity. Her grieving, Hunt added, merely "detain[ed]" her mother's "spirit" when it sought to "disengage itself from its earthly abode" (210).

Kezia Hunt died on April 21, 1847, at the age of seventy-six.[14] Despite her belief that Kezia's spirit lived on in heaven, Harriot was devastated by her death. She claimed that her grief was greater than Sarah's. "Orphanage means one thing to a married, another to an unmarried child," she emphatically declared. A woman who has a husband and children to care for, Harriot added, is "unavoidably occupied" by the many "claims" and "duties" of family life. But there was no respite from grief for an unmarried woman like herself. Harriot noted that after her mother died she lived for a time "in the past . . . in dreams and reveries" (211).

It is revealing that even though she was forty-one when her mother died, Hunt repeatedly described herself as an orphan. When she contrasted her bereavement to Sarah's, she intimated that hers had to be more intense and prolonged because as an unmarried daughter she had "never been any thing but a child" (211). Such comments illuminate Hunt's continued emotional dependence on her mother, a dependence that one would expect from a child but not a middle-aged adult who had established a successful career for herself. Hunt's remarks bring to mind her earlier admission that in many respects she remained "childlike, resting on a mother" (137).

Hunt also seems to have had ambivalent feelings about her younger sister. On the one hand, she claimed that her love for Sarah became "stronger" and that she was "now my all" (214). Yet Harriot also seemed to resent the fact that Sarah had other "claims" and "duties." What she omitted to mention but probably recognized was that the Wright family cushioned the blow of Kezia Hunt's death for Sarah. Unlike her elder sister, Sarah Wright had a husband and children who not only made demands on her but also loved and comforted her.

Harriot Hunt conveyed the sense of loneliness, abandonment, and desolation she felt after her mother died when she quoted an uncited passage: "'Alone we enter the world—alone we launch forth upon eternity, and between these two periods, there is many a moment when we are compelled to feel that we are utterly alone'" (212). Elizabeth Cady Stanton echoed similar comments in her last presidential speech before the annual meeting of the National American Woman's Suffrage Association in 1892. But Stanton delivered her "Solitude of Self" talk as a way to urge women to become self-reliant and fight for their rights.[15] Although Hunt shared Stanton's sentiments and would soon campaign for woman's rights, she despaired of life in 1847. She was caught in the maw of loneliness and depression.

Sarah Wright recognized her sister's despair and tried to help by repeatedly urging Harriot to live with her family (214). The offer must have been tempting for Hunt, promising as it did respite from her living alone and unhappily. But ultimately she decided to continue living on her own and to concentrate on her medical career. In this respect Hunt was very unusual. Most single women in antebellum middle-class families lived with relatives and remained dependents.[16]

Yet if she was unusual in many respects, Hunt still operated in a society that circumscribed the role of women, especially spinsters. Many unmarried middle-class women sought to contribute to society not only by caring for relatives but also by dedicating themselves to the betterment of humanity. Seeking a vocation where they could help others, many of these women became teachers, missionaries, or reform activists. Yet a life of "single blessedness," even for women from affluent families, was not for the fainthearted. Such a life often entailed hardships and slights as "old maids." What enabled many single women to persevere was viewing themselves as engaged in "noble work" allegedly ordained by God.[17]

This belief is what nurtured Harriot Hunt and gave her the courage to forge a new life for herself after her mother died. She viewed her medical practice as a holy mission—in a sense she sacralized her work, which was evident when Hunt recounted her decision not to live with the Wright family. Convinced that her practice required "a separate home," she declared: "My profession seemed hallowed to me; my patients were my family; and a new purpose to labor more effectively for woman, seized my soul. . . . I must be wedded to Humanity" (214).

Hunt's sense of mission made her determined to gain both expertise and professional recognition from Boston's medical establishment. In the late fall of 1847 she petitioned Harvard Medical School to attend lectures there. The rejection of her request underscored how discriminatory the practice of medicine was in antebellum America. Yet Hunt's reaction to this rebuff—tending to ailing women in various Shaker communities and offering public lectures on women's health issues—highlighted her resilience and commitment to medicine.

Hunt made her request to study at Harvard in a letter dated December 12, 1847, and addressed to Dr. Oliver Wendell Holmes, dean of the medical school. Although the tone of her letter was deferential and supplicatory, Hunt also carefully stated her reasons for seeking admission to the medical lectures. Portraying herself as a mature and experienced medical practitioner of forty-two who adhered to the highest ethical standards, she emphasized that in 1835 she began practicing medicine in "a very quiet, unpretending manner" and "gradually and steadily" built up her practice, rejecting "every immorality" and embodying "respectability." After offering this character portrait, Hunt admitted that she needed formal training to serve her patients best. She sought "scientific light" to be in "harmony" with her "professional duties" and to be "worthy of the trust" her patients placed in her. Toward the end of her letter Hunt alluded to the fact that "one lady" was studying at the "Geneva Medical College." The implication was clear: if the latter school accepted Elizabeth Blackwell, then Harvard Medical School should allow Hunt admission into its lecture hall.[18]

Holmes supported Hunt's petition. In his letter to Harvard's president, he declared that Hunt's gender would not distract male students since she was a woman of "mature age." He also intimated that she was not very attractive: she might be "dobly [sic] trusted, so far as appearances go." Perhaps most important, Holmes stressed that Hunt was "full of zeal for science" and therefore worthy of admission.[19]

Despite Holmes's comments, Harvard Medical School rejected Hunt's petition. The faculty minutes for December 27, 1847, tersely declared that it was "inexpedient" to reconsider their exclusion of women from medical lectures.[20] The school's response angered and embittered Hunt. The use of the word "inexpedient" infuriated her because it revealed Harvard's inability or unwillingness to own up to the fact that they refused her admission simply on the grounds of gender. The school was obfuscating its reasons, equivocating, and Hunt publicized this fact in her autobiography: "That word inexpedient I had always abhorred—it is so shuffling, so shifting, so mean, so evasive.... Any kind of a reason might have been accepted, but this '*inexpedient*' aroused my risibles, my sarcasm, my indignation." Hunt stressed that her patients were also indignant at how Harvard treated her. In response to those who told her that it was "contemptible" for Harvard to use such "a doubtful expression" as "inexpedient," Hunt replied that the institution did this because it was a "safe and non-committal" expression to use (219).

Snubbed by Harvard, Hunt persevered as a physician. She also sought out communities that experimented with new ways of organizing society and rejected established gender roles. One such group that especially attracted Hunt was the United Society of Believers in Christ's Second Appearing, better known as the Shakers. Now best remembered for their ecstatic dancing and simple, beautiful furniture, the Shakers were a vibrant and growing religious sect in antebellum America, one that embraced celibacy and Christian communalism.

By 1840 they had 3,627 members living in over twenty Shaker villages, most of them located in Upstate New York and New England.[21] Various factors promoted equality of the sexes in Shaker communities. Mother Ann Lee, their late eighteenth-century founder, claimed to be Jesus's "deputy" on earth. In 1796 a devout Shaker named Lucy Wright assumed leadership of the community, and during her twenty-five-year rule she increased the sect's membership and geographic reach. Although they often assigned men and women different work roles, the Shakers insisted that both sexes did labor of equal value. Wright and other Shaker leaders boldly maintained that God was both male and female. Of course, their belief that Lee had embodied the spirit of Christ promoted an androgynous view of God.[22]

Although they were initially wary of nonbelievers, the Shakers increased their interactions with mainstream American society in the 1840s and 1850s. The sect's growing involvement with the nation's capitalist economy likely promoted their greater accommodation to the outside world.[23] Shakers welcomed numerous visitors to their villages, especially after the mid-1840s. These included such celebrities as Charles Dickens, Ralph Waldo Emerson, Bronson Alcott, and James Fenimore Cooper. Although some of these guests condemned Shaker beliefs and rituals, many praised sect members for their piety, chastity, industry, and commitment to a communal order, one that rejected the competitive individualism of society.[24]

Hunt was one such visitor. She recalled traveling to her first Shaker community, the one in Shirley, Massachusetts, in the summer of 1848 (219). The Shakers described Hunt as "the celebrated Female Physician of Boston."[25] Hunt regularly visited the Shirley and Harvard settlements during the late 1840s and 1850s, traveling by train from nearby Boston.[26] At times she took friends with her. One such person was the English traveler and writer Marianne Finch, who toured Harvard and Shirley with Hunt in the spring of 1851. Finch praised the Shakers for their hospitality as well as their orderliness, cleanliness, and concern for others, especially the aged. Sect members sang to her and Hunt, read them poetry, and gave them an extensive tour of their facilities. According to Finch, Hunt regaled her Shaker hosts with "lively" conversation and "bursts of merriment" and at one point led the elder sisters in song. Not surprisingly, Finch stressed that Hunt was a "great favorite" with the Shakers.[27]

Hunt's visits were particularly welcomed because she tended to ailing Shakers (220).[28] Finch remembered that when Hunt visited the Shakers, she came "in the twofold capacity of friend and physician."[29] Each Shaker community, Hunt emphasized, designated a woman as a "physician" because they believed that women had "a peculiar gift in that direction" (230). Hunt often worked with such female healers. She stressed how "delightful" it was to "put on a Shaker apron" and prepare herbal medicines while a Shaker "sister who officiated as nurse and doctor was with me" (228).

When the Shakers traveled to Boston they often enjoyed Hunt's hospitality. She housed and fed these visitors, helped them tour the city, and also introduced them to numerous reformers. In the early 1850s, for example, Shakers appreciatively noted Hunt's many kindnesses during their trips to Boston. At her home they met such noted reformers as the phrenologist Lorenzo Fowler; his wife, Lydia Fowler, the second woman to earn a medical degree in the United States; and Paulina Wright Davis, a leading woman's rights activist. Hunt also arranged for her Shaker guests to visit Boston's "home for aged females" and to attend lectures related to women's health. Seeking to repay Hunt's hospitality, female Shaker guests sewed for their hostess.[30]

Several aspects of Shaker life attracted Hunt. First, she commended this religious community for "their care of the aged" (229). When Hunt traveled to Shaker villages she often visited and doctored "the aged sisters."[31] No doubt Hunt's own devotion to her mother and grief over her death made her particularly sensitive to the plight of these elderly women and appreciative of the care the Shaker community gave them. Hunt also stressed the Shakers' love of Ann Lee, their "spiritual mother," and praised their piety and "purity" (229). Somewhat sheepishly, Hunt admitted that the Shakers' indefatigable work ethic at times made her feel inadequate: "Their unceasing industry tired me, for I have lazy moments" (229).

But what most impressed Hunt about the Shakers was their commitment to gender equality. As she admiringly declared: "The equality of woman with man is recognized in every department of Shaker life. The duties and responsibilities of ministers, elders, and caretakers were *equally* shared by *both* sexes" (229–30). Hunt became friends with "many noble women" in the Harvard and Shirley communities (220). Shaker women appreciatively shared her autobiography among themselves shortly after it was published. Elder sisters also discussed their theology with Hunt.[32]

One woman who might have done so was Roxalana L. Grosvenor, a prominent Shaker administrator and church elder living in Harvard, who became friends with Hunt. A maverick like Hunt, Grosvenor would be expelled from the Shaker community in 1865 because she had rejected their doctrine of celibacy and urged the procreation of children conceived through "pure love," not lust. For Grosvenor, the act of giving birth was a unique female function that empowered women and therefore should be valued.³³ But when Hunt formed her friendship with Grosvenor during the summer of 1849, she was still a prominent Shaker in good standing. In her autobiography Hunt described Grosvenor as "one of the loveliest, noblest women" and noted her "deep interest in the sick, her subdued, chastened bearing,—her deep devotional earnestness,—[and] her humility." She also approvingly stated that Grosvenor was a minister, a position that confirmed for Hunt the Shakers' progressive attitudes toward women (228).

Visits to the Shakers exposed Hunt to a way of life that gave women greater authority and equality than in mainstream America. They showed her a successful religious experiment that subordinated the interests of individuals to the welfare of the community and homage to God. Through the Shakers, Hunt also learned the tragic life stories of many female converts. These women's "heart histories" led Hunt to recognize that the Shakers performed a crucial function in antebellum America: they offered one of the few sanctuaries for women fleeing abusive, tyrannical husbands. Since there were "no convents in New England," Hunt declared almost wistfully, "*many women*" desperately needed "an asylum." She poignantly illustrated this point when she recounted the story of a woman who fled her husband after suffering "a depth of agony." This wife "retired from the world" and joined the Shakers when she was "broken in health, crushed in spirit, [and] unable to care for her children" (229–31). Unfortunately, her husband, after they divorced, refused to let her see their children.³⁴ There were countless other "brave, earnest, thoughtful women" living in Shaker communities, stressed Hunt, who suffered "equally mournful" experiences (232–33). Their plight made it all the more praiseworthy that "our Shaker brethren and sisters have opened their villages as *cities of refuge*" where women can heal their "bleeding hearts and broken constitutions" (234).

Harriot Hunt came to have great respect and affection for the Shakers. Their religious community gave her an opportunity to practice her healing skills and also alleviated the sadness and isolation she experienced after her mother's death and rejection from Harvard. She admired the Shakers for their willingness to provide refuge to women fleeing unhappy homes and for their care of the elderly and sick. The fact that the Shakers seemed to accept her as a friend was important to Hunt; as she noted with obvious satisfaction: "My professional position placed me . . . into their innermost; so that it is not too much for me to say that I understand them better than any one who has not lived in a Shaker village" (230). Of course, Hunt's boast may well have reflected wishful thinking on her part rather than an accurate description of how far the

Shakers actually allowed her to penetrate their society. But what is important is that Hunt *believed* she had been able to enter the inner circle of the Shakers. Her visits to their communities nurtured her. They "opened new chapters of life to me" and "I was so happy to find myself useful," she joyfully declared (228).

Yet despite her close association with the Shakers, Hunt never converted to the religion. Her flourishing medical practice and ties with Sarah's family anchored Hunt to her Boston life. She stressed that when she returned from visiting the Shakers, her patients in Boston "welcomed" her return. Hunt was heartened to see that they followed her advice; their "obedience to physical laws" allegedly improved their health. Her patients kept her busy and she spent a great deal of time visiting the Wrights. Sarah and Edmund's children were "quite a fascination," she declared (221).

Hunt's objections to some of the Shakers' beliefs and customs also made it unlikely that she ever seriously considered joining their community. Hunt described the Shakers' "costume and language" as "quaint" and stated that their manners had "a tendency to *chill* one." More significant, Hunt declared: "*My perception of freedom was wholly different from theirs.*" Although she quickly added that this fact did not "hinder" her from "perceiving *their* stand-point, and respecting it," Hunt recognized that she had fundamental disagreements with the Shakers (230). She could visit and befriend them, tend to their illnesses, but she could not join their religious order. In the end, Harriot Hunt remained in Boston.

Shaker recollections and those of Marianne Finch suggest that Hunt made a wise decision. Her assertive personality, boisterous laugh, and exuberance upset some Shakers. Finch recounted that Hunt's merriment and loud conversation in Shirley led one older Shaker man to enjoin: "*Make less noise—you disturb me.*" This rebuke, noted Finch, mortified the Shaker sisters, while Hunt's face temporarily "lost all its rotundity."[35] Hunt also seems to have irked some Shakers from the New Lebanon, New York, village who met her in 1850 when they visited Harvard. While recalling this meeting, an unidentified Shaker declared that the "Boston doctress," while "very friendly to Believers," was too chatty and loud: "She is a great talker and an immoderate laugher."[36] As these comments suggest, Hunt probably would have found it very difficult to bend to the communal discipline the Shakers required, especially when she asserted herself as an independent woman who cherished the freedom to act, speak, and laugh in a way some deemed "immoderate."

Although she seemed to have a full life in the late 1840s, Hunt remained restless. In 1849 she embarked on an ambitious project—she became a public lecturer on women's health issues. She joined a growing number of women who spoke to female audiences about various matters, including the importance of temperance, diet, and exercise as a way to promote good health. Although popular male lecturers, such as William Alcott and Sylvester Graham, offered similar advice, their female counterparts tackled issues that particularly concerned women, lecturing about the female anatomy and discussing such issues as menstruation, childbirth, and menopause.[37] Noted female speakers included Paulina Wright Davis and Mary Gove Nichols, the water-cure advocate who became notorious when she espoused free-love principles in the 1850s.[38]

Women became health reform lecturers for personal as well as professional reasons. They sought not only to educate their sex about their own bodies and improve female health but also to forge a career for themselves and earn badly needed money. One such lecturer was Sarah Coates, who toured various Ohio towns in 1850. She offered a particularly revealing account of her motivations in letters she wrote to her friend William Darlington, a retired Pennsylvania physician and amateur botanist, noted for his friendships with scientifically inclined women.[39]

Coates stressed to Darlington her commitment to improving women's health by educating her audience about "the importance of pure air, invigorating exercise, wholesome food, ... comfortable dress, ... & most of all cleanliness." But Coates's letters also conveyed how her public speaking offered her a needed escape from a narrow, frustrating life. She confessed how limiting women's role to the domestic sphere was "death to both soul & body. ... [W]omen were not made for puppets & doll-babies, to be set upon a damask cushion in the parlor & there to vegitate [sic]." Despite the obvious differences between men and women, asserted Coates, they were alike in one key respect—"they must labor or die—The activities must have vent. ... This death of the soul from unemployed powers is almost worse than death of body by starvation—I must fill a place in life. ... I pant—I smother, if compelled to an aimless life." Financial considerations also prompted Coates to lecture on women's health. She noted that lecturing enabled her not only to pay all the expenses she incurred during her travels but also to clear $75. Lecturing was a profitable as well as a fulfilling experience for Coates, and she reluctantly gave it up only when she moved to a rural area in Minnesota and later married.

As for Hunt, several reasons motivated her to become a public lecturer. First, she sought to educate women about their bodies and the need to live in accordance with nature's alleged laws. Second, she also sought to stave off loneliness by traveling and meeting new people. As she poignantly declared in *Glances and Glimpses*: "Hours of loneliness were often spent in my solitary home, and I might have sunk under the blow, had not the angel of mercy visited me, and inspired me with the thought of endeavoring to enlighten my sisters on the subject of the 'laws of life'" (222). Hunt saw herself as "a minister in the grand work of diffusing a knowledge of hygienic laws." (221). What did not seem to motivate her, however, was the need for money. Hunt noted that her talks were free (222).[40]

But if her lectures were not financially lucrative for Hunt, they were nevertheless essential to her well-being. Lecturing and traveling, she stressed, meant "the opening of a new life" for her, just as ministering to the Shakers had. The work of preparing and delivering the lectures mitigated her continued grieving for her mother: "The clouds of sorrow, the selfishness of grief was exchanged for the cheerfulness of hope, the garments of heaviness for the vestments of praise" (222, 223). Hunt conceded that Harvard's rejection of her request to attend medical lectures "strengthened" her resolve to educate women about health matters (224–25).

Hunt delivered her first lecture in late February 1849 in a Boston chapel, gratefully remembering that many of her friends and fellow congregants from the New Church were there to support her. These lectures had a profound impact on Hunt. She recalled that they put her in "more intimate relations with the laboring classes" (223). Her talks encouraged wage-earning women to reveal their life stories to her. These "heart histories" echoed what she had heard from the working-class patients she saw in her practice. They poignantly detailed how women's lack of education, few job opportunities, and low pay ravaged them and their families. Hunt heard from "broken-hearted widows" who had to "break up their homes" owing to lack of money. She heard stories about young girls who had to leave the "protection" of their homes to provide for "aged or afflicted parents" and "helpless brothers and sisters" (224).

Learning firsthand about the experiences of destitute women nurtured Hunt's commitment to woman's rights. But so too did ministering to women who suffered in other ways—those who had been hurt by male doctors and their "heroic therapies"; those who were trapped in miserable, even abusive, marriages; those who had lost their children when they joined the Shakers; and finally, those who felt desperate despite living privileged lives as the spouses of affluent husbands. Hunt heard the "heart histories" of these women; she treated them and witnessed their anguish. Their plight evoked not only Hunt's compassion but also drew her to the woman's rights movement. As she proclaimed in *Glances and Glimpses*, "My bereaved spirit felt more than sympathy and veneration for those noble women who had struggled at fearful odds against injustice, poverty, and oppression; new life, fresh vigor were infused to strengthen my purpose to meliorate the condition of my sex, and elevate woman to the platform of humanity, to the enjoyment of human rights" (224).

But bearing witness to the agonies of others can be a wrenching experience. Hunt also kept a grueling work schedule—she delivered multiple lectures at different places while maintaining her regular medical practice. Her autobiography also suggests that a friend betrayed her trust, although Hunt did not offer details about this matter other than to note that a "false friend" caused her "mental distress" (225).

In May of 1849, Hunt became seriously ill. She diagnosed herself as suffering from "a bilious fever" which "prostrated" her. But her symptoms suggest that she had an emotional as well as physical breakdown. She became "sleepy, morbid, weak" and was unable to continue lecturing. Overwork and exhaustion were probably major causes of Hunt's illness. In an especially revealing comment she conceded that when she was unable to lecture and had to retire to her sick room, she felt relieved, even happy: "I wept for joy that I had a right to lie down and rest.... The couch and the night dress are real luxuries" (225).

Illness provided Hunt with much-needed respite from work. She also basked in the attention and sympathy of family, friends, and patients, relishing her patients' gifts of flowers and fruit and most of all their "kindest notes" (225). Hunt could now be the patient and enjoy the earnest attention of her physician. Best of all, she enjoyed the care of her sister, Sarah. The latter's "faithfulness and tenderness," she remembered, were "like our mother" and offered her the "sweetest solace." In early June the Wright family moved Hunt to their home. There she was "surrounded by family loves" and nursed with "tender . . . sweet . . . ministrations" (225–26).

Hunt obviously enjoyed her time as a patient. Her recollection of the care she received from Sarah and the Wright family makes it sound as if she was immersed in a warm, nurturing cocoon. It seemed like a return to her childhood when her parents, especially Kezia, enveloped her in a loving domesticity. Her words describing her illness and convalescence are both revealing and poignant: "I seemed to realize a second babyhood, so passive, so quiet,—this is favorable to recovery, I owed much to this childlike feeling" (226). As she lay in her sickbed, Hunt remembered her "childhood's happy days." Her vivid memories were crucial to her recovery, she insisted. They enabled her "to refresh and fortify the soul" (227).

Hunt's illness, at least partly psychosomatic in nature, allowed her to regress to a helpless, childlike state. Although she stressed that she missed her mother's "hand upon [her]" and "her voice of kindness" (226), Harriot had the next best thing when she became ill in 1849—Sarah ministered to her with great tenderness. Sickness enabled Harriot Hunt to withdraw from her many duties and to avoid living alone, at least for a while. Most of all, it gave Hunt the excuse she needed to focus on herself, to be coddled, babied.

Hunt was not unusual when she did this. During the antebellum era, many women found respite from caring for others when they themselves became ill, often the only way that women could justify leaving their families and spending weeks, even months, in water-cure establishments that catered to their needs.[41] When Hunt was on the mend in early July, she traveled to Hopkinton Springs, where she found the baths there to be "quite a tonic" (228). Her illness, she said, offered "a needful pause in [her] life"; it provided her with an opportunity to take "stock" of her "profession" and to think "more deeply" about the need to educate women about their bodies and health (227).

But after several months Hunt was ready to resume her medical career, lecturing, and traveling to Shaker communities. As she picked up the threads of her life again, Hunt formed a friendship with Fredrika Bremer, the well-known Swedish novelist whose popular writings promoted her Christian socialist views.[42] In September 1849, Bremer began an extensive tour of the United States which lasted until 1851. Hunt met Bremer while she was in New York City that November, and the Swedish writer later stayed in Hunt's home in Boston (235–38). Bremer offered a complicated portrait of Hunt in her 1853 account of her travels to America entitled *The Homes of the New World*. She recalled that initially she was reluctant to leave the very comfortable home of her friends to stay with Hunt, but "Miss H. seized upon me with her might," and the visit "turned out much better than I expected." Yet Bremer at times offered a patronizing and unflattering description of Hunt. She repeatedly referred to her hostess as "my little doctoress" and declared that she was a "very peculiar individual," a person who needed "better manners" and "more tact." Bremer also described Hunt as a physically unattractive woman: "The round, short figure has wholly and entirely an earthly character." The only physical attributes that Bremer liked about Hunt were her "small, beautiful, and white hands, as soft as silk," and her "glance," which was "peculiarly sagacious and penetrating."[43]

If in some ways she found Hunt off-putting, Bremer also expressed genuine respect and affection for her. She stressed that one could not find a person with "a better heart" and "more practical sagacity" than Hunt. Admiringly, the

Swedish writer also noted how Hunt helped countless patients suffering from myriad diseases. Her "little human doctoress" was also "a benefactor to the women of the lower working classes" by not only treating their ailments but also educating them through her lectures on physiology. Bremer recalled that she developed "a high opinion" of Hunt's "powers of mind" after she heard some of these lectures: "There was an earnestness, a simplicity, and an honesty in her representations, integrity and purity in every word; the style was of the highest class, and these lectures could not but operate powerfully upon every poor human heart." If Hunt at times discomfited Bremer, she also impressed her as a dedicated, intelligent, and kind woman. Bremer ultimately gave Hunt unstinting praise: "I was really delighted with her, and now for the first time fully saw the importance of women devoting themselves to the medical profession."[44]

Hunt nurtured in Bremer a commitment to reform activism. Bremer noted that her Boston friend taught her a great deal about the Shakers and that the two women planned to visit the Shaker community at Harvard. Although illness prevented Hunt from making the trip (237), Bremer did go and credited Hunt's many friends there with making her visit both pleasant and educational.[45] Shortly before leaving the United States, Hunt and Bremer visited the North American Phalanx, a community founded on the utopian principles of the French socialist Charles Fourier (237). This community and the Shakers exposed Bremer to societies that redefined traditional gender roles and urged more freedom for women.

Hunt also introduced her Swedish houseguest to leading reformers. Bremer seemed somewhat amazed to meet women who were public lecturers on controversial political topics. She noted that at Hunt's home she met "'emancipated ladies'" who "speak in public" about "anti-slavery" and other controversial causes. She was particularly impressed with Paulina Wright Davis, a woman whom she described as a "picturesque beauty" with a "pale noble countenance" who combined "perfect gentleness and womanliness" with the "manly force of will and conviction."[46] As her words suggest, Bremer subscribed to many of the gendered stereotypes popular in her day. But the reformers she met in the United States, especially Hunt and her activist friends, helped her become a woman's rights advocate.[47]

After her return to Sweden, Bremer wrote her most influential novel, the bestseller *Hertha*. Published in 1856, the book narrated how a young girl became a strong, independent woman who challenged patriarchy and espoused feminist principles.[48] After this novel's publication, Bremer wrote to Hunt asking for information about the progress of the woman's rights movement in America.

Bremer told her friend that she now recognized that "the true liberation of mankind" depended on "the elevation of woman." Although they were an ocean apart, Bremer regarded Hunt as a friend and fellow activist in an international woman's rights movement. She asked Hunt to tell her what she was doing "for the great cause in America" and promised to respond in kind: "I will tell you by and by what I try to do and want to do for it in Scandinavia."[49]

And how did Hunt view Bremer? Almost seven years later Hunt could recall the details of her first meeting with the Swedish writer. The morning was "bright and bracing," and Hunt felt "at once" that she had found "a kindred spirit." "My inmost was alive," she gushed, and it seemed natural to urge Bremer to stay with her in Boston: "I felt that I was only inviting her to what was partly hers already" (235). With Bremer, Hunt felt she did not have to articulate her ideas to be understood; Bremer seemed almost to intuit them. According to Hunt, they shared "those movements, those looks that electrify the soul without the utterance of a word" (237).

Part of the reason that Hunt felt so close to Bremer was that they shared a common misfortune. "Her mother, too, has passed away—she is an orphan," emphasized Hunt. She also suggested that Bremer offered her a needed role model as she scrambled to regain her footing after her recent personal and professional setbacks. Bremer seemed to have achieved what Hunt sought to do. This Swede's "harmony with nature had wedded her to humanity," claimed Hunt, and therefore "her loneliness was only external" (236). Bremer was also a person in whom Hunt could confide, someone to whom she could tell her "heart history."

But Bremer did not just provide solace and sympathy; she also spurred Hunt on as she created a nonconventional life for herself, one rooted in serving others, especially women in need. For these reasons, Hunt's lifelong friendship with Fredrika Bremer had a major impact on her. This was evident when Hunt wrote in *Glances and Glimpses* that "Fredrika had a mission for me, my womanhood needed rousing . . . . [Bremer's] visit was to my soul as dew upon the mown grass. . . . I have enjoyed a sweet correspondence with her since, and know that the soul has feelers, and in sympathy we may breathe a prayer though oceans roll between [us]" (235–36).

Hunt's account of her friendship with Fredrika Bremer underscores the kinship she felt with this woman. But at times it seems as if Hunt were writing about a lover rather than a friend. Her references to the excitement she felt at meeting Bremer and to exchanging looks with her that "electrify the soul" suggest that she felt a sexual attraction and possibly romantic love for Bremer. There is no evidence that Hunt ever had a romantic involvement with a man. The only time that she overtly expressed any romantic feelings for another human being was when she recalled that as a girl she formed "many love attachments" with fellow "school-girls" and would correspond with them, sometimes anonymously (21).

Given the lack of evidence about Hunt's sexual or romantic life, we can only speculate about the true nature of her feelings for Bremer. But the fact remains that, throughout her life, Hunt formed intensely close friendships with other women, ones that sometimes displayed a homoerotic dimension. She was probably what historian Judith Bennett has described as "lesbian-like," a woman who enjoyed "intimate friendships" with other women that were "erotically charged," even if they did not involve genital or other overt sexual contact.[50] Women like Hunt and the relationships they formed with members of their own sex highlight how fluid the lines were between homosexuality and heterosexuality in mid-nineteenth-century America.[51]

The closest, most emotionally intense friendship Hunt forged was with Sarah Grimké.[52] Like Hunt, Grimké was an older, unmarried sister who was extremely close with her younger sibling, even after the latter became a wife and mother. Like Hunt, Grimké also remained emotionally dependent on her mother, even after the latter died in 1839. Sarah Grimké's letters to Hunt make clear that she drew strength from allegedly communing with her mother's spirit. Probably aware of her friend's lifelong closeness with her own mother, Grimké was confident that Hunt was one of the "few" to whom she could confide how she spent her Sabbaths—alone in her room in "sweet retirement," relishing the spirit of her "dear mother" appearing "so lovingly, so angelically."[53] Another similarity between Hunt and Grimké was that both rejected conventional Protestantism and belonged to churches committed to reform. By the end of the 1820s, Sarah and Angelina had become Quakers, a religious sect stressing the equality and dignity of every human being. This action promoted the Grimkés' opposition to slavery and support for woman's rights.

Their political activism, especially their public speaking about the horrors of slavery, attracted widespread condemnation. In late July 1837, the General Association of Massachusetts Congregational Churches issued a pastoral letter denouncing women who abandoned their "appropriate" sphere and wrongly assumed "the place and tone of man as a public reformer" and as "public lecturers and teachers."[54] Although the ministers did not explicitly name the Grimkés, they were clearly the major target of the ministers' reproach.

Sarah Grimké responded by publishing a series of letters that articulated the major principles of feminism in nineteenth-century America. In her *Letters on the Equality of the Sexes*, published as a book in 1838, Grimké asserted the innate equality of all human beings and berated men for subjugating women and depriving them of their God-given and natural rights. No longer a Quaker by the time she penned the *Letters*, Grimké asserted that God was androgynous, both male and female. She also argued that the Bible had been misinterpreted by men to justify their misogyny. Men, she stressed, had benefited from their domination of women throughout the centuries and then blamed females for their alleged inferiority. Grimké bristled at women's lack of educational and economic opportunities and the legal submission of wives. She boldly asserted that "men and women were CREATED EQUAL; they are both moral and accountable beings, and whatever is *right* for man to do, is *right* for woman."[55]

Grimké's ideas had a profound impact on Hunt's views on woman's rights and shaped how she wrote her 1856 autobiography.[56] But Sarah Grimké was a close friend as well as a mentor. As Gerda Lerner, the Grimké sisters' biographer, has noted, Hunt became Sarah's lifelong confidante.[57] Unfortunately, most of Hunt's letters to Sarah and her family have disappeared, but Sarah's letters to Hunt as well as the latter's autobiography highlight the close bond between the two women.

The friendship apparently began in the latter half of the 1840s. By then Sarah was living in Belleville, New Jersey, with Angelina, now married to fellow abolitionist Theodore Dwight Weld, and their children. She helped the Welds run a school they had established.[58] Her letters addressed to Hunt during this time show that she already treasured her Boston friend and shared all kinds of concerns with her. Grimké repeatedly addressed Hunt as "beloved Harriot," and at times her letters suggest that she felt more than friendship for Hunt.[59] At one point, for example, Grimké wrote Hunt: "Your heart meets mine, dear Harriot. Sometimes I say, to myself, what is to come of this new but fervent love—*Be patient* is the only answer." Grimké added that she hoped they would soon be able to see each other.[60] In another letter, written shortly after she had visited Hunt in Boston, Grimké stressed that it had been "very pleasant" to receive her friend's "innocent love" and "childlike confidence" and then declared: "You welcomed me to your heart, nestled me closely there ... love me Harriot-I will love you."[61]

Irrespective of whether Sarah Grimké loved Hunt in any romantic way, what is clear is that she confided in her, which was already evident in the letters she wrote to Hunt during the 1848–50 period. To Hunt she repeatedly shared her worries about Angelina's health. The latter seemed to suffer from a displaced uterus which often incapacitated her. At one point Sarah Grimké asked Hunt if she could diagnose her sister from afar and prescribe an appropriate treatment.[62] Grimké also confessed her sadness and sense of inadequacy in fulfilling her numerous duties at the school in Belleville.[63]

But she did not use her correspondence with Hunt merely to vent about her life. She supported Hunt in her endeavors. This was evident when Grimké congratulated Hunt for sending her petition to Harvard Medical School and urged her to persevere in her struggle to gain entrance into this institution's medical lectures. Grimké made clear both her admiration for Hunt and her frustration with women's subordinate status when she declared: "It is a great blessing to see our way clear, & feel energy & perseverance to pursue the path of duty—thousands of women are perishing around us, for want of something to do."[64]

In the spring and summer of 1850, Grimké and Hunt drew closer together as they visited each other. Grimké supported Hunt when she undertook a series of free lectures in the North End that spring. It was an important event for Hunt—she saw again many of her parents' former neighbors and friends and felt that they could now judge for themselves whether she, "the North End girl," had "lived an aimless, useless, and fashionable life." Hunt recalled that the lectures went well, that many in her audience "welcomed [her] back," and that several of the women gave her a gift (247). The lectures ended with Sarah Grimké making closing remarks. But these talks may have been less successful than Hunt claimed. While still in Boston, Sarah Grimké wrote Angelina, telling her how "depressed" she and Hunt were at the public reception to the first lecture. Angelina wrote back words of encouragement, which Sarah shared with her friend. Hunt, affirmed Angelina, was doing "a good work" and should not be "discouraged" as she would eventually "triumph."[65]

That summer Hunt traveled to Belleville and had a lovely time. She was effusive in her praise for the Grimké sisters and Theodore Weld. Their "truth-loving spirit," she declared, infused their home with beauty and, more important, furthered the cause of reform. Hunt also pointedly recognized that it was the Grimkés who had "paved the way for woman as public speaker, and every lover of freedom owes much to them" (248).

In the 1850s Hunt built on what the Grimké sisters had begun—she became a prominent public figure in the woman's rights movement, participating in major conventions, petitioning repeatedly for woman's right to vote, and demanding other reforms to empower America's female citizens. Hunt also again petitioned Harvard Medical School to let her attend medical lectures. The 1850s, then, saw Hunt battling on several fronts for her rights and those of all women.

Chapter 4

Battling Harvard Medical School, Becoming a Woman's Rights Activist

n early June of 1854, the *New York Daily Times* reprinted a snide commentary by the popular British magazine *Punch* regarding "Dr. Harriot Hunt" and her recent lectures in New York City. Her talks on "Woman as a Physician," stated *Punch*, brought to mind Walter Scott's "hackneyed lines":

> Oh woman! In our hours of ease,
> Uncertain, coy, and hard to please
> When pain and anguish wring the brow
> A ministering M.D. thou.

The editors at *Punch* declared that they "prefer the original 'angel.'"[1]

Such remarks reflected the public's disapproval of women who became physicians and thereby transgressed traditional gender roles. But they also illustrated an important fact about Harriot Kezia Hunt: by the mid-1850s she had become a public figure, one who attracted the attention of not only major American newspapers but also British publications. During the last decade before the Civil War, Hunt engaged in a whirlwind of activity that thrust her into the public spotlight. Her second application to attend lectures at the Harvard Medical School embroiled her in controversy that was widely reported in the press. Her participation in various reform conventions, especially those on woman's rights, and itinerant lecturing about the need for health reform and female doctors also attracted significant news coverage. So, too, did her annual public protests regarding several matters, especially the fact that she had to pay taxes but could not vote. Finally, Hunt garnered publicity when she published her autobiography, *Glances and Glimpses.*

Such high-profile activism took Hunt away from her medical practice and the patients who relied on her. In *Glances and Glimpses* she seemed defensive about her extensive travels and lecturing. She stressed that these activities were neither indulgent nor unfocused. Instead, they served one overarching goal—promoting the cause of human rights by advocating for women, particularly their inalienable right to an education. Hunt insisted that her travels, lectures, and speeches were crucial in "calling attention" to the "importance and propriety" of women "entering the medical profession" (311).

Hunt's campaign to open the field of medicine to women promoted her own career as well as human rights. Frequent travels also provided a needed respite from a taxing and at times frustrating medical practice. Hunt conceded that she traveled because it seemed to be "the best means of restoring strength to the physical and of renewing the power of the mental." She added that when she was not "vigorous," she soon felt "an indescribable *shabbiness*, a lack of interior power" which "prevent[ed]" her from giving to her patients "all that they require and have a right to demand from a physician" (311).

Hunt was always a woman who sought challenges. By the early 1850s, her career as a Boston physician who primarily treated women by listening to their "heart histories" no longer seemed as fulfilling as it once had. She needed a larger stage to implement her ideas about women's health and education and also to keep herself engaged as a physician and reformer. By 1850, however, Hunt had both the money and the time to travel widely and participate in various reform activities. By 1860 she had real estate appraised at $24,000 and a personal estate valued at $12,000.[2]

Following the advice that she always gave her female patients—become knowledgeable about financial matters and always handle your own affairs rather than trusting men to do this (71, 73, 79, 372, and 396)—Hunt was wealthy by the time she died in 1875. Her will shows that she made bequests to numerous family members, friends, and different charitable organizations in the thousands of dollars. This document also reveals one major source of Hunt's income: investments in rental property.[3] One newspaper in 1862 noted that Hunt owned "valuable property in Boston."[4] This fact, coupled with a successful medical practice, gave her the financial means she needed to pursue an independent life by the time she was in her late forties. No wonder, then, that Elizabeth Cady Stanton remembered Hunt as a "woman of wealth and position."[5]

Hunt's financial success was a remarkable accomplishment for any person, male or female, in antebellum America, especially one who came from a working-class family. Despite the popularity of countless tales of rags-to-riches success stories, prosperity was an elusive dream for the majority of Americans during the first half of the nineteenth century. Utilizing the census of 1860, historians estimate that only 60 percent of free adult males had personal estates valued at more than $100, and no more than 40 percent of them owned real estate. In 1860, unskilled laborers earned about $200 to $400 annually, while craftsmen and other skilled male workers earned from $400 to $800 a year. The overall average income for nonfarm workers in 1860 totaled $363. Not surprisingly, only one-fifth of American men achieved a "middle-class" life, earning $800 to $5,000 a year. The rich, who comprised less than 1 percent of the population, were those who had annual incomes of over $5,000.[6]

Wage-earning women were considerably worse off financially than their male counterparts. Comprising less than 15 percent of paid workers in 1860, most of these women toiled as domestic servants, seamstresses, laundresses, and mill and factory workers.[7] They earned only a fraction of what men did. As Alice Kessler-Harris has noted, throughout most of the nineteenth century "women's wages customarily ranged from one-third to half those of men." Much of this disparity was because "starting wages in the least skilled men's jobs paid more than those earned by highly skilled and experienced women." The low wages and limited economic opportunities for most women workers meant that they often lived in poverty. As Kessler-Harris poignantly concluded in her study of antebellum female laborers, the hope that wage work would enable women to achieve "a proud independence" remained a quixotic goal; most women labored long and hard to stave off destitution.[8]

Although marriage to a prosperous man might bring a minority of women financial security, it did not confer on them a "proud independence." Following English common law, the American judicial system declared a woman legally dead when she married; her legal identity was subsumed under that of her husband's. The feme covert status of wives deprived them not only of rights over their persons and children but also over whatever property they inherited and monies they earned.[9] As Sarah Grimké grimly declared, marriage subordinated a wife to the power of her husband, and one result was to make it impossible for her to retain control over "her own honest earnings," acquired through "great industry" and careful savings.[10]

These facts highlight how unusual, even extraordinary, was the financial success of Harriot Kezia Hunt. She was a self-made, professional, single woman who earned good money and amassed a considerable estate independent of male control. Hunt's affluence, coupled with her status as an unmarried, childless woman, freed her to travel, lecture, and write. She was also fortunate to live in Boston. Known as the "Athens of America," antebellum Boston was a center of political activism, religious liberalism, and cultural ferment.[11] It was a city where a maverick such as Hunt could forge a career for herself and find a community of activists committed to improving women's lives. A brief review of antebellum female reformers offers a needed context for analyzing Hunt's participation in the struggle for woman's rights during the 1850s.

During the 1820–60 period, numerous women, especially those who were middle-class Anglo-Americans, mobilized against various ills, including intemperance, prostitution, poverty, and slavery. As they addressed these problems, women defied efforts to limit them to the domestic sphere. They did this when they asserted their right to petition legislators, to speak to "promiscuous" or gender-mixed audiences, and to attend and even organize reform conventions.[12]

Although these public activities, traditionally gendered masculine, attracted widespread condemnation, many women continued to participate in them. This was especially true for female abolitionists. During the 1830s, for example, Sarah and Angelina Grimké persisted in speaking and writing about the horrors of slavery even when prominent New England clergy condemned them.[13] African American activist Maria Stewart also braved public opprobrium when she lectured in public about the evils of slavery and racial discrimination in Boston during the early 1830s.[14] By the end of that decade, black as well as white women had formed numerous female antislavery societies throughout the North and organized national Antislavery Conventions of American Women. They successfully demanded membership in all-male state and national abolitionist organizations, especially the American Antislavery Society. These activists also flooded Congress with thousands of antislavery petitions. Such actions enabled countless women to forge a collective, political role for themselves, one where they asserted their right to equal citizenship.[15] Through such actions, women challenged their nation to expand the public, civic sphere to include themselves as well as people of color.[16]

As numerous historians have shown, female abolitionists were the political leaders of the woman's rights movement.[17] Antebellum feminists boldly challenged their fellow Americans to recognize that limiting full citizenship only to white men contradicted the nation's professed beliefs in democracy and liberty.[18] They demanded rights for women, including the right to vote. Citizenship should not be gendered, they insisted. Attacking patriarchy, these reformers demanded that women be granted "co-equality" with men, seeking to achieve "self-sovereignty" and "self-protection" for women.[19] As they waged this struggle, advocates for the rights of women demanded an end to coverture in marriage. Wives, they stressed, should retain their legal independence and not be subjugated by their husbands. They should have the right to retain custody of their persons, their children, their earnings and properties.[20]

One of the most crucial ways that antebellum feminists publicized their ideas in the 1850s was through annual national woman's rights conventions held in different northern states, especially Massachusetts, New York, Pennsylvania, and Ohio. These conventions served a number of crucial purposes. First, they enabled woman's rights supporters to articulate and clarify their multifaceted struggle against patriarchy and their vision for a more egalitarian society. The annual meetings also became a way for activists from different parts of the country to forge regional and national networks of reform. Participants also honed their public speaking and writing skills, gaining invaluable experience for the long struggle to gain their rights. These conventions also publicized the cause of woman's rights throughout the United States. There was extensive press coverage of these meetings, and although much of it was negative, these gatherings nevertheless helped disseminate the feminist agenda. Often timed to coincide with the calling of state constitutional conventions, annual woman's rights meetings challenged politicians to grant basic rights to women in revised constitutions.[21]

National conventions on woman's rights also helped American activists link up with feminists in other countries. This was apparent during the first two and arguably most important of the conventions, both of which were held in Worcester, Massachusetts, on October 23 and 24, 1850, and October 15 and 16, 1851, respectively. News of the first convention spurred Harriet Taylor Mill, wife of the noted philosopher John Stuart Mill and a reformer in her own right, to publish in 1851 an essay entitled "Enfranchisement of Women" in the influential British journal, the *Westminster Review*. Her work soon became required reading for feminists in Britain, America, and other countries.[22]

The calling of the second convention in Worcester heartened the noted French feminists Jeanne Deroine and Pauline Roland, who were imprisoned for their activism on behalf of the failed revolution in 1848. In a long letter read at the convention, Deroine and Roland praised their American "sisters": "Your courageous declaration of Woman's Rights has resounded even to our prison, and has filled our souls with inexpressible joy." They urged feminists in the United States to continue the struggle to "break the chain of the most oppressed of all—of Woman, the Pariah of humanity."[23] As these comments suggest, the American national woman's rights conventions played an important role in promoting the international feminist movement during the first half of the nineteenth century.

Harriot Hunt was in the thick of this struggle. She recalled that friends tried to dissuade her from attending the first convention held in nearby Worcester. They warned her that she would look "ridiculous" by associating with the "motley crew" who would attend such a gathering. Some of them "scolded" and "entreated" her not to go; others claimed she would "lose caste" and soon regret her decision (250). Such comments suggest that there was a class dimension behind the objections of Hunt's friends. They seemed to fear that she would lose status as a "lady" by attending a convention filled with women who transgressed the boundaries of respectable femininity.

But, for Hunt, the convention was an opportunity not to be missed. By 1850, Hunt's life experiences had made her a feminist. The hostility she faced from licensed male doctors and her inability to attend lectures at Harvard Medical School made her realize how gender discrimination thwarted her career. Hearing the tragic "heart histories" of countless women who lacked education, economic opportunity, and legal rights also drove home to Hunt a key point: constricted gender roles marred women's lives. As she pointedly asserted in her autobiography, "the false position" of women had "much to do with their diseases" (159).

Hunt stressed that the calling of the first national woman's rights convention made the year 1850 "a prospective epoch" for her (251). She experienced tremendous joy when she learned that this meeting would occur in her own state: "My whole being rejoiced. . . . That call [for the convention] was bread and water to my soul—it electrified me." It promised to fulfill her "unuttered hopes" and "half formed desires." What especially excited Hunt was the prospect of participating in a movement dedicated to woman's "RIGHTS as an *individual*, and her FUNCTIONS as a *citizen*" (249-51).

Participation at this convention was a turning point for Hunt for several reasons. First, she joined the community of leading activists who formed the first major woman's rights movement in the United States. She recognized how critical the Worcester Convention was: "This is the first national historic act of woman to ask the why and the wherefore of her political nonentity in this glorious republic. It was the voice of liberty struggling for utterance" (254). Hunt knew some of the major participants at the convention, such as the noted Unitarian minister and reformer William Henry Channing and abolitionist Wendell Phillips, men whom she praised for "consecrat[ing] their talents to the elevation of humanity" (253). She also met for the first time a number of renowned Bostonian reformers. These included William Lloyd Garrison, the controversial editor of the *Liberator*, who by 1850 espoused not only abolitionism and racial equality but also a form of Christian anarchism known as "nonresistance." The belief in the inviolable rights of every human being led Garrison to become a staunch advocate of woman's rights. A somewhat bemused Hunt recalled that those who vilified Garrison as a "terrible" and "wicked person" would have been amazed to see him "so placid, so benignant" at the convention (253). Hunt also recounted meeting Dr. Josiah Foster Flagg, the noted dental surgeon and homeopath with whom she formed a lasting friendship and who collaborated with her on future efforts to educate women (254).[24]

But it was the women at the convention whom Hunt most remembered. Her excitement was palpable as she recalled meeting the founding mothers of America's woman's rights movement—Paulina Wright Davis, the president of the convention, Lucy Stone, Antoinette Brown, and Clarina Howard Nichols. Hunt also admired Ernestine Rose, the Polish émigré now best remembered for her efforts to gain legal rights for married women. Rose, she declared, was an "ardent, eloquent, intellectual" woman whose "foreign accent added interest to the truths she uttered" (252).

The woman who most impressed Hunt, however, was the noted Quaker minister, abolitionist, and feminist Lucretia Mott. Underneath her gentle Quaker demeanor was a steely commitment to human equality and rights for all, irrespective of race or gender. Even the *New York Herald*, a paper notoriously critical of woman's rights and other reform movements, grudgingly described Mott with respect and even admiration—this "elderly lady" was "all bone, gristle, and resolution" and as "indomitable as Caesar."[25] For Hunt, Mott embodied a number of admirable qualities and roles. As a minister she was a "teacher of religion and of morals." Yet she balanced this role by "fulfilling her maternal duties" as wife, mother, and grandmother. But what Hunt most admired about Mott was her devout Christian faith. According to Hunt, Mott had a "religious chastened expression [that] proved the ascendancy of the spiritual over the intellectual, [and] her full earnest eye spoke of light within, her radiant smile said 'Trust in God, all will be well.'" In Lucretia Mott, Harriot Hunt met a woman who fulfilled her ideal of what a human being should be (252).

The first Worcester Convention allowed Hunt to network with a remarkable and committed group of reformers dedicated to furthering human liberty. But it also provided her with a public forum that she used to make an eloquent and forceful appeal for women's education in medicine. Her "Address on the Medical Education of Women" was very long, even by the loquacious standards of the times, and therefore the convention proceedings unfortunately provided an abridged version of the speech. But this extant version shows that Hunt marshaled all sorts of arguments to demand that women be educated as doctors. She began her talk in an Emersonian vein, urging her listeners to question "old established customs" and to discard those which thwarted individual freedom and human progress. "We are living in a struggling age, in a transition age," she declared, and the time had come to rejuvenate the "*heart*" of a stagnant society by "demand[ing] equal freedom of development, equal advantages of education, for both sexes."[26]

Hunt then sought to assure her listeners that she possessed the credentials to tackle the issue of medical education. She stressed that she spoke "from the experience of many years" as a "PHYSICIAN." For "fourteen years in the city of Boston," she continued, she had been a "physician for my own sex and for children." She had initially faced "ridicule" and the "ill nature" of those who rejected her practice. The fact that she had successfully weathered such criticism, helping numerous patients, believed Hunt, made her uniquely qualified to speak out now on behalf of women physicians.

Such comments were an early example of what literary scholar Carolyn Skinner has called "professional witnessing." Nineteenth-century women physicians used "public rhetorical acts," such as speeches and writings, to establish their credentials as "objective medical professionals."[27] These women physicians invoked qualities that were gendered both female and male in nineteenth-century society. They sought to convince a skeptical public that women could be competent physicians because they possessed the allegedly masculine qualities needed to cope with the rigors of medicine—scientific expertise, toughness, and resiliency. To allay the anxieties of those who feared that they had "unsexed" themselves, female doctors emphasized that they still retained the supposedly innate feminine characteristics of sympathy, virtue, and delicacy.[28]

These attributes, combined with their medical expertise, they argued, made them particularly well suited to treat women and children. They also qualified women physicians to "prescribe" for an ailing society by tackling various public health problems and vices such as prostitution and intemperance. So nineteenth-century women doctors portrayed themselves as not only competent physicians but also reformers, as ones best prepared to purge their nation of moral as well as physical illness. Not surprisingly, many pioneering female doctors became active in the woman's rights movement, including the suffrage struggle. For them, gender equality not only empowered women but also promoted needed reform activism.[29]

Hunt pioneered in creating a professional ethos among nineteenth-century women physicians. Her lectures, speeches, and published writings were rhetorical acts designed to gain public acceptance for women in medicine and to promote gender equality.[30] Hunt's 1850 address at the first national woman's rights convention in Worcester illustrates how she did this.[31] She repeatedly cited prescribed views of femininity, popularized by the mass media of her day, to make the case for female doctors.[32] How could anyone, Hunt asked, oppose female physicians, given "how strong is the religious element in woman?" These doctors' pious "dependence upon the Lord" made them well suited to minister to ailing women and children. So, too, did women's "intuitive" nature and innate "sympathy." Given these qualities, Hunt wondered what could be "more delicately feminine, more truly womanly," than "to take the hand of a sister, afflicted in body and mind" and "to lead her by kind sympathy and wise advice" to good health.

Through such comments Hunt implicitly criticized male doctors; she suggested that they lacked the requisite delicacy and sympathy to effectively treat women. Although she did not out rightly accuse male physicians of sexual misconduct as did her former mentor Elizabeth Mott and other alternative health practitioners, Hunt suggested that it was particularly inappropriate for men to treat girls on the cusp of womanhood. Women physicians, she insisted, could act as necessary moral sentinels as well as healers when girls needed medical attention. They could "guard the young girl[s]" against corrupting influences and teach them to reverence and protect their bodies. Such mentoring, stressed Hunt, ensured "true delicacy and refinement" and thereby safeguarded the "moral character of society."

Traditional notions of femininity permeated Hunt's address to the Worcester Convention. Paradoxically, she also insisted that women could become doctors because gender was irrelevant to the practice of medicine, given that the mind had no sex. Therefore, the qualities deemed essential for effective doctoring—rational, analytic ability, scientific expertise, emotional resiliency and toughness—were not innately masculine, and women as well as men could possess them. Hunt issued the following challenge: "that the medical colleges may be opened to MIND, not to *sex*, that the whole of human nature may aid in promoting the well being of humanity."[33]

Hunt sought to have it both ways. Even as she claimed that women made good doctors because of innately feminine qualities, she denied that medicine was a gendered activity. Her use of both arguments no doubt reflected her willingness to use multiple, at times contradictory, strategies to convince the public of the need for women doctors. She had one last card to play. Hunt asserted that medical schools must accept women because irrespective of whether they were trained, women were already acting as physicians. She developed this argument in the context of claiming that there was a "great increase of quackery" and that it had already "produced a distrust of physicians." Although Hunt blamed mostly male doctors for this disturbing development, she conceded that there were "kind but ignorant women . . . traveling through the country, advertising to cure all diseases."

Acknowledgment that there were female "quacks" who practiced medicine and hurt patients was a dangerous argument for Hunt to make. It undercut her claims that women were natural healers and thus particularly suited as physicians. It also undermined her efforts to forge a professional ethos for women doctors that trumpeted their competency and expertise. Yet, ultimately, Hunt thought it best to confront facts already known to the public: women as well as men could be guilty of "quackery." She also stressed that the numbers of female physicians, whether they were competent or not, would inevitably grow because most ailing women preferred to "consult one of [their] own sex." She hoped these developments would force medical schools to admit women in order to protect the reputation of their profession as well as the welfare of patients.

Hunt used her address before the 1850 Worcester Convention to present herself as a professional physician, one who was unlike the many "quacks" she derided. But despite her claim that the practice of medicine had "no sex," Hunt fashioned a medical career that was gendered. She specialized in the treatment of female patients. She embraced a "mind-cure" approach to medicine that sought to heal women by listening to their "heart histories." This was a therapy gendered feminine in antebellum America. In the end, Hunt believed that female physicians were best suited to treating sickly women. It therefore angered her that she and other women were denied formal medical training.

Hunt used her address before the 1850 Worcester Convention to publicize the wrong she felt Harvard Medical School had done her when the faculty rejected her 1847 application to attend lectures there. She read the letters that she sent to Dean Holmes and that she received from him. She also recounted how Harvard Medical School lamely rejected her on the grounds that it was "inexpedient." As she rehashed this incident, Hunt settled scores—she exposed Harvard's gender bias against not only her but also all aspiring women doctors.[34] No doubt she was gratified when the delegates passed a resolution declaring that women deserved admission into all educational institutions, including medical colleges, based solely on their "abilities" and "capabilities."

Although addressing a large assembly and speaking for the first time to a gender-mixed audience gave her momentary stage fright, Hunt remembered that she soon forgot her "embarrassment" when she focused on "the truths" she had come to promulgate (253–54). For her the first national woman's rights convention was an unalloyed success, and she described its proceedings as a sort of religious awakening or revival: "Honesty, justice, truth, laid their offerings on the altar—absorbing interest was evinced by large, thoughtful audiences, and a cloud of incense, the prayers, and blessings of absent spirits, o'ercanopied the assembly. The success of this convention was the deep recognition of its need, its electrical power was felt through every class of society" (254).

But if Hunt's response to the feminist gathering was one of joy and satisfaction, the public reaction was mixed. Several newspapers offered respectful, even positive, reports on this meeting. Not surprisingly, the *Liberator* praised it as a "highly intellectual and moral assembly," characterized by "an eloquence, a philanthropy, an impressiveness, and a power that inspired . . . a fresh hope of humanity."[35] The *New York Daily Tribune*, edited by Horace Greeley, a staunch supporter of various reform causes, also lauded the convention. It singled out Hunt for praise, stating that she delivered "a very forcibly written address" in "an impressive manner."[36]

But such favorable accounts of the Worcester Convention and of Hunt were in the minority. The majority of newspapers excoriated this event and denounced its female participants as unnatural and ungodly women—they were "screeching," "gabbling," "clamoring," "unsexed . . . amazons" and "hybrids." Male participants were allegedly emasculated or effeminate "Aunt Nancy men."[37] Hunt was often in the crosshairs of newspapers' attacks against the convention. The *Boston Daily Mail*, for example, used sarcasm to deride her.[38] Referring dismissively to Hunt as "Mrs. H," this paper alleged that she nonsensically described her era as "a kind of cross between the unicorn and the 'sea-sarpint' [sic]." Her speech, fumed the reporter, was a "pathological" and "inexplicable harangue," designed "to give her business of female doctoring a very barefaced puff" and to promote "female ascendancy." It was also so long that its end was "anxiously looked for as dinner time to a very hungry man [presumably the writer referred to himself]."[39]

The *New York Herald*, edited by Greeley's rival and noted opponent of reform James Gordon Bennett, was also vitriolic in denouncing the Worcester Convention. It described the meeting's participants as a "motley gathering of fanatical mongrels, of old grannies, male and female, of fugitive slaves and fugitive lunatics" and their platform as "the most horrible trash" which proselytized "the most monstrous and disgusting principles of socialism, abolition, amalgamation, and infidelity."[40]

This paper targeted Hunt for particular abuse. Like the *Boston Daily Mail*, the *Herald* addressed Hunt as "Mrs." and attacked her in several ways. Patronizingly describing Hunt as "a regular brick," the *Herald*'s reporter mocked her assertion that women made good physicians. Such a claim, he groused, ignored "the fact that every old woman in the country is a quack doctor, and always ready, with her all healing nostrums of sage tea, yarbs, salves, and lotions." This writer also portrayed Hunt as a person who outrageously exaggerated women's abilities when she allegedly proclaimed that "woman was adapted in a superior degree to wrangle with the lawyers—to delve into matters of science—and to conduct the affairs of legislation in the most splendid style. In regard to science, she sustained the argument of sister [Ernestine] Rose, yesterday, in which the scientific capacity of woman was proved from the fact, that a young lady had discovered a comet, with the aid of a telescope."[41]

These comments make one wish that the Worcester Convention *Proceedings* had included all of Hunt's address. Did she discuss women scientists and lawyers? Did she argue that women could be not only doctors but also attorneys and scientists? Did she refer to the arguments of fellow feminists such as Ernestine Rose? These are questions that must remain unanswered owing to the lack of a complete transcript of her address. But the *New York Herald*'s diatribe unwittingly suggests that Hunt offered a broader challenge to her society than the abbreviated version of her talk shows. She may well have urged that women be educated for all sorts of professions, including those of law and science.

Newspapers' condemnation of Hunt underscores the tremendous animosity that the national woman's rights conventions provoked in the popular press. But the vitriolic hyperbole and almost hysterical denunciations of convention speakers, including Hunt, suggest the insecurities of their critics. Fearful that the woman's rights movement might touch a resonant chord among Americans, these writers sought desperately to disparage feminists by any means possible.

And how did Hunt respond to the hostile press coverage? In *Glances and Glimpses* she recalled feeling initially "astonished" and later disheartened by the public outrage against the convention and the widespread caricature of its principles: "It was laughable and yet sad . . . to hear the invective and contempt that was poured out on this gathering of earnest thinkers. . . . The idea of the subjugation of man, instead of the elevation of woman, appeared to have taken possession of the public mind." Almost as an afterthought she declared that one of the papers had "noticed" her in an "amusing" article (256). Of course, Hunt may have been trying to put on a brave face as she recalled being subjected to public ridicule and attack.

But she seems to have recognized a crucial fact that other feminist leaders also grasped: any publicity, even if it was negative, was better than none. Diatribes against the Worcester Convention, no matter how vicious, inadvertently brought the issue of woman's rights to the public's attention. As Hunt revealingly declared, the daily papers, with their increasing coverage of woman's rights, forced growing numbers of Americans to grapple with issues that "angered, annoyed, puzzled" many of them but that could not be ignored. Publicity about the subjugation and discrimination women faced meant that the public could "not shut their eyes, or close their ears," to the fact that feminists discussed grievances that needed redress (256).

The Worcester Convention ratcheted up Hunt's activism in the woman's rights movement. Participation in this convention as well as the success of her medical practice made her more assertive and confident, more willing to challenge restrictive gender roles. It also made her more determined to obtain formal medical training. Hunt, however, rejected applying to the New England Female Medical College or the Female Medical College in Philadelphia. She denigrated the former school by noting that "its standard has never been such, as to induce the highest minds to *graduate* there." Although she praised the female medical school in Philadelphia, it was too far away from her home and practice for her to attend. Hunt also noted that separate female medical colleges were at best a stopgap measure but not a substitute for allowing women the opportunity to attend medical schools alongside men as their equals. She firmly believed that "separate institutions of *all kinds*" were only "*transitional*" (271–72). For these reasons, Hunt decided to reapply to attend lectures at the foremost medical school in the nation, Harvard.

Her November 12, 1850, letter to Dean Holmes was much more assertive than her first request. Hunt now claimed that public opinion was turning in her favor. "Public sentiment," she declared, increasingly recognized how "delicacy, propriety, and necessity" required women to be treated by female physicians. According to Hunt, the school's gender restrictive policies were unfair as well as outdated. She reproached the Harvard faculty's rejection of her earlier petition as "unjust" and urged them to have the "clearness of vision, strength of purpose, and high justice" to recognize that "mind," not "sex," should determine admission to medical lectures.[42]

By the time it received Hunt's letter, Harvard was grappling with another challenge to its admission policies. In October 1850, three African American male students also requested admission to the lectures. Two of these students were sponsored by the American Colonization Society to serve as missionaries in Liberia, and the third petitioner was Martin R. Delany, now best remembered for his abolitionist work and calls for free blacks to emigrate to Africa.[43] Faced with racial as well as gender challenges to its admission policies, Harvard Medical School initially decided to allow both Hunt and the three African American men to attend lectures. This meant that all four prospective students could buy the tickets required to hear lessons from particular professors. Yet in their November 30, 1850, minutes, the faculty stressed that Hunt's attendance at the lectures did not mean she could obtain a medical degree from Harvard.[44]

The decision to accede this time to Hunt's petition indicated Harvard's recognition that it was time to end their opposition to female students. In his letter to President Jared Sparks, Holmes noted that the faculty should recognize changes that had occurred since Hunt's 1847 request. During the past three years, stressed Holmes, several women had attended medical lectures at "respectable schools" in the United States, Elizabeth Blackwell had earned a medical degree, and the New England Female Medical College had been established in Boston to educate female doctors. Such developments, noted Holmes, showed that "general opinion" had "somewhat changed" regarding the "propriety" of women practicing medicine.[45] His remarks indicate that Hunt was right to think that a growing public acceptance of female physicians would force Harvard to accept her second petition.

Although Hunt must have been heartened by Harvard's response, illness prevented her from immediately purchasing her tickets to attend the medical lectures (268). By the time she was well enough to do so, a firestorm of protest from Harvard's medical class, comprised solely of white men, had begun. On December 10, 1850, the student body passed a series of resolutions protesting their faculty's decision to allow both Hunt and the African American men to attend lectures. Although the students claimed that they were "not opposed to allowing woman her rights," they stressed that admittance of women into the medical school was an egregious violation of prescribed gender norms. The male students asserted that "no woman of true delicacy" would want to be in the same room as men when subjects related to the human anatomy were discussed. They strenuously objected to "having the company of any female forced upon us, who is disposed to unsex herself, and to sacrifice her modesty, by appearing with men in the medical lecture room." Harvard students also argued that the admission of women into the lecture hall would not only threaten their "self-respect" but jeopardize the "dignity" of the school and even its "very existence."[46]

The overwhelming majority of the student body of the Harvard Medical School, approximately sixty men, also remonstrated against the admission of the three African American men. Their language highlighted their racial animosity: "We cannot consent to be identified as fellow students with blacks, whose company we would not keep in the streets, and whose society as associates we would not tolerate in our houses." Student protestors suggested that if African Americans were allowed to attend lectures, then Harvard would lose many "respectable *white* students." Indeed, they predicted that their numbers would soon be in "inverse ratio to that of *blacks*" and the school's reputation would decline.[47]

The student resolution opposing Hunt's admission into the lecture hall passed almost unanimously; only one student dissented.[48] By contrast, not all students at the Harvard Medical School opposed the admission of black male students. Twenty-six dissented. In a letter to the medical school faculty, this minority admitted that "their prejudices" caused them to wish that blacks would not attend their school, but they felt that it was a "far greater evil" to refuse admission to an "unfortunate class" who sought the "privileges of education."[49]

The controversy revealed Harvard's different levels of racial and gender prejudice. The overwhelming majority of the medical students mobilized to exclude both women and blacks. Yet, in the end, more than one-third of the students were willing to accept male African Americans, whereas nearly all were opposed to women's admission. This strongly suggests that gender prejudice was more deeply ingrained than racial bigotry.

Members of the Harvard Medical School faculty, whose salaries depended on pupils buying tickets to attend their lectures, responded quickly to the student remonstrations. Their December 13, 1850, minutes noted that the "female student" who sought to attend medical lectures had withdrawn her application on the "advice of the Faculty" and no further action was needed about the matter of women's admission.[50] Harvard's medical faculty soon also decided to stop admitting "colored students" after the present term since "the intermixing of the white and black races in their lecture rooms" was so "distasteful to a large portion of the class & injurious to the interests of the school."[51] Students ramped up the pressure on the faculty when fifteen of them sent a petition threatening to withdraw from the medical college if they were forced to attend lectures with blacks.[52]

Although the controversies over the admission of Hunt and African American men to Harvard's medical lectures seemed to run on parallel tracks, they were intertwined, which was evident in a December 17, 1850, article in the *Boston Daily Journal*, authored by "Common Sense," a writer who praised Harvard's medical students for refusing to "fraternize" with the "inferior . . . negro race" and protesting with "indignation" when they heard that "a *woman* had taken tickets for the lectures!" This author began his article by stressing the crucial point that when students opposed allowing Hunt and African American men into the lecture hall, they were protesting "against this amalgamation of sexes and races."[53] For this author, as for many other white Americans, the prospect of allowing Hunt and blacks to study at Harvard did not simply upend the college's long-established policies but also raised the frightening possibility that white women and black men would mingle socially, perhaps even sexually.

Fears of racial amalgamation had long haunted the imaginations of white Americans. As the abolitionist movement gained momentum in the 1830s, pro-slavery forces sought to discredit it by claiming it promoted a racially integrated society characterized by sexual relationships between black men and white women. This charge fueled antiabolitionist riots throughout northern cities, including New York, Cincinnati, and Philadelphia.[54] Abolitionists counterattacked by arguing that it was white slaveholders who promoted interracial sex. They depicted a licentious South where slave masters regularly raped and impregnated their slaves, creating "dreadful amalgamating abominations."[55] Sometimes their descriptions of slave owners' sexual abuse was so graphic that it smacked of "voyeuristic abolitionism."[56] The word "amalgamation" was sexually and racially charged in antebellum America, a word that evoked deeply ingrained fears in the white majority.

Hunt was painfully aware of how sexual and racial anxieties scuttled her hopes for a medical education. When she recounted the controversy later in *Glances and Glimpses*, she repeated the phrases "Common Sense" had used in his article. She stressed that the student body had vehemently protested against what they perceived as the "amalgamation of sexes and races" (271). As she concluded discussion of this controversy in her autobiography, Hunt noted that a terrible injustice had been perpetrated against her and other women who sought to practice medicine. "The class at Harvard in 1851," she bristled, had earned for themselves "a notoriety" that they would regret in years to come. She turned the tables on those male students who argued that admitting women into the medical lecture hall would be improper—it was they who grossly violated propriety when they "irreverently" and "irreligiously" mishandled the bodies of "a sister in the dissecting room" and when they, later as doctors, subjected women to examinations "*too often unnecessary*" (271).

Hunt was not the only one angry at Harvard's treatment of her. In March 1851, the *Liberator* reprinted an article from a Rhode Island paper that denounced the medical students who opposed Hunt's admission to their lecture hall. The author claimed that the majority of these men were "most gross and vulgar" and lacked "half the brains," the "perseverance," and the "common sense" that Hunt had. Harvard's medical class, stressed this writer, reeked of elitist privilege and immaturity as well as misogyny. They were "upstart dandies" whose "impudent puppyism" and "arrogant assumption of the kid glove and standing collar" thwarted the educational pursuits of a woman who had proven her commitment to medicine. The article ended by asserting that Hunt should have "insisted on her right" to attend medical lectures.[57]

But Harriot Hunt did not renew her efforts to study at Harvard. Instead, she pursued her career without benefit of formal education. In January of 1853, the Female Medical College of Pennsylvania conferred on her an honorary medical degree.[58] Hunt noted this honor in her autobiography and added with satisfaction that for "many years" a great number of her patients had addressed her as "doctor," a sign of their "respect" for her ability. Yet, in the end, all of this was not enough to reconcile Hunt to the basic fact that because she was a woman, the nation's major universities refused to allow her to study or to earn a medical degree. Bitterly she asked, "How many males are practicing on an *honorary* degree? Did they wait as many years for it?" (272).

———

Hunt's anger at Harvard shaped the tone of her speeches at national woman's rights conventions in the early 1850s. She was especially active at meetings held at Worcester, Massachusetts, on October 15 and 16, 1851; at West Chester, Pennsylvania, on June 2 and 3, 1852; and at Syracuse on September 8 through 10,

1852. Unlike her talk before the first convention in 1850, Hunt's later addresses offered much more pointed, extensive criticisms of the medical establishment and more expansive views about the role of women doctors. This was especially apparent in her speech at the second Worcester Convention. Hunt depicted the state of medicine as being in crisis. There was a "vast and serious increase of quackery," as male doctors and druggists hurt patients by dispensing harmful medicines. The medical profession, she fumed, also focused on merely curing rather than preventing disease. Echoing Swedenborg's ideas, Hunt insisted that doctors must counsel patients about how "communication between soul and body" ensured good health.[59]

She gendered the practice of preventive medicine as feminine. Gone were her earlier pronouncements that the "mind" had "no sex." Rather, Hunt emphasized idealized views of femininity to argue that women were best suited to medicine. The "virtuous, high-toned woman, supported by medical knowledge," she claimed, had the "sympathy" and "domestic nature" to advise other women and their families about how to avoid illness. Hunt was so confident that women physicians' practice of preventive medicine was a panacea for the nation's health crisis that she somewhat cavalierly asserted, "We would give to man most cheerfully the Curative department and to woman the Preventive."

In her second Worcester address, Hunt also offered a more ambitious public role for women doctors. They were to cure, regenerate, society of vice and corruption. They were to be the guardians of the nation's morality as well as its health. "We need a moral police, a moral vigilance committee, a moral reform society, based upon medical knowledge," declared Hunt, to "enter the haunts of vice, places of assignation, desecration, and prostitution and fear nothing." Only women physicians, she continued, could use their "maternal element—so potent, so touching—and blend it with her medicines" to "heal" their "sisters" who were prostitutes.

Hunt's comments occurred when growing numbers of reform-minded Americans were alarmed about prostitution and the plight of female sex workers. This issue had already emerged as an important theme at woman's rights meetings. In fact, the prostitute had become an iconic image for antebellum feminists, one that symbolized the degradation of women at the hands of predatory men.[60] Concern about the plight of prostitutes, for example, was a prominent theme at the first Worcester Convention, where such major speakers as William H. Channing and Abby Price addressed this issue. So too did the noted reformer and author Caroline Wells Healey Dall in a long letter that convention president Paulina Wright Davis read before the audience. Dall urged her fellow feminists to speak out against the evil of prostitution and to help the "miserable creatures," engaged in this trade, often out of economic necessity.[61] A particularly moving presentation at this convention occurred when Lucretia Mott paid tribute to the successful businesswoman and feminist Sarah Tyndale for her efforts to aid prostitutes in Philadelphia.[62] The Syracuse conventioneers also excoriated prostitution when they praised the efforts of reformers who tried to clean the "vilest sinks of infamy" in New York City and sought to help the "thousands of women ... driven to a life of pollution" owing to destitution.[63]

But Hunt did not merely reiterate the concerns of her fellow feminists about prostitution and the degradation and immorality it allegedly entailed. She offered her listeners a solution to the vexing problem of the sex trade—women physicians were to be in the vanguard of purging America from vice as well as ill health. The belief that female physicians had a "holy mission" to regenerate America made the refusal of medical schools to admit women all the more egregious. Hunt used this line of argument to lambaste medical schools, including Harvard, and to assert that it was inappropriate for male doctors to treat women.

These points were especially evident in her addresses at the West Chester and Syracuse Conventions in 1852. In the first convention, for example, she offered a resolution that declared that denying women the "same educational advantages" men enjoyed under the "pretext of delicacy" revealed the "impropriety" of male doctors ministering to women. Her second resolution declared the need to support women who entered medicine so that they could attack "the strongholds of vice." Perhaps most significant, however, was Hunt's third resolution at the West Chester Convention, in which she excoriated medical colleges that closed their doors to women applicants. She bitterly recalled that owing to the "false delicacy of the students," Harvard had found it "inexpedient to receive one who had been in successful practice many years." Although Hunt added that such actions would not dissuade her or other women from following their "duty" and practicing medicine, Harvard's treatment of her still rankled.[64]

The resolutions Hunt proposed at the Syracuse Convention were even more explicit in associating male doctors and medical schools with immorality. If man insisted on treating woman in her "sick chamber," declared the first resolution, then he must be "prepared to meet her in the Lecture Room," since an unwillingness to meet her "*there*" suggested "a low state of morality in our Medical Colleges." The second and third resolutions Hunt presented at Syracuse asserted that the "present low standard of morals" highlighted "the need of a new medical infusion, through the woman element."[65]

That the Syracuse Convention unanimously adopted all Hunt's resolutions underscores the support her ideas enjoyed among her fellow feminists.[66] So, too, did the fact that Hunt was asked to serve on key committees, such as the Business Committee, along with leading feminists like Lucy Stone, Paulina Wright Davis, and Ernestine Rose.[67] Not surprisingly, however, Hunt and other woman's rights advocates attracted public opprobrium. The *Syracuse Daily Star*, for example, apologized to its readers for publicizing the "mass of corruption, heresies, ridiculous nonsense, and reeking vulgarities" which the "bad women" at the convention "vomited forth."[68] The *New York Herald* condemned the Syracuse woman's rights meeting as a "farce," filled with unattractive "old maids" or unhappily married women who have "much of the virago in their disposition." Feminists were allegedly "mannish women, like hens that crow," and displayed "boundless vanity and egotism." They were also "flimsy, flippant, and superficial." Not content with these criticisms, the *Herald* ridiculed feminists, including Hunt, by invoking their procreative abilities: "What do the leaders of the Woman's Rights Convention want? They want to vote, and to hustle with the rowdies at the polls. . . . They want to fill all other posts which men are ambitious to occupy—to be lawyers, doctors, captains of vessels, and generals in the field. How funny it would sound in the newspapers, that Lucy Stone, pleading a cause, took suddenly ill in the pains of parturition, and perhaps gave birth to a fine bouncing boy in court! . . . Or, that Dr. Harriot K. Hunt, while attending a gentleman patient for a fit of the gout or *fistula in ano*, found it necessary to send for a doctor, there and then, and to be delivered of a man or woman child—perhaps twins."[69]

This derisive tirade illuminates the anxieties that the emergence of the woman's rights movement provoked in patriarchal men. The editor's focus on women's capacity to bear children is a mantra still today invoked by opponents of woman's rights—women are ultimately slaves to their bodies, to their reproductive organs, and are therefore incapable of fulfilling any public role or occupation. The improbability of Hunt, an unmarried woman then in her late forties, producing a child or the inaccurate claim that she treated men highlights not only the author's misogyny but also his own fears. Ultimately, his shrill denunciations and false claims reflected the rants of a man who feared he might be on the losing side of history.

Despite press denunciations, Hunt continued her activism. Participation in the national woman's rights movement enabled her to hone her public speaking and writing skills. It also allowed her to meet and collaborate with numerous feminist leaders. Finally, it provided Hunt a needed public forum in which to promulgate her ideas about the need for women physicians and their right to education in medical schools. But even as she continued to participate in these conventions, Hunt began to use other public venues to articulate her ideas. She also expanded the demands she made on society, urging her fellow Americans to empower women politically by granting them the right to vote. The struggle for the female franchise would increasingly consume Hunt's energies and complement her crusade to educate female physicians.

Chapter 5

Seeking Political Power, Gender Equality, and Female Friendship

Newspaper obituaries on Harriot Kezia Hunt highlighted two key facts about her: she was a pioneering female physician, and she annually published petitions, addressed to the assessors and citizens of Boston, in which she protested paying taxes while denied the right to vote.[1] Her protests against "taxation without representation" first appeared in newspapers in October 1852 and continued until at least 1866.[2] She reiterated this demand at national woman's rights conventions and lambasted the Massachusetts Constitutional Convention in 1853 when it refused to enfranchise its female citizens.

Even as she battled to empower women politically, Hunt worked to emancipate them in other ways. She advocated for female education by campaigning for the establishment of girls' public high schools and the opening of colleges to women. She challenged patriarchal power by participating in temperance conventions and supporting the ordination of female ministers. While engaged in these multiple activities, Hunt continued her medical practice, traveled as a public lecturer and tourist, deepened her friendship with Sarah Grimké, and forged an ever-widening network of reform-minded women. Hunt led an unusually busy life during the early to mid-1850s, one that nurtured, challenged, and at times exasperated her. Discussion of reformers' efforts to gain suffrage for women offers a needed context for understanding her commitment to promoting gender equality during this era.

Antebellum feminists knew that they were stirring up a hornet's nest when they advocated for women's right to vote. It was a particularly radical demand for various reasons: it viewed women first and foremost as individual citizens rather than as wives and mothers; it challenged male monopoly of the public sphere of politics; and it declared that women must rely on themselves and not depend on the much-vaunted notion of male protection. Perhaps most important, the struggle for the female franchise was part of a larger battle: one to gain for women all the educational, legal, economic, and political rights that men had long enjoyed.[3]

As feminists fought the suffrage battle, one that they did not win until 1920 with passage of the Nineteenth Amendment, they challenged antebellum Americans to broaden their idea of citizenship. But it was a grueling, uphill battle, characterized by many defeats. As numerous historians have documented, antebellum Americans increasingly gendered and racialized the notion of citizenship. Paradoxically, the democratization of electoral politics in the early Republic was built on the exclusion of racial minorities and women from political power. This process continued throughout the nineteenth century as states increasingly limited the full rights of citizenship only to white men. People of color and women, as well as many disabled white men, were systematically excluded from the "borders of belonging" in the American polity.[4]

Constricted notions of citizenship invariably led to suffrage restrictions. Even as antebellum American society extended the franchise to abled white men it limited or disallowed it for other groups. In one northern state after another black male citizens saw their right to vote curtailed and often revoked during the 1820s-1850s era.[5] Meanwhile antebellum Americans' association of citizenship with qualities traditionally gendered masculine—citizens must be rational, independent, able to defend the nation—worked to exclude women from the governing structure and to rationalize their disenfranchisement.[6] As historian Rosemarie Zagarri has argued, the first two decades of the nineteenth century saw the ascendancy of an ideology that consigned women to the private, domestic sphere and proscribed her involvement in politics. This development represented a conservative backlash against brief efforts in the 1790s to allow women political rights and a public voice in the new Republic. By 1830, women who ventured into political activity were vilified as unnatural, unfeminine.[7]

Recognition that women were losing political rights even as growing numbers of white men gained theirs angered antebellum feminists. In an effort to politically empower women, they petitioned their state legislatures and constitutional conventions to grant women basic rights, including the franchise. In August 1846, for example, female petitioners from Upstate New York demanded that their state's constitutional convention enfranchise women.[8] Two years later, at the first woman's rights convention, held in Seneca Falls, New York, Elizabeth Cady Stanton insisted on including the demand for the female franchise in the *Declaration of Sentiments and Resolutions*. Many of those present feared that such a radical measure would alienate the American populace. Even Stanton's own husband and fellow reformer told her that the suffrage plank would "turn the proceedings into a farce."[9] But despite this initial dissent, organizers of future woman's rights conventions committed themselves to demanding the franchise. They realized that gaining the vote was a critical way for women to finally become full-fledged citizens.[10]

Such organizers also urged the minority of women who were property owners to risk public opprobrium and legal prosecution by refusing to pay their taxes.[11] At the third national woman's rights convention held in Syracuse in 1852, for example, Lucy Stone counseled her audience to not pay taxes even if it resulted in "the loss of friends" and "property." According to Stone, there were "fifteen millions of taxable property, owned by women of Boston," and their "revolt" was necessary to force the public to recognize the "self-evident truth that 'taxation and representation are inseparable.'"[12]

Clearly Harriot Hunt was not alone when she protested the injustice of women paying taxes when they could not vote. But she was the first woman to issue such a public protest in the state of Massachusetts.[13] She was also a rarity in her society: a single, self-supporting woman with property whose only reason for disenfranchisement was her gender. Hunt repeatedly began her petitions by stressing that she was a "physician, a native and permanent resident of the City of Boston, and for many years a taxpayer." Her presentation of herself in these terms was an effective rhetorical ploy, one designed to highlight how unfair it was to deny her rights that she surely would have enjoyed if a man. Depiction of herself as a professional, taxpaying, native-born Bostonian helped establish her credibility and her right to protest against "the injustice and inequality" of forcing women like herself to pay taxes when they could not vote (294, 308, 339).

Like the feminists who drafted the Seneca Falls Declaration, Hunt invoked the republican principles of the American Revolution to argue that she and other female citizens had an inalienable right to the franchise. Her repeated use of the phrase "no taxation without representation" deliberately echoed that used by Americans during the 1760s and 1770s to justify their protests and eventual rebellion against British rule. So, too, did her cry in her 1853 petition that "taxation *without representation* is tyranny" (309).

The fact that Boston had been at the epicenter of the American revolutionaries' protests against British oppression made Hunt's argument particularly compelling. Massachusetts abolitionists, both white and black, effectively invoked this revolutionary legacy to mobilize their state against slavery during the antebellum era.[14] Feminists like Hunt sought to emulate this strategy when they pointed out that denying American women the right to vote violated their Republic's historic commitment to democracy and liberty. This belief was a common refrain throughout Hunt's annual petitions: "The present system of taxation is . . . a violation of republicanism" (308, 1853 petition); "the noble spirit of our forefathers" holds that "taxation and representation" are "coextensive" (340, 1854 petition); the state legislature must grant to women the "*right*" they "crave," namely, the right to vote, "just as our fathers craved it of the British government, when *they* protested against 'taxation without representation'" (370, 1855 petition).

But Hunt also offered another argument for the female franchise in her annual protests during the first half of the 1850s. She stressed how unfair it was to deny upright, hardworking American women the right to vote but then grant it to unsuitable men. "Even drunkards, felons, idiots, or lunatics of *men*," she bitterly noted, "may still enjoy the right of voting, to which no woman, however large the amount of taxes she pays, however respectable her character, or useful her life, can ever attain" (294, 339).

Such language illustrates how aggrieved, humiliated, Hunt felt at being denied the franchise simply because of her gender. Antebellum feminists had an acute sense that they belonged to "a disabled" or "an inferior caste," which recognition gnawed at them. Repeatedly, feminists stressed their feelings of "degradation" and "humiliation" over their lack of rights and freedoms.[15] At times these feelings caused even leading woman's rights advocates to wish they were men. Stanton stated such late in 1859, shortly after the execution of the abolitionist revolutionary John Brown. Exasperated by the setbacks both the abolitionist and feminist struggles were then experiencing, she bitterly confessed to Susan B. Anthony, her longtime partner in the movement for woman's rights: "When I pass the gate of the celestial city and good Peter asks me where I would sit . . .

I shall say 'Anywhere, so that I am neither a negro nor a woman. Confer on me, good angel, the glory of white manhood so that henceforth, sitting or standing, rising up or lying down, I may enjoy the most unlimited freedom.'"[16]

Hunt's annual protests offer a revealing case study of how feelings of humiliation and degradation motivated the activism of antebellum suffragists. Exacerbating her sense of grievance was the belief that women had lost ground since the post-Revolutionary era, that in earlier times they had enjoyed more political rights and freedoms but were now increasingly disempowered. Hunt particularly made this point when she recalled in *Glances and Glimpses* her mother's "strong love for politics" and then revealingly added: "Those were days when women were not stigmatized for having an interest in the National housekeeping, as well as the domestic!" (4).

Nativism also intensified Hunt's resentment at being denied the right to vote. She emphasized that what finally prompted her to publish her first protest was visiting the assessor's office in October 1851 and seeing the naturalization papers of an Irish youth that made him an American citizen and thereby enfranchised him. Hunt's resentment was palpable as she described the "pale, thin, waxy, tall, awkward, simple Irish boy" with a "vacant stare" and "shuffling manner" who could now vote, while she, "a Bostonian by birth, education, and life, paying taxes without representation," was disenfranchised and thereby "*insulted*" by her nation (293). In several of her annual petitions Hunt harped on the injustice of denying the franchise to native-born, educated, and respectable American women while readily granting it to "aliens," most of whom supposedly lacked either an "interest" or "knowledge" in American institutions (294, 341).

Hunt reiterated these sentiments at the national woman's rights convention held in New York City in September 1853, where she played a prominent role, both as a featured speaker and a member of the Business Committee.[17] Her bitterness was palpable when she recollected seeing that "thin, weak, stupid-looking Irish boy" able to vote while "thousands of intellectual women, daughters of the soil, no matter how intelligent, how respectable, or what amount of taxes they paid, were forced to be dumb!"[18]

Such comments highlighted how Hunt wove together nativist, class, and gender grievances to articulate her rage at women's disenfranchisement. Other leading antebellum suffragists did so as well; even Elizabeth Cady Stanton, a woman committed to promoting human rights for all, periodically invoked such views. In a September 1848 address, for example, she resentfully claimed that all men in the United States, including "the most ignorant Irishman in the ditch," enjoyed full citizenship, whereas native-born, educated, white women like herself remained disenfranchised. When she stressed that such men had merely "muscular power," Stanton suggested that they were stupid as well as ignorant. She also lumped Irish immigrant males with men who had moral or physical defects. It was "grossly insulting to the dignity of woman," fumed Stanton, to have the rights of "drunkards, idiots, horse-racing, rum selling rowdies" as well as "ignorant foreigners" be "fully recognized" while American-born, intelligent women remained excluded "from all rights that belong to citizens."[19]

Alternately plaintive, reproachful, and angry, suffragists such as Stanton and Hunt hoped to shame their nation into granting women the right to vote when they stressed how male citizens, even if they were "vicious," "ignorant" "foreigners," could do so (341). Such arguments illustrated the toxic brew of nativism and class prejudice then prevalent in mainstream America. These sentiments especially roiled Bostonians, as the Irish, many of them destitute and uneducated, flooded into the city during the 1840s and 1850s. Census figures show that by 1850 over 40 percent of Boston's population were foreigners, most of them Irish. Many native-born Bostonians feared and hated the Irish. To them, these immigrants represented an alien, subversive force, one characterized by drunkenness, criminality, ignorance, poverty, and allegiance to "popery," or Catholicism.[20]

Like many other antebellum suffragists, Hunt portrayed Irish American male voters in ways that reflected as well as reinforced the prejudices of her society. There was also a class, ethnic, and racial dimension to how she depicted disenfranchised American women. Hunt repeatedly bemoaned the fact that it was women like herself—white, native born, educated, propertied, and "respectable"—who deserved the vote. But she never discussed the injustice of denying the franchise to less privileged groups of American women, including those who were impoverished, recent immigrants, or members of religious or racial minorities.

Hunt's omission illustrated how class and racial prejudice marred the antebellum suffrage struggle. But this fact should not obscure a crucial point: during the 1850s, Hunt braved public opprobrium to champion a cause that most Americans scoffed at. She redoubled her efforts on behalf of female suffrage when the Massachusetts Constitutional Convention convened in May 1853. Like many activists throughout the state, Hunt saw this convention as a welcome opportunity to advocate for major legal reforms in Massachusetts. She and other suffragists especially hoped to convince the convention to delete the word "male" from a constitutional amendment listing the qualifications for voting, which would enfranchise female citizens in Massachusetts.

Twelve petitions with over two thousand signatures were submitted to the Constitutional Convention urging this reform. Hunt's name was among the signatories.[21] She also submitted a petition requesting that propertied women either be allowed to vote or be "excused from paying taxes" (299–300).[22] But convention delegates, by a vote of 108 to 44, rejected these petitions and also refused to change the existing suffrage qualifications, declaring it "inexpedient" to do so.[23] There was that word again—"inexpedient," as used by Harvard Medical School to reject Hunt in 1847.

Not surprisingly, Hunt excoriated the convention when she issued her annual protest in November 1853. "No permanent good" could result from the convention, she angrily stated, as the "great central element of justice was, by the committee on our petitions, winked into 'expediency.'" With obvious bitterness, Hunt added that no act at the convention "vindicated or even recognized the right of woman, on the *real basis of representation—humanity*" (309).

The passage of time did not ameliorate Hunt's bitterness. In her November 1854 protest she seemed even angrier at the men who ran her state and predicted that eventually the "party factions, political intrigues, and the selfish cabals of scheming politicians" would be "abolished" and "the people" would finally return to "first principles" and "realize the enormity of depriving one half the citizens of Boston of rights secured to them in the parchments of a republic." Hunt defiantly added: "*We are strong in the right*, and we bide our time" (341). Her words are revealing. Like other feminist leaders, Hunt believed that the fight for woman's rights would inevitably succeed because it was based on eternal notions of truth and justice and also reflected the democratic principles on which the United States was founded.

Hunt's campaign to enfranchise women attracted widespread newspaper coverage. The *Liberator* regularly printed and praised her annual protests, proclaiming her 1853 petition, for example, a "righteous protest," one that correctly recognized that "taxation without representation is fundamentally antirepublican."[24] When the Massachusetts Constitutional Convention rejected Hunt's suffrage petition and those of other feminists, editor William Lloyd Garrison angrily declared: "Shabby business this for a Reform Convention!"[25]

A minority of newspapers in the mainstream press offered a mixed verdict of Hunt's suffrage efforts. The *New York Daily Times*, for example, described her as a woman who allegedly created a "sensation" at a convention promulgating "woman's rights mania"; she was also "a real, genuine, strong-minded woman" who gave the "tax-gatherer fits last year, and now she is into him again with renewed vigor." At a time when women were to be gentle, retiring, and accommodating to men, the latter description was a particular jab at Hunt. Yet this paper did refer to Hunt as a doctor with no hint of sarcasm. Most important, the *New York Daily Times* told its readers to "hear" Hunt's message and then printed her 1853 protest.[26] The *National Era*, a leading paper in Washington, D.C., also gave Hunt a respectful hearing. It described her as "a lady who is distinguished as a physician" and who enjoyed an international reputation "as an advocate of the rights of her sex." The paper "recommend[ed]" Hunt's protest to its readers, describing it as "a clear and forcible statement, which can be more easily attacked with sneers than answered with arguments."[27] Similarly, a Michigan paper disapprovingly described Hunt as "one of the 'strong-minded women' of the day." Despite this criticism, it reprinted her claim that as an "independent American woman" she should have the right to vote just as a male citizen did and that "taxation without representation is tyranny."[28]

Yet many papers sought to discredit Hunt and the suffrage movement she espoused. One newspaper condescendingly referred to her as "a smart little woman" who thankfully would fail in her efforts to stoke "hatred and strife" by having women exercise "political suffrage."[29] Another paper excoriated Hunt for violating "*God's truth*" that women were subordinate to men. It then opined that "the woman who mounts the rostrum, or walks the public area . . . is unfaithful to the possession of a true womanly nature." The "woman's movement," added the writer, "crushed and trampled" the "delicate, sensitive nature" of the "ideal woman," the "true woman."[30]

Such sentiments provoked efforts to stop Hunt and other suffragists from speaking publicly about their cause. During the 1853 national woman's rights convention in New York, a minority attended in order to disrupt the proceedings. As the *New York Daily Tribune* reported, there was "hissing, yelling, and stamping, and all manner of unseemly interruptions." One of the speakers who was booed and hissed was Hunt, especially when she invoked the Declaration of Independence to claim her constitutional right to vote and denounced as tyrannical the practice of taxing disenfranchised women.[31]

Hunt was in the crosshairs of those committed to maintaining the status quo. In her autobiography she made light of many of the criticisms her annual protests triggered, claiming that it was "very amusing" to read newspaper articles that misrepresented or caricatured her demands for the franchise and answered her arguments with "spite and slang." Yet some attacks evidently rankled Hunt. She took particular exception to an editorial published in a Cleveland paper which stated that if she wanted to get involved in politics, she had better be prepared to participate in "*brandy smashes and blackguardism*" and also a "*timely drink, or a smutty repartee.*"[32] Hunt retorted by invoking an argument that became prominent in the late nineteenth-century suffrage movement—when women finally got the vote they would purge politics of decadent, rowdy behavior and use it for "high and noble purposes" (342).

Despite public criticism, Hunt continued to issue her annual protests denouncing the injustice of taxing women while denying them the franchise. She also used these declarations to protest women's lack of educational opportunities. Why, she asked in her 1852 petition, was there no "public provision" for the education of girls beyond primary school but two public high schools, including the Boston Latin School, provided a college preparatory program for boys? She also pointed out that there were "a great multitude of colleges and professional schools for the education of boys and young men" but none for female students. This educational disparity rankled Hunt. She referred to her own rejection from Harvard to try to shame city officials into establishing a public school for the girls in Boston: "The fact that our colleges and professional schools are closed against females, of which your remonstrant has had personal and painful experience . . . [shows] why the city should provide at its own expense, those means of superior education [for female students]" (294, 295). The following year, Hunt ramped up her campaign for state-supported education for girls and women when she petitioned the Massachusetts Constitutional Convention "to secure to females equal educational rights with males, and especially to make provision for a People's College, at which females may be as completely educated as males" (299).

But Hunt devoted most of her efforts to urging Bostonians to establish a female public high school. She especially marshaled various arguments to support her case in her 1852 annual petition—secondary education would give girls an opportunity to develop their intellect; "save them from lives of frivolity and emptiness"; "open the way to many useful and lucrative pursuits, and so raise them above that *degrading dependence*, so fruitful a source of female misery" (295).

These comments warrant extended analysis because they illuminate what propelled Hunt into the woman's rights movement. For her the struggle to gain women the right to vote and access to higher education were two halves of the same whole. Each demand reflected her determination to emancipate women from "degrading dependence" and to establish them as coequals with men, enjoying the same rights of citizenship. Hunt was in good company when she advocated such an agenda: the above-stated goals were central to the antebellum woman's rights movement in the United States.[33]

But these goals had particular resonance for Hunt. Her status as a professional, single woman made her feel especially aggrieved that she could not vote. Meanwhile, advocating for girls' higher education dovetailed with Hunt's other agenda—promoting the admission of women into medicine. Obviously females could not become physicians if they were unable to pursue their schooling beyond the primary grades. Given her own struggles, Hunt knew better than most women the rewards education offered her sex: it enabled them to become professionals; to engage in lucrative, interesting work; and to achieve financial independence and status without relying on men.

Finally, Hunt's comment that education would liberate girls from lives of "frivolity" and "emptiness" reflected a belief articulated by leading woman's rights advocates. In her *Letters on the Equality of the Sexes*, Sarah Grimké, for example, groused that too many girls from affluent families obsessed about fashion, dances, and pursuit of a suitable mate. Regretfully, she admitted having done this in her youth. She had lived "among the butterflies of the *fashionable* world" where women who sought to develop their minds were "generally shunned." Instead, they were trained to be "pretty toys" or "instruments of pleasure." But education, stressed Grimké, was crucial if women were ever to achieve their potential and promote a more just and egalitarian society.[34] By midcentury, history had already begun to vindicate Grimké's hopes for the power of education. As Mary Kelley has documented, educated women in antebellum America took the lead in forging a civic, public voice for their sex and in spearheading the first stage of the feminist movement.[35]

Hunt's demand for the establishment of a girls' public high school in Boston reflected her hopes for the future emancipation of women. But it also revealed her frustration and anger with her fellow Bostonians, especially city officials. Although the cultural and intellectual mecca of antebellum America, Boston had retrogressed in its commitment to female education. In 1825 the Boston school committee established a girls' public high school, which quickly attracted 286 applicants. Unfortunately, many could not attend because they were academically unprepared. The one-room school also had to turn away many prospective students owing to limited space. Nevertheless, the high school flourished, and numerous girls sought admission. But in a sad irony the school's success was its undoing. The mayor and other Boston leaders feared that the school would soon expand and become too expensive—it cost the city eleven dollars a year to educate each girl.

Nativist, gender, and class issues soon led to a public outcry against continuing the "experiment" in publicly funded higher education for girls. As growing numbers of working-class students, many of them Irish, matriculated, the school became a lightning rod for controversy. Many Bostonians objected to spending tax dollars to educate the children of the immigrant poor, especially when they were girls. Some voiced concerns that educating Irish American girls would unfit them for domestic service. The school was discontinued in 1827. In 1852, Boston did establish a normal school for girls, an institute designed to train them as primary grade teachers, and several years later this became the Girls' High and Normal School. But this school focused on offering students preparation for one occupation only—teaching young children. Female students in Boston had to wait until January 1, 1878, with the opening of a girls' Latin School, before they had access to a rigorous, publicly funded secondary education in Boston.[36]

The dissolution of the girls' public high school in 1827 undoubtedly reinforced Hunt's belief that women were losing ground in the early Republic, that rights and opportunities they had enjoyed earlier were now disappearing. Determined to reverse this tide, Hunt used several strategies to pressure Boston officials to reestablish the high school for girls. She gave public lectures explicitly linking the woman's rights movement to the cause of female education. In April 1853, for example, she delivered a talk in Boston titled "The Woman's Movement, Educationally Considered." She also helped gain signatures for petitions addressed to the mayor and aldermen demanding a high school for girls.[37] These petitions struck a resonant chord with many Bostonians as approximately twenty-seven hundred people, Hunt stressed, signed them (309, 340). But in the end, Boston school and city officials refused to reestablish a girls' public high school.

Hunt's bitterness at this response was evident in her 1853 and 1854 annual protests. She accused the school committee of defying the public's wishes when they rejected petitioners' demands. She also reiterated a point she had made in her speech before the first Worcester convention on woman's rights and to the Harvard Medical faculty—authorities should stop "*sexualizing education*" (309); there should be "equal advantages of education for mind not sex" (340).[38]

The intransigence of Boston city officials did not stop Hunt from repeating her demands and making new ones. Her 1854 protest demanded that Massachusetts establish a college for women and that it allow them to vote and even serve on school committees. Was it fair, angrily asked Hunt, to force women to pay school taxes but then give them no say in how those taxes were spent? (340–41). In her 1855 protest Hunt raised another issue that highlighted the injustice of "sexualizing education": Why were women teachers in Boston's public schools paid considerably less than their male counterparts? Why were their salaries based on "*sex, not capacity*"? (370). Hunt's memories of the paltry salaries she and her sister, Sarah, received when they were schoolteachers likely made the persistent gender disparity in teachers' pay particularly galling to her.

Another issue that galvanized Hunt's activism on behalf of woman's rights was temperance reform. During the 1840s and 1850s, women, especially those who were middle-class evangelical Protestants, assumed an increasingly major role in this movement. They argued that abusive drinking by men caused a litany of horrors, including domestic violence and poverty, which threatened women, children, and the home. Female temperance advocates played a prominent role in producing and disseminating the popular plays, novels, short stories, and other texts that dramatized how men's drinking destroyed their lives and those of their families. By the mid-nineteenth century they were also engaging in increasingly political and at times confrontational actions to wage the temperance crusade. Women marched in temperance parades, physically attacked saloons, and sent thousands of petitions to state and national governments demanding prohibition. Many also became suffragists as they sought political power to pass prohibition laws at the state and the federal level. By the late nineteenth century, the Woman's Christian Temperance Union, demanding total prohibition of alcohol, had become the most popular and influential female reform organization in the United States.[39]

Concern for the welfare of women and children drew Hunt to the temperance movement just as it did so many other female reformers. Listening to the "heart histories" of patients married to abusive drinkers and visiting families blighted by alcohol brought home to her how this "everyday vice" threatened the lives of women and children. "Life has brought before me serious cases," she sadly recollected. Images of the "unfortunate victim[s]" of drunken men, their "worn out, anxious, haggard wives" and "sad, wretched, frightened children," haunted Hunt. As she poignantly stated, they "peopled my brain" (119). No wonder, then, that Hunt favored women leaving their husbands "in cases of intemperance and personal abuse" (231). For her as for other temperance advocates, the former evil often led to the latter one.

Hunt was well within the mainstream of temperance discourse when she focused on how abusive drinking by men hurt their wives and children. But she also tackled an issue that many other reformers avoided—drunkenness by women. Hunt stressed that she was "first arrested by the horrors of intemperance" when she visited the home of a family whose children attended her school and saw their alcoholic mother in withdrawal. Watching this woman in the throes of "delirium tremens," she remembered, was "a fearful shock to my nervous system. "Dishevelled hair, glaring eyes, partial nudity, in one of my own sex, was terrific to me" (119). Feeling both pity and revulsion, Hunt distanced herself from this female alcoholic by identifying her as "a foreigner." Although Hunt did not specify the woman's ethnicity, she was probably Irish, a group with a reputation for abusing alcohol. For Hunt, the gravely ill mother she saw was an alien in several ways. She was not only an immigrant but also a woman who violated prescribed codes of femininity in a particularly egregious way.

The only other cases that Hunt noted of women being problem drinkers was when she discussed how many employers inadvertently contributed to the ruin of female servants when they exposed the latter to liquor, especially wines. The servant who had been "addicted to intemperance, but with a giant effort, had conquered the appetite" and found gainful employment now began drinking again with predictably terrible consequences. Her "old appetite broke its chain, and vanquished the will," and soon her employer dismissed her and her life became a downward spiral of poverty and desperation. Reproachfully, Hunt asked her readers, "How far are you responsible for her [the servant's] ruin?" (167).

Through this anecdote Hunt challenged her readers to examine their class privilege and to recognize that employers could destroy their servants' lives when they exposed them to alcohol kept in affluent homes. By the 1850s most female servants in Boston were Irish, thus Hunt's story reinforced the stereotype of the drunken Irish. But she pointed out the culpability of affluent Anglo-Americans for this evil. In a sense Hunt suggested that the burden of protecting lower-class immigrant women from the horrors of alcohol rested with middle- and upper-class people.

In 1853, Hunt's participation in two temperance conventions vividly illustrated how many male reformers, especially the clergy, worked to scuttle women's prominence in the movement to prohibit alcohol. Their actions brought home to her the need to link the temperance struggle with the one for woman's rights. The first Whole World's Temperance Convention, which began in New York City on May 12, 1853, quickly became a contentious affair. Many protested recognizing women as delegates and refused to let them speak. They also objected to appointing Susan B. Anthony, a leading temperance as well as woman's rights activist, to the Business Committee.[40]

Their actions echoed those who protested women's equal participation at the American Anti-Slavery Society's annual convention in May 1840. These developments helped to rupture the abolitionist movement and led to the formation of the American and Foreign Anti-Slavery Society which advocated a more limited, subordinate role for women activists.[41] Thirteen years later efforts to marginalize women's involvement in temperance reform provoked similar controversy.

Clergymen from mainstream Protestant churches led raucous protests against women in the Whole World's Temperance Convention just as they did against the female delegates at the American Anti-Slavery Convention in 1840. Their successful efforts to deny women recognition as delegates fractured the former convention just as it did the latter. Many female delegates and their male supporters, such as the noted Unitarian minister and reformer Thomas Wentworth Higginson, angrily left the Whole World's Temperance Convention. Most of the mainstream ministers welcomed their exit. The Reverend John Chambers of Philadelphia, for example, stated that those assembled could now focus on the temperance issue since they were "rid of the scum of the convention."[42]

But the women delegates and their male supporters quickly delivered an effective rebuke to their critics. They called for another Whole World's Temperance Convention, one which would welcome women as both delegates and speakers. When the latter convention met in New York City on September 1 and 2, 1853, women played prominent roles. Susan B. Anthony was president; other prominent feminists, such as Angelina Grimké Weld and Frances D. Gage, were among the vice presidents. Attended by approximately three thousand people, the convention featured such speakers as Lucy Stone, Antoinette Brown, and Thomas Wentworth Higginson who denounced the previous meeting for its treatment of female delegates.[43]

Harriot Hunt enthusiastically participated in these events. She was one of the people who seceded from the first convention and signed the petition calling for the second; she was also a vice president at the latter convention.[44] Hunt was both scornful and angry when she recalled the abuse women suffered at the first temperance convention. "That women were *ejected* from the one-sided convention" by "coarse and unmanly remarks," such as "women in breeches" and "a disgrace to their sex," she fumed, only showed how critical it was for women to increase their public activism (302). Only women could rescue men from their "coarse and rowdy-like behavior" and lead them to "a perception of true manhood" (303). Hunt also voiced contempt for the role the clergy played in the first convention. If these *"reverend gentlemen"* were *"glad"* to get rid of the women, she stressed, *"we* were equally glad to retire from their presence, and breathe a purer atmosphere" (302–3).

Hunt's comments ironically underscored her embrace of traditional views of femininity. Even as she battled the notion of gendered spheres, she still articulated the belief that women were generally "purer" than men, that only they could redeem their society from immorality. Such ideas were crucial themes in nineteenth-century American culture. Indeed, by the early 1830s they had become staples of popular discourses on religion, reform, and politics.[45] Hunt was therefore well within the mainstream of her society when she associated virtue and moral redemption with femininity.

She also embraced an evangelical model of manhood, one that became increasingly popular in antebellum America, especially among the middle class. This model prescribed piety and self-discipline for men and demanded that they reject traditional masculine pastimes such as drinking, carousing, and brawling.[46] In her riposte to the conservative ministers who condemned female participation in temperance and other reform movements, Hunt stressed that many of them still needed to embrace the reformed model of masculinity. By depicting these clergymen as coarse and rowdy, she hoisted them with their own petards. Her withering rebuke of them suggested that many of America's ministers had to practice what they preached and stop behaving like louts and become "true" men.

If Hunt and other woman's rights advocates excoriated the misogyny of many male reformers, their own temperance convention provoked public censure and derision. One Massachusetts newspaper, for example, disapprovingly noted that "women as well as men, blacks as well as whites," were "participants" and "speakers" at the second Whole World's Temperance Convention. After stressing that "ladies" served in prominent offices like the vice presidency, the paper issued a diatribe: "This whole world's convention resolved itself into every conceivable form of humbug and charlatanry. It enacted its strange orgies, on different nights, and in different halls, under the name of Abolition meetings, [and] Vegetarian banquets." Through such remarks the newspaper sought to discredit the second temperance convention as both a radical and foolish venture. And by using the word "orgies," it suggested that gross immorality characterized a meeting where the two sexes interacted as equals.[47]

On September 15, 1853, Hunt participated in another event that quickly provoked a howl of protest—the ordination of Antoinette Brown as a Congregational minister of South Butler, New York. Brown became the first woman to be ordained in a mainstream Protestant denomination in the United States.[48] Although "the storm raged," declared Hunt, she was determined to see Brown ordained a minister. She recognized that this was a milestone for women, one that augured a new role for them in American society: "Even an equinoctial tempest could not detain me from being present, on an occasion so momental to the cause of woman; there was something grand and elevating in the idea of a female presiding over a congregation, and breaking to them the bread of life—it was a new position for woman, and gave promise of her exaltation to that moral and intellectual rank, which she was designed to fill" (304).

Brown's ordination represented a major challenge to men's monopoly of the ministry. Antebellum feminists recognized that the regular Protestant denominations and clergy thwarted their efforts to emancipate women from patriarchal control. Repeatedly, ministers from mainline churches told women that they had to accept their subordinate status and that they defied God's law when they attempted to function in the public sphere. The denunciations ministers leveled against female delegates at antislavery and temperance conventions were part of this larger clerical crackdown on activist women. So, too, were ministers' earlier diatribes against women like the Grimké sisters, who dared to lecture publicly on the evils of first slavery and later patriarchy.

But antebellum feminists persistently challenged their clerical critics, denouncing the mainline churches as stagnant sects that no longer had the genuine spirit of Christianity. Gerrit Smith, a noted abolitionist and woman's rights advocate as well as cousin of Elizabeth Cady Stanton, spoke for many feminists when he declared in 1840 that a number of churches were now merely "soul-shrivelling enclosures of a sect."[49] In opposition to such churches, feminists increasingly gravitated toward "free churches" or "people churches." These latter institutions rejected traditional, hierarchical church structures and promoted all sorts of reforms, including rights for women.[50]

These developments help contextualize Brown's ordination in 1853. Her ministry was yet another volley in the struggle feminists waged to democratize American churches, to make them more responsive to the disempowerment faced by female congregants. Hunt was in the thick of this struggle. Her own unorthodox religious activities—her upbringing as a Universalist, involvement with the Shakers, and conversion to Swedenborgianism—contributed to her willingness to challenge mainline churches.

Hunt also admired the Quakers, the religious sect whose egalitarian principles led them to support woman's rights and accept female preachers. In her autobiography she recounted how seeing Quaker minister Lucretia Mott and other activists take a prominent lead in the national woman's rights conventions "impressed" her "deeply" (251–52). That the Grimkés had been Quakers also drove home the crucial role this religious group played in the struggle for woman's rights.

Hunt's respect for Quaker women deepened when she attended their gathering at the Yearly Meeting of Friends, held in Philadelphia in the spring of 1851. It "was worth the whole journey," she remembered, to see "one thousand women assembled to transact the business of their society," and it was a particular "privilege" to hear Lucretia Mott address "her own people." Hunt emphasized that it was a "revelation" to see "the order, the quiet, the solemn silence" when these women "retired within themselves before a word was spoken." But also impressive was to see these women "legislating clearly and consistently." This moment was pivotal for Hunt: "I shall never forget this gathering—it impressed me with the power and capacity of woman, and convinced me that she was able to legislate for herself" (274).

Hunt's attendance at Brown's ordination reflected her religious unorthodoxy, her alienation from mainstream Protestant churches with their all-male clergy. It also highlighted her long-held belief that the roles of doctor and minister were intertwined. If women could act as physicians, then surely they should be able to become ministers given that both nurtured the souls of their patients/congregants. The resonance Hunt saw between these two vocations made her embrace of female ministers a logical consequence of her support for women physicians. As she revealingly noted while describing the Brown ordination: "The union of the clerical and medical life had long been a beau ideal with me, and the installation of one of my sex as pastor over a church, seemed one step toward its realization" (305). The fact that Brown weathered the storm of criticism she faced after her ordination and spoke effectively at a national woman's rights convention in Ohio heartened Hunt. Although she did not attend the latter conference, Hunt proudly noted that Brown "ably but calmly vindicated her rights as a human being" (306).

Hunt was unable to attend the Ohio convention because she was on a lecture tour in Upstate New York. Her attendance at national woman's rights conventions had not stopped her from continuing her public presentations on the need for women doctors and health reform. One talk she regularly gave was "Woman as Physician" (285).[51] When she traveled first to Niagara Falls and later to Buffalo, she floated the idea of establishing "medical parishes" where people paid doctors to keep their families healthy. No sooner did she finish this lecture tour than she was off to New York City, where she spoke at the Five Points Mission (307).[52]

Hunt's commitment to educating the public about women's health also led her to ratchet up her involvement in the Ladies' Physiological Institute. By the early 1850s she had become one of this organization's regular and most popular lecturers. Institute minutes for October 30, 1850, for example, noted that "Miss Hunt" delivered "an exceedingly interesting" lecture on the subject of "the Temperaments" in which she discussed how mothers should best manage their children. Although the minutes did not elaborate further on the subject of Hunt's talk, it must have made a very favorable impression on the institute's members since on November 2 they passed a resolution formally thanking Hunt and urging her to reprise her lecture in the future when "teachers and others" could attend.[53] Hunt gave another lecture on January 29, 1851, on the nervous system that was also well received and that members requested she repeat.[54] Later that year institute members singled out Hunt and several other women lecturers for their thanks and declared that "the voice of woman is needed to be heard, to call her sisters' attention to the general dangers threatening them from their blind adherence to false customs, from their stupid submission to the requirements of fashion, against the dictates of their own taste and sense."[55]

Despite her hectic schedule and numerous activities, Hunt seemed to enjoy generally good health during the 1850s. One way that she promoted her well-being was by dancing. In a widely reprinted newspaper article, Hunt declared that for many years she had enjoyed this "life-cheering exercise" and testified to its "healthful" as well as "recuperative power." Eager to dispel the popular association of dancing with the "late hours," "indecency," and "vulgarism and excitements" that allegedly characterized the "ball room," Hunt insisted that dancing was a "beautiful, graceful recreation" as well as a remedy for ill health. She clearly relished this pastime and readily prescribed it to her patients and readers.[56]

Hunt also enjoyed traveling, especially for pleasure. During the 1850s she took several memorable trips to Niagara Falls, a place that had a powerful impact on her: "Heart language, soul music has found no exponent of this sacred place. My first sensation was a *new birth*—I felt all lungs—as though I had never breathed before—a pulsation pervaded my whole being" (287). Hunt added that the "awe-inspiring influence" of the falls "render[s] you spellbound. . . . The mystic element of my being was fed for the first time, and like the wee child, *more* would have been greater than I could bear" (288).

Such language is redolent of words used by countless visitors to Niagara Falls during the latter eighteenth and nineteenth centuries. By the 1850s, this site had become the "icon of the American sublime." It frequently evoked in tourists an almost overwhelming sense of power, majesty, and beauty. These visitors often sacralized the falls, viewing them as the embodiment of God's creative force. Often their tributes to Niagara Falls verged on pantheism.[57]

The fact that Hunt's rapt description of these waterfalls echoed what innumerable other tourists said did not make her response any less heartfelt. Her effusive descriptions of Niagara Falls were in sharp contrast to her brief and rather patronizing portrayal of the Native Americans she encountered there. Although Hunt appreciated that the "Indians" were "very kind" to her, especially after they learned that she was a "Medicine Woman," she gave them short shrift, merely noting that they had her "deepest sympathy" (289–90). Presumably Hunt felt sorry for their dispossessed and impoverished state. But as Joan Burbick has stressed, Hunt was very different from well-known women writers such as Lydia Maria Child and Margaret Fuller, who noted how European colonizers devastated Native American societies. Unlike these authors, Hunt did not use her published writings to elaborate on the plight of native peoples or to urge redress for their grievances.[58]

For Hunt what was important about Niagara Falls was not the indigenous people who lived there but rather the sublime beauty and power of the natural environment. The falls acted as a tonic for her, reviving her spirits as well as physical well-being. No wonder, then, that Hunt returned to Niagara whenever she could. As she declared in her autobiography: "As the pilgrim with his staff wends his way to Mecca, so I went to Niagara;—the music of the heavenly orchestra soothed and harmonized the soul. . . . I needed the tone of the air, the bracing power of the sounds to arouse and make me feel that work was still to be done" (301). These comments highlight the religious as well as healing powers that Hunt ascribed to Niagara Falls. But they also show that she used her visits there to recommit herself to her multifaceted career.

Work was critical to Hunt. Her labors as a physician, health reformer, and woman's rights advocate anchored and nourished her. So too did living in one of antebellum America's most vibrant cities. Despite her extensive travels, Hunt always remained a Bostonian. Even though she had not lived in the North End for many years, it retained a particularly strong emotional hold on her. This was evident when she recalled delivering lectures at the "Bethel," or church for sailors, in January 1852. Although Hunt did not state what topics she discussed, she did note that her talks were well attended by "hardy mariners" and their families. She also stressed that the opportunity to lecture to Boston seafarers was crucial for her because it brought back precious childhood memories—morning walks with her father on the wharves where he told her stories about "the sailor's life." No wonder, then, that she retained vivid memories of the nights she spoke at the Bethel: "I gave three lectures there. To me it was epochal—it seemed as though the tears and smiles of childhood with incomparable art and power had beautifully prepared for me a mantle of protection; and my North End life was lived over again" (282).

Hunt's words reveal her persistent nostalgia and yearning to return to an idealized childhood life. They also suggest that, despite her hectic schedule, she still felt lonely and continued to mourn the loss of beloved parents and their home in the North End. No doubt Hunt visited her sister Sarah and the Wright family whenever she was in Boston, but one wonders how close she was with them, especially given her frequent travels. Perhaps her increasingly itinerant and busy life was a way for her to escape the loneliness she faced when she was in her Boston home.

Fortunately, Hunt's public activism introduced her to a wide circle of activists, some of whom befriended her. She became close to the Unitarian minister Samuel J. May and also Gerrit Smith, both of whom Hunt met at the 1852 Syracuse national woman's rights convention; she regularly visited them and even stayed at their homes, sometimes for weeks at a time (291, 304, 311, 319).

Hunt also socialized with Lucretia Mott and Elizabeth Cady Stanton. She stayed with the Mott family when she attended the West Chester, Pennsylvania, national woman's rights convention in June 1852. There she happily experienced the "order," "economy," and "ceaseless industry" of the Mott household and also came to know another houseguest and leading feminist, Frances D. Gage (286). Later that year Hunt visited Elizabeth Cady Stanton at her home in Seneca Falls, New York. She had a "delightful" time, she recalled, and felt fortunate to get to know Stanton, whom she described as "a woman of rare intellect, logical power, [and] keen perception." Fortunately Hunt was able to lecture at the Wesleyan Chapel in Seneca Falls, the site of the first woman's rights convention in 1848. To be able to discuss women's "wrongs and rights" in such a historic place, recollected Hunt, was "indeed a privilege" (290).

Hunt's closest friendships continued to be with other women. The kindness and hospitality of Shaker women nurtured her. So too did her correspondence with Fredrika Bremer, whose letters from Sweden encouraged Hunt to "follow thy genius" and continue her work as a physician and activist (238). But Sarah Grimké remained Hunt's closest friend. Grimké repeatedly encouraged Hunt, praising her work, especially in woman's rights. In April 1853, for example, she wrote Hunt: "God bless thee my noble friend" for "thy lecture" in the "cause of woman" or rather "I ought to say in the cause of humanity."[59] Grimké later praised Hunt for her efforts to prod the Massachusetts Constitutional Convention to treat its female citizens more equitably: "I greatly rejoice to find that you are circulating a petition to secure if possible equal rights under the new Constitution."[60]

Hunt's writings had a powerful impact on Grimké. After one of Hunt's visits, where she read one of her lectures, Grimké wrote how deeply it affected her: "That lecture did my soul good, yet it sunk into the depths of my being, kept me from sleeping & haunted me. While you sat by me reading it, a soft calm, a sweet repose covered my spirit. I lay motionless, gushing tears struggled to flow."[61] Hunt's lecture apparently provoked strong, contradictory emotions in Grimké. Although it initially calmed her, it later haunted her, kept her from sleeping. Irrespective of which complicated set of emotional reactions ultimately dominated, Grimké clearly felt Hunt's words very deeply.

Grimké increasingly seemed to live vicariously through Hunt. She repeatedly peppered her Boston friend with questions about woman's rights conventions and other public events that Hunt would or had attended. Shortly after the second national woman's rights convention in Worcester, for example, Grimké asked Hunt to give her a full account of the proceedings: "Tell me, whatever you find to tell me, about the spirits who were prominent in the Convention."[62] Early in January 1852, Grimké eagerly asked Hunt if it was true (it was not) that she would soon address the Massachusetts State Legislature on the need to recognize that "woman's rights are coequal with man's, based on the ground of Human Rights."[63]

Grimké's letters suggested dissatisfaction with her life. As her biographer, Gerda Lerner, has documented, the early to mid-1850s were a difficult time for Sarah Grimké. She felt inadequate as a teacher, and increasing tensions with her sister Angelina led her to temporarily leave the Weld household in 1854.[64] For our purposes, what is important is that Grimké looked to Hunt to continue the woman's rights struggle during a time when she no longer felt capable of doing so. Late in 1854 Hunt sent Grimké a copy of her latest annual protest and apparently asked her to submit an article to the *New York Tribune* arguing for woman's rights. Grimké praised Hunt's protest as "excellent" but then declared that she was "incapable of writing anything fit for the Tribune." Hunt, she stated, would "have to fight this battle [of woman's rights] alone," but perhaps this was for the best because Hunt would "grow stronger by the contest."[65] It is sadly ironic that the author of the brilliant *Letters on the Equality of the Sexes* did not feel capable of writing an article for a newspaper. But if Grimké seemed to have lost confidence in her own abilities, she was convinced Hunt could continue the struggle for woman's rights.

The above letter also highlights advice that Grimké repeatedly offered Hunt—rely on yourself; do not depend on others. When Hunt became ill, Grimké expressed sorrow that she was unable to nurse her but then quickly added that it was better this way: "Perhaps we should spoil each other . . . and not stand up like independent women."⁶⁶ Grimké's personal problems, particularly her painful efforts to forge a life for herself independent of Angelina and her family, probably fueled these comments. But she may also have sought to warn Hunt against her deeply felt yearning to be a child again, to be as protected and dependent as she had been in her idealized early life.

Grimké also offered Hunt advice about how to conduct herself as a reformer. In 1853, while querying whether Hunt would speak at the forthcoming woman's rights convention in Ohio, Grimké urged her friend to resist the temptation to resort to anger or sarcasm when faced with "the Ninnies & Drunkards & wicked men of all sorts" who opposed the cause of female equality. She then emphatically stated that "while we claim for woman the Rights of Humanity, let us do it in a spirit that shows that we do not vaunt ourselves but deeply feel that it is the God in us, who does whatever is done, that is lovely and of good report."⁶⁷ Grimké had earlier criticized Elizabeth Cady Stanton for allegedly lacking this spirit. Although "in many respects a noble woman," Stanton showed too much "antagonistic feeling" toward men, which "deeply injure[d] our cause," she asserted.⁶⁸

One wonders how Hunt reacted to her friend's advice and implicit criticisms. Did she resent them? Did she appreciate Grimké's comments, even if she did not always follow her advice? Given the paucity of evidence, one can only speculate about these questions. But the warmth and regularity of Grimké's letters to Hunt suggest that theirs was a steadfast friendship which weathered whatever differences they might have had.

This friendship provided Hunt with a needed confidante. She shared with Grimké details about her work and also used her as a sounding board to gauge the effectiveness of her lectures and speeches. Hunt also allowed Grimké to see her when she was "worn, exhausted, body, soul, & spirit, lying on the sofa, spent with the intensity of feeling."⁶⁹ In short, Grimké was one of the few people who saw the toll that Hunt's hectic life took on her.

Perhaps the most important role Grimké played in Hunt's life was to reassure her that her hard work and sacrifices were invaluable, that she was doing God's work. No matter how ill or exhausted Hunt became, Grimké proclaimed, the "majesty of God" would give her the "strength" to continue her medical practice and reform activities and "fulfill thy mission."⁷⁰

Grimké admired, respected, and loved her dear friend. But what did she think about Hunt not being involved in what was undoubtedly the leading human rights cause of her era, the antislavery struggle? During the 1840s and early 1850s, as this movement gained momentum, especially in Boston, Hunt did not mention any participation in this crucial reform. In her autobiography she somewhat sheepishly admitted that as of 1850 she "had never even been at an anti-slavery meeting" (250). That many of her reform colleagues and friends were prominent abolitionists made her noninvolvement in the antislavery crusade all the more curious.

But there were probably several reasons why Hunt did not become active in this struggle until the mid-1850s. In the 1840s she was still trying to establish herself professionally and her time was limited. Perhaps Hunt also realized that she needed to conserve her energies—she had to focus on issues that might be lost in the swirl of numerous reform activities. While leading Bostonians dedicated themselves to abolition, she committed herself to the cause of enfranchising and educating women. Hunt's upbringing as a Universalist might also have dissuaded her from becoming active in abolitionism. As noted previously, most Universalists, despite their opposition to slavery, rejected abolitionists' shrill condemnations of slaveholders as "sinners" and resented their hostility toward their church.[71] Whatever the reason, Hunt steered clear of involvement in the antislavery struggle during the 1840s and early 1850s. But in 1854 her personal experiences as well as national developments forced Hunt to confront the evil of slavery and embrace the abolitionist cause.

Chapter 6

Forging New Connections in the Mid-1850s

Hunt's Involvement with Abolitionists, Western Feminists, and Female Doctors

During the years 1854 and 1855, Harriot Hunt remained as busy as ever. She traveled several times to Ohio, where she lectured and drummed up financial support for women seeking to study medicine. During her stays in Ohio, Hunt established a friendship with a leading feminist from that state, Caroline Severance. She also reached out to the next generation of female doctors, many of whom had received professional medical training. Hunt became active in the abolitionist movement as the sectional controversy over slavery intensified. Yet she had to confront a crucial question that bedeviled her compatriots: Would the nation tolerate the expansion of slavery? Soon Hunt and her fellow Americans were caught in the maw of civil war as they struggled to answer this question.

In mid-January 1854, Hunt left Boston and headed toward the nation's capital. She stayed for three weeks in the Washington home of Gerrit Smith who was then a congressman elected by a coalition of antislavery supporters (311, 319). While there Hunt socialized with fellow reformers and friends. Sarah Grimké, then visiting Washington, eagerly anticipated having "uninterrupted hours together" with her "dear H."[1] But Hunt's primary purpose in visiting Washington, D.C., was to educate herself about different institutions. She had a "delightful" time visiting a "school for colored girls," run by a teacher allegedly characterized by "untiring zeal, energy and benevolence." Hunt also attended Sunday services at a Swedenborgian church and praised its minister as a "man of catholic spirit and enlarged mind" (316).

But the main institution Hunt investigated while visiting Washington was the United States Congress. She recognized how crucial this body was for the future of the nation. It was there, "the seat of government," where politicians "discussed and settled questions which make or mar the happiness of millions," and Hunt determined to study it firsthand (317). She visited Congress during a time when the sectional controversy over slavery roiled the political landscape. The territories acquired from the Mexican-American War forced Americans to determine if the "peculiar institution" would spread to the West. The Fugitive Slave Act of 1850 exacerbated sectional tensions when it expanded the federal government's responsibility to track down runaway slaves and required all citizens to aid in this effort. This act triggered widespread protests throughout the North and struck fear among escaped slaves who had been living for years as free men and women and now faced recapture and reenslavement in the South.

When Hunt began her visit, Congress was grappling with yet another controversial bill designed to contain the explosive sectional divisions over slavery. The Kansas-Nebraska Bill voided the Missouri Compromise of 1820, which had prohibited slavery above the southern border of Missouri. By permitting the people in the Kansas and Nebraska territories to decide whether to enter the Union as free or slave, this bill theoretically allowed the "peculiar institution" to expand even as far as the Canadian border. Although the northern territory of Nebraska quickly barred slavery, Kansas, situated nearer the Mason-Dixon Line, was soon wracked by violence as pro- and antislavery forces fought bitterly for control of this land. Far from defusing sectional conflict over slavery, the Kansas-Nebraska Act stoked sectional divisions and violence. By 1856 the violence in "Bleeding Kansas" had precipitated a realignment of political parties: the Whig Party imploded; the Democratic Party split along sectional lines; and the Republican Party emerged, pledging to stop the expansion of slavery in the territories.

Harriot Hunt watched with great interest but growing disgust Congress's debates over the Kansas-Nebraska Bill. As she noted in *Glances and Glimpses*: "I was glad to be in Washington at this time. I learned more than I should have during a quiet session." But she then revealingly added: "The funeral pile of liberty was lighted in Congress" (320). Like so many Americans in the North, Hunt felt angry and betrayed when Congress passed the Kansas-Nebraska Act. The Fugitive Slave Act, especially its abrogation of the Missouri Compromise, also infuriated her. In 1856, as Kansas exploded in violence, Hunt angrily declared: "In Congress the very men who *passed* the fugitive slave law, to preserve the Union (so they said), are now *disturbing* the Union by endeavoring to increase slavery and counteract a compromise upon which every lover of freedom has rested" (315).

Hunt was also disgusted with the way members of Congress conducted themselves. With few exceptions, she declared, most members seemed to have "*no* appreciation of the dignity and solemnity of their position as representatives and legislators—*no* conception of their high and momentous duties. My heart was pained by a sense of the superficiality, heartlessness, and disorder of our national assembly" (313).

According to Hunt, one of the major reasons why Congress lacked both morals and dignity was because it was an all-male body. The "house" of Congress, she fumed, "looked as if it was kept by *men*, . . . tobacco juice, awkward positions, and incessant noise, reminded one of a parcel of school-boys who had no respect either for their teacher or *themselves*." Hunt contrasted congressional meetings with those held by the Women's Yearly Meeting of Friends in Philadelphia. When the Quaker women met, she declared, they were a "perfect model of dignity, propriety, and reverend, patient attention to the business before it. . . . *their* assembly [was] controlled by the principle of truth, not by a noisy and obstreperous *majority*" (313).

The contrast with Congress could not have been greater. For Hunt, Congress was a raucous, vulgar, and immoral place where men regularly betrayed both democratic principles and Christian ethics. Like other suffragists, Hunt proclaimed that the only way to redeem Congress was to elect women to this legislative body. "Cleanliness and godliness will come into Congress hand in hand with woman," she asserted. The presence of women would also promote the election of "virtuous, high-minded men" (314, 313).

Hunt pointedly excluded Gerrit Smith from her withering portrayal of Congress. She praised him as a man of unflinching principle who hated slavery and was committed to serving his country with "honesty, faithfulness, and love." As politics became more acrimonious, Hunt stressed that Smith practiced "charity" toward his opponents. Despite "abhorring slavery," he still spoke kindly of the "unfortunate slaveholder." Hunt used her descriptions of Smith to excoriate the rest of Congress: "Yes, Gerritt [sic] Smith is a member of the House of

Representatives, *yet not of them*. His sphere raises him above them" (311). By the time Hunt published these remarks in her autobiography, Smith had long left Congress. Dismayed by Congress's passage of the Kansas-Nebraska Act, he resigned his congressional seat in August 1854 and returned to his home in Peterboro, New York.[2]

But fortunately for Hunt, Gerrit Smith was a hospitable host in his Washington home during the short time he served in Congress. She was therefore able to witness the historic and contentious debates over the Kansas-Nebraska Bill, which left a lasting impact on her. Hunt's travels after she left Washington also brought home to her the horrors of slavery. Her trips to Richmond, Baltimore, and then the border state of Ohio were eye-opening experiences for her. "For the first time," she recalled, she found herself in "the midst of [slavery]." Seeing racially mixed people in the streets of the southern cities she visited made her realize how "slavery ruthlessly ruptured *all* family relations between the slaves." This institution also ruined slave masters' families. White men, she fumed, often violated their "sacred" marital vows and "blasted the happiness" of their wives when they sexually abused female slaves and fathered numerous "illegitimate children" (324, 325).

Hunt's comments reveal how complicated attitudes about race and racial identity were in antebellum America. She echoed the remarks of many abolitionists who dramatized the evil of slavery by publicizing how it violated the institution of marriage and family life. Like them, Hunt invoked the specter of miscegenation to discredit the "peculiar institution" and urge its destruction.[3] But her emphasis on how racially mixed slaves had become also suggested her repugnance about interracial sex.

What also perturbed Hunt was that people who appeared to be white were enslaved. This was a concern that haunted antislavery discourse in antebellum America. Harriet Beecher Stowe's bestselling novel *Uncle Tom's Cabin* particularly conveyed the plight of such slaves, especially when she narrated the story of the light-skinned, beautiful Eliza who made a daring escape to the North to save her young son from slave traders or that of Cassy, the quadroon brutalized by the cruel, lustful Simon Legree. It was such stories about "tragic mulattos" that garnered the most sympathy and concern from whites critical of slavery.[4]

Hunt had her own story about a "tragic mulatto" when she recounted meeting at the Smiths' Washington home "a very fine looking man" who was "no darker than a Spaniard." Hunt stressed that he was a refined man. In fact, he was so well mannered that she wished "some of our aristocrats had half the refinement he had." This gentleman, she pointedly noted, was also a devoted husband and father. But he was in terrible straits—he was a slave and desperate to find the money to buy his wife and baby before their master sold them to traders. Fortunately, Gerrit Smith helped this man financially and hopefully enabled him to buy his family's freedom (314).

While recounting this slave's anguish, Hunt conveyed her own racial and class biases. To dramatize the horrors of slavery, she focused on an extremely atypical slave, one who embodied the qualities of a Victorian gentleman: he was well spoken, polite, and devoted to his family. Perhaps most important, he was so light skinned with Caucasian features that he appeared to be white. What snagged Hunt's sympathy and concern for this enslaved man was that he fit her model of masculinity. One wonders how much sympathy she would have felt for a slave who was dark skinned, labored on a cotton plantation, was illiterate, and lacked the manners and diction of a gentleman. She probably would have felt pity for black field hands, just as she did for the dispossessed indigenous people of Niagara Falls, but it is doubtful that she would have empathized with them as she did with the slave who was "refined" and appeared to be European.

Like many other white, middle-class reformers, Hunt racialized as well as gendered the concept of virtue.[5] Her descriptions of a white wife's "blasted happiness" and her "bitterness and woe" at her husband's adulteries with female slaves reinforced a deeply entrenched view in antebellum America: it was *white* women who were paragons of moral virtue; it was therefore they who especially suffered when their husbands "desecrate[d] the *homes* of the South" (326).

Hunt did not reserve all of her sympathy for the unhappy wives of adulterous southern planters but also felt compassion for female slaves who were sexually exploited by their masters. Her anger was palpable when she described how such women and their children were often expelled from the master's home just as the biblical character Hagar suffered banishment with her son, Ishmael. Hunt emphasized the injustice and cruelty of a discarded slave woman "cast out—*not* into the wilderness, where in freedom [she] might roam, but sold into other States, perhaps to be seduced and cast out as a nuisance again and again." Such a woman, she bitterly noted, had no control over her life. Instead, she was "frequently bartered for gold" and at the mercy of not only her master but also his "outraged legal wife" who demanded that she be sent away (326).

Through such comments, Hunt highlighted how ultimately both slave women as well as white wives were at the mercy of lustful, mercenary masters who readily sacrificed their families, no matter what their color or legal status. Like other abolitionists, she also illustrated how the institution of slavery corrupted genteel white women. Their jealousy and rage at their husbands' transgressions made them condemn female slaves, who were powerless to protect themselves and their children.

Shortly after her return home, Hunt and her fellow Bostonians had to confront the terrible impact the Fugitive Slave Act had on runaway slaves living in their city. On May 24, 1854, an escaped Virginia slave named Anthony Burns was arrested, and proceedings began to return him to his master. Boston quickly erupted: mass protests ensued against Burns's recapture and rendition; an unsuccessful armed attack to free him was made; the government was forced to send marines and soldiers to maintain order. In the end Anthony Burns was reenslaved and returned to Virginia.

Although there had been other publicized cases of northern citizens protesting the recapture of slaves, the Burns case quickly became a cause célèbre. The capture and rendition of Anthony Burns created a "pocket revolution" in Boston, one that radicalized many of its leading cultural and intellectual figures, such as Ralph Waldo Emerson and Henry David Thoreau. The Burns case mobilized not only the people of Boston but also countless other northerners against the "peculiar institution." The fact that Burns's recapture occurred only several days after passage of the Kansas-Nebraska Act convinced many that the "Slave Power" had to be fought if American liberty was to survive. Perhaps Amos Lawrence, a member of the wealthy family of textile manufacturers, best expressed the impact the Burns case had on him and countless other Bostonians when he declared: "We went to bed one night old fashioned, conservative, Compromise Union Whigs and waked up stark mad Abolitionists."[6]

As federal troops marched a manacled Burns to the wharf to board his Virginia-bound vessel, thousands thronged the streets to protest his reenslavement. Many screamed at the troops: "Kidnapper! Slave Catcher! Shame! Shame!" Many Bostonians also hung funeral crepe on storefronts and other buildings; they covered American flags in black crepe. The crowd also carried through the streets a huge, black coffin with the word "Liberty" on it. Church bells rang out a funeral dirge.[7]

The day that Anthony Burns was sent back to Virginia was when the New England Woman's Rights Convention began in Boston—June 2, 1854 (334).[8] Hunt played a prominent role in this convention; she was one of the vice presidents and served on the Business Committee.[9] The mass protests over the Burns rendition predictably overshadowed the woman's rights convention. The *Anti-Slavery Bugle*, for example, stressed that it was difficult to "turn aside for a moment" the "intense interest" over the Burns affair to discuss this convention. But the author declared that it was important to do so because "Woman's

Rights" had "equal, if not paramount importance, to freedom to the colored man." Although Boston was "in an incipient state of civil war" with federal troops sent to escort Burns back to bondage, the woman's rights convention showed that Bostonians remained defiantly committed to promulgating "universal humanity and justice as well as . . . our Constitutional bill of rights." The author praised leading organizers of the convention, including Harriot Hunt, who discussed her views in "her thorough and convincing style."[10] In a similar vein, the *Liberator* stated that most of the "earnest men and women" who assembled for the woman's rights convention shared the feelings of those protesting the sad fate of Anthony Burns. Their commitment to feminism, however, caused them to proceed with the meeting.[11]

The delegates reiterated demands that they had made at earlier meetings—that women be given the vote; that wives receive basic legal rights, including "custody of [their] own person" and that of their children; that society stop forcing women to live in "dependent idleness" and grant them a "right to earn their own bread." But many of the resolutions assumed a particular force because they resonated with the demand for human rights that was occurring in the streets of Boston when Burns was led back to Virginia. The first resolution pointedly declared that "no accident of birth can determine the sphere of any mortal." When the delegates urged states to grant their female citizens the right to vote, they alluded to the Burns tragedy and the growing sectional controversy over slavery, claiming that only the participation of women in politics could save the nation from the dreadful conflict that threatened to tear apart the Union. Because "the political influence of woman is especially needful in this trial hour of our country, now convulsed with passion, and oppressed by force," and since the moral force of women would be "needed still more in the coming crisis," it was imperative to enfranchise them.[12]

When Hunt wrote to her friend Anna Parsons shortly after the convention ended, she noted that delegates frequently made antislavery remarks which ordinarily would have been "out of place" but which were appropriate given the terrible event occurring in Boston. Anthony Burns, she declared, was a "human being" whose "bright, beautiful life" was "outraged, taken in bondage." As for Congress, she claimed that members needed to clean their house after "passing the Nebraska Bill." Despite her anger over the Burns affair and congressional passage of the Kansas-Nebraska Act, Hunt was pleased with how the woman's rights convention went. "I hear many converts were made," she happily wrote her friend. She also praised convention leaders, especially Lucy Stone, who "did nobly." As for herself, Hunt regretted that she was not able to attend the evening part of the convention and was often "behind the scenes." Apparently she had suffered an accident and was temporarily lame with bandaged ankles.[13]

Hunt healed and resumed her travels and numerous other activities. Ultimately, the Burns affair resonated with her and other antebellum feminists because they not only recognized the injustice of slavery but also drew parallels between the plight of fugitive slaves and that of runaway wives. By the mid-1850s, growing numbers of feminists were campaigning against laws that severely penalized wives who ran away from husbands, even if the latter were tyrannical brutes. Such women faced the loss of all financial support, custody of their children, and any property they had brought to the marriage. Some husbands used the courts to try to recapture their wives, much as masters did their slaves. The notion of a husband's "marital custodianship" over his wife still remained, and a woman who fled her husband was an "orphan lady." Given these facts, it is not surprising that feminists increasingly argued that wives were legally no better off than slaves. As Ohio feminist Adeline Swift asserted: "The husband can compel his wife to leave her home and children, or he can compel her to return; and if she refuses to go with him, he can call men to aid him to securing her, and she has no redress unless she can prove extreme cruelty. Does not that show the husband is master of the wife?"[14]

That Hunt shared this perspective was evident when she prominently reprinted in *Glances and Glimpses* a brief notice that appeared in an Edgartown, Massachusetts, newspaper in July 1854. A contrite husband declared: "Whereas I posted my wife, Augusta M. Austin, on the 5th of January last—this is to counteract that act and make it void, as I did it *without* provocation, I being at the time in a *passion*, for which I am sorry." Hunt stressed to her readers how this statement illustrated the terrible "wrongs" wives endured: "Now this is in Massachusetts, in 1854, and shows how entirely a woman is at the mercy of her husband, to be cried up or cried down as passion moves him" (337). Hunt implicitly suggested that a wife was much like a slave—totally dependent on the will and passions of her husband/master. The fact that such incidents as the above occurred even in one of the most progressive states in the country underscored how pervasive was women's disempowerment.

Women's subjugation and exploitation haunted Hunt. Committed to ending this state of affairs, she waged a multifaceted campaign to empower women and end the discrimination they suffered. Although some of her proposed reforms, such as her demand for the female suffrage, earned her widespread criticism, her advocacy for more women doctors increasingly struck a resonant chord with growing numbers of her fellow citizens. Discussion of shifting public sentiment on this latter issue warrants extended investigation, because it offers a needed context for understanding the different strategies Hunt used in the mid-1850s to increase the number of professionally trained female physicians in the United States.

———

By the early 1850s, growing numbers of Americans were asserting that female physicians, not men, should treat women and children. As this view gained momentum, so too did the belief that women had to receive a medical education. A particularly important turning point occurred when Sarah Hale, the editor of *Godey's Lady's Book*, the most popular woman's magazine in the country, published a series of editorials extolling the need for female physicians.[15] In August 1851, for example, she declared that it was "self-evident" that women "by nature" were "better qualified than men to take charge of the sick and suffering." They were also the only "proper attendants for their own sex in the hour of sorrow" and best suited to treating children. Hale praised the career of Elizabeth Blackwell. She stressed how well qualified Blackwell was as a physician, having received a "full degree, Doctor of Medicine, the first ever bestowed on a woman in America." Blackwell, pointedly noted Hale, had "well won" her degree and was treated with the "greatest courtesy and respect" by the "most eminent physicians" in London and Paris where she continued her studies. She urged American male doctors to follow suit; they needed to encourage "their own countrywomen who are preparing to enter on this important mission of 'female physicians for their own sex.'" Hale approvingly added that several women had recently graduated from medical schools in Rochester and Syracuse and praised the opening of medical schools for women in Philadelphia and Boston. Boldly, she argued that half the physicians in the United States should be women.[16]

Other influential public figures echoed Hale's views. One such person was Catharine Beecher, the author of best-selling works on domesticity, health reform, and female education. In her popular 1855 work, *Letters to the People on Health and Happiness*, she championed women in medicine and criticized male doctors. The poor health of Americans, especially women, asserted Beecher, was partly due to the harsh remedies prescribed by male physicians. She claimed that her own ailments worsened when the "most celebrated regular physicians" dosed her with harsh drugs such as "sulphur" and "carbonate of iron." By contrast, Beecher touted the benefits of water cures where female caregivers sympathetically ministered to ailing women.[17] She herself benefited from such therapy when she repeatedly visited her brother, the Reverend Thomas Beecher, at his home in Elmira, New York, to frequent the nearby Gleason water cure.[18] In her *Letters* Beecher singled out this institution as one of the best water cures in the nation owing to the excellent care Rachel Gleason provided her female patients. Gleason, stressed Beecher, recognized that "a well-educated female physician" should be the one to treat sickly women.[19]

Beecher also credited Dr. Elizabeth Blackwell with helping her regain her health. Blackwell gave Beecher books published in Europe that touted the importance of preventive medicine, the need to exercise, to frequent water cures, and to follow "a strict obedience to *all* the laws of health."[20] When Beecher prescribed a health regimen for women, one advocating the importance of comfortable clothing, frequent bathing, a spare diet, and regular exercise, she relied heavily on Blackwell's *The Laws of Life*, a series of lectures delivered to "ladies" in New York in 1852.[21]

During the 1850s, newspapers debated the wisdom of allowing women to become doctors. What is most interesting about this debate is how many newspapers supported this development. Numerous editors, especially from New England and the West, approvingly noted that more women were becoming doctors and ably ministering to ailing members of their sex and children. The *Bangor Daily Whig and Courier*, for example, declared that there was "no doubt" that women could be capable, caring doctors. It therefore welcomed efforts to educate female physicians and women in general through free lectures on "the laws of health."[22] In a similar vein, the *Cleveland Herald* was "gratified to learn" that there were "nine Ladies attending Lectures at the Homoeopathic College in this city," instead of only two as the paper had mistakenly noted in an earlier edition. "The more [women] the better," opined the editor.[23] Meanwhile a paper in Warren, Ohio, happily declared that the female medical college in Philadelphia was "flourishing" and asserted that when women were "well fitted for the office of a physician," they performed admirably.[24] The *Lowell Daily Citizen and News* articulated similar views when it approvingly quoted the words of a male physician and naturalist who praised the Boston Female Medical College and stressed that women doctors were best suited to treat "diseases incident to parturition."[25]

Paradoxically, allegiance to prescribed views of femininity bolstered arguments for women physicians. One newspaper in Lawrence, Kansas, for example, stated that female physicians were "one of the best innovations of the age" since the "gentle and womanly care of a doctress" best treated sickly women and children. The author proclaimed that a woman was not "out of her own sphere" when she practiced medicine. This profession, he reassured readers, "demands no unsexing" like that which allegedly occurred when women embraced "Bloomerism" or "the ballot-box." Instead, medicine "leaves to the [female] sex all that ever made it charming and would only add to the attractions of Venus the grave wisdom of Pallas [the ancient Greek goddess of wisdom]."[26]

By the early 1850s, some major newspapers were writing as if it were inevitable that there would soon be significant numbers of women doctors. The *New York Daily Times*, for example, stated in 1853 that "it is not worth while [sic] to fight against fate—to struggle against destiny." Although the editor recognized that it would be "terrible hard work" for male doctors to admit women as colleagues, he stressed that they could not stop the future. "Better meet it manfully," counseled the author, and recognize that the "lady-physician" was here to stay and well suited to her task.[27]

Even the *Boston Medical and Surgical Journal*, the flagship journal of the city's medical establishment and long opposed to female doctors, began suggesting that it was time to reconsider male physicians' entrenched opposition to women colleagues.[28] An 1853 editorial, for example, noted with concern that women physicians were making "serious inroads" in the "obstetrical business, one of the essential branches of income to a majority of well-established practitioners." Yet the writer challenged his readers' prejudice against female doctors in several ways. First, he pointed out that "female physicians" were "establishing circles of good practice, in spite of the jeers, innuendos and ridicule of us lords of creation." Second, he argued, these women's insistence that in a "civilized society" they had as much right as men to practice medicine was "not a matter to be laughed down, as readily as was at first anticipated." He also wondered how much longer the medical establishment could exclude women when the "female medical colleges" had charters from the "same sources from which our own emanate and the law is no respecter of persons, whether dressed in tights or bloomers, in affairs purely scientific and intellectual." Finally, this author claimed that public sentiment was turning against those who intransigently opposed female physicians. If state medical societies continued to exclude women doctors who "can show that they are properly educated," he warned, then "public sympathy will assuredly be a shield for their protection, and we shall be denounced as a band of jealous monopolists."[29]

Significantly, the editorial began by noting that "Miss Harriet [sic] K. Hunt" had recently been given an honorary degree from the Female Medical College of Pennsylvania. With grudging admiration, the writer noted that "this lady is no every-day body. She demands her rights, and is determined to have them too. While paying taxes into the treasurer's office, in this city, last season, Dr. Hunt handed over the money, under a protest that must have made the treasurer's ears tingle." Clearly this editor recognized that Hunt did not fit the prescribed model of womanhood, but rather than denounce her as unfeminine or unnatural, he expressed respect for her grit and determination. Note how quickly he changed from calling her "Miss" to "Dr. Hunt."

By the mid-1850s, Hunt had become a public figure increasingly respected by many, even some in the Boston medical establishment. But her ambition, restlessness, and energy led her to travel out West in an effort to expand her overlapping campaigns for female physicians, health reform, and women's political rights. In December 1854, she embarked on an extensive tour of Ohio, one which lasted at least two months.[30] While there she urged financial support for women studying medicine. As she toured different medical colleges, Hunt met and often befriended the upcoming generation of professionally trained female physicians. She also forged a network with leading western feminists. Hunt's experiences in Ohio ultimately offered her a new perspective on the challenges feminists and women doctors faced in the East.

When she first traveled to Ohio, Hunt stayed with a woman whom she met at the 1852 Syracuse national woman's rights convention, Caroline Severance, a pioneering Ohio feminist (291). The two women quickly became friends as well as collaborators on many feminist projects. There were similarities between Severance and Hunt. Although married and the mother of five children, Severance was originally from Boston and, like Hunt, a religious nonconformist. She and her Ohioan husband, Theodoric Cordenio Severance, established a nondenominational Christian church in Cleveland, one which advocated antislavery and other reforms. By the early 1850s Severance was attending woman's rights conventions and had become a feminist leader in Ohio. In the spring of 1853 she presided over the first annual meeting of the Ohio Woman's Rights Association. When her family returned to Boston in 1855, Severance quickly gravitated toward the religious liberalism of the Reverend Theodore Parker and also continued her work for woman's rights.[31]

One of the major reasons why Hunt traveled to Ohio in May 1854 was to support Caroline Severance when she presented a memorial on behalf of the Ohio Woman's Rights Association to the state senate. Severance urged a number of reforms on behalf of the women of her state, including that wives have custody of their children when they divorced and that they retain their rights to inherited property and earnings, even though married. The memorial also urged that female citizens of Ohio be granted the right to vote.[32] Hunt noted that she attended Severance's presentation with "peculiar pleasure" and that the male legislators listened to her friend with the "most quiet and earnest attention" as she "pleaded the cause of humanity" (323).

When Hunt returned to Ohio in January of 1855, she stayed with the Severance family in Cleveland, and the two women often traveled together throughout the state (350–51).[33] Hunt used her time in Ohio for several purposes. First, she sought to learn about the state of education and feminism in the western state by visiting various institutions. She and Caroline and Theodoric Severance, for example, visited Oberlin College, the first institution of higher education to matriculate female as well as black students. Such feminist leaders as Antoinette Brown and Lucy Stone graduated from Oberlin.

Although Hunt looked forward to visiting what she called "the first Woman's Rights College," she confessed that Oberlin disappointed her. This college struck her as a dour, constrictive place, one where students diligently prayed and studied under the watchful eye of President Charles Grandison Finney, the renowned revivalist minister of the Second Great Awakening. "The sphere at Oberlin seemed to me one of constraint; I queried whether the soul had *free play*, whether there were amusements enough to recreate and unbend the mind" (352).

One aspect of Oberlin that especially bothered Hunt were Sunday religious services. Because Finney was temporarily absent from the campus, Hunt could not listen to this dynamic preacher. But the religious meeting she attended disheartened her: "To my joyous nature there *seemed* to be a lack of cheerfulness" (352). Later that year, when she was back home, Hunt gave a humorous account of the grim Presbyterian services that she and Caroline Severance had to endure as the guests of an Oberlin professor. Reformer Sallie Holley recalled that Hunt regaled her and others during an evening social with what occurred when the professor began his weekly "Presbyterian Sunday" ritual. When he announced that there would be extensive family religious services sandwiched between two long sermons and evening lectures at the church, Caroline Severance excused herself, claiming that "she was a Quaker in regard to prayer, praying silently." As for Hunt, she told her host that she was a Swedenborgian, and "we never use any other than the Lord's Prayer." After repeating "doleful selections from the Bible," the family then turned to Hunt and asked her to participate. Hunt drolly recounted what came next: "When it came my turn, I thought I should be suffocated with the awful solemnity if I didn't do something to turn the tide of lugubrious sentiment; so I must out with 'Bless the Lord, O my soul, and all that is within me bless his holy name!' If a cannonball had been shot through the room the effect could not have been more startling."[34]

Hunt shocked members of the Oberlin faculty with her religious liberalism, and they exasperated her with their mournful piety. But her visit to Oberlin did have its bright spots. She was "delighted" when she attended student recitations and saw how well the "colored students" performed. But she was also concerned to see how prescribed ideas about femininity undermined women's academic performance. "One thing struck me as singular," she recalled, "the *male* pupils delivered their compositions from memory, the females *read* theirs; it might be this statue-like exhibition was thought feminine or *lady-like*, but it detracted wonderfully from the interest of speaker and piece." Despite her disappointments with Oberlin, Hunt remained confident that the school would "be open to progress, all in good time" (352).

Not surprisingly, Hunt was primarily interested in visiting Ohio schools that educated women in medicine. She was pleased to see that the state seemed especially receptive to alternative health care therapies. Her visit to the Eclectic Medical Institute particularly pleased her. The dean of the faculty was Joseph R. Buchanan, one of the leading practitioners of an "eclectic" approach to medicine. The school offered a grab bag of therapies, many of them reflecting its founder's faith in spiritualism, phrenology, mesmerism, and other mind-cure approaches to medicine.[35] Although Buchanan had no medical degrees and boasted about this fact, Hunt called him a doctor. The fact that the school then had ten female students pleased Hunt; so too did conversing with Buchanan about the "laws of the mind." Hunt quickly struck up a friendship with Buchanan and visited his family home in nearby Kentucky (359).

Hunt's rapport with Buchanan and approval of his school underscored her commitment to an eclectic approach to medicine. Despite this belief, Hunt enthusiastically visited medical colleges in Ohio that stressed a scientific approach to health care and admitted women. In Columbus she toured and later attended the commencement exercises at Starling Medical College. During a conversation with the faculty dean, Hunt learned that many of his colleagues were reluctant to admit women yet ultimately they were "too honorable to sexualize science" (358).

Hunt also visited the Western Reserve Medical College in Cleveland, which trained a number of leading female doctors, including Emily Blackwell. During her visit Hunt achieved a long-sought goal—she finally attended lectures at an accredited medical school, even if only for a day. She recalled that the lecture dealt with diseases "peculiar to women." It heartened her that men and women studied this topic together in the same hall and "not one shade of levity or impropriety" marred the classroom.

After the lecture Hunt spoke with the professor, and he proudly told her that Ohio was "more democratic" than Massachusetts when it came to making medical schools coeducational. It was a bittersweet moment for Hunt. Although she "rejoiced greatly" that progress on female medical education was occurring out West, Hunt's tour of Ohio highlighted how intransigent and backward her own state was when it came to admitting women into established medical colleges. She recalled that she felt "like hanging [her] head" over the fact that her home state and city, the "Athens of America," had been "eclipsed by a younger sister" (350).

Throughout her stay in Ohio, Hunt lectured on her favorite topics. She talked about the need for female physicians and also the importance of practicing preventive medicine by following physiological laws. Newspaper accounts of Hunt's Ohio tour noted that although she primarily lectured to women, she also addressed large, gender-mixed audiences.[36]

As her tour continued, Hunt began to lecture on a new topic—the need to support the Ohio Female Medical Loan Fund Association, which was established in Cleveland in October 1852. Its primary purpose was to financially assist prospective female students by granting them interest-free loans. As its constitution stated, this association would consider only applicants who "furnish[ed] testimonials of a past upright life," had a "good rudimental education," and "a sufficiently robust constitution ... to endure the course of study" (349). Recipients of the loans would be required to repay it once they received their medical degrees and had established their practice. Another purpose of the association was to educate women throughout the state about how to preserve their health and those of their families. As one Ohio newspaper approvingly noted, the association and its auxiliaries established in different towns and cities aimed "to form a sort of nuclei of physiological centers whence the rays of hygienic and medical knowledge may radiate and enlighten ... every mother and daughter in the Buckeye State."[37]

Hunt traversed Ohio drumming up support for the loan association and establishing auxiliary societies (351–60). Although her audiences were generally receptive to her lectures, Hunt occasionally faced a hostile listener. This occurred in Tiffin, where, while lecturing to a "packed" hall on the need for women doctors, Hunt seemed almost to invite several attending male physicians to challenge her. She peppered her talk by saying "my medical brother can answer this or that." After she finished, some of her listeners urged physicians in the audience to respond to Hunt's comments. One doctor admitted that there were medical cases where a "woman was needed." Not surprisingly, Hunt described his response as "true and manly." But another physician sarcastically declared that women could never be physicians because they could "not cultivate a moustache." His disparaging remark provoked "an uproar" from the audience and a speedy rebuke from Hunt. She indignantly reminded him that there had not been "a single vulgarism" in her lecture and that she would "tolerate none" now. The audience supported her, and the offending physician was silenced (354–55).

As this incident suggests, Hunt generally enjoyed public support during her Ohio tour. Her lectures were well attended, and she received favorable press coverage. Ohio papers depicted Hunt with respect, even admiration; they stressed her qualifications and good reputation; they urged their readers to attend her talks. The *Cleveland Morning Leader*, for example, noted that "Dr. Harriet [sic] K. Hunt" was a Boston physician whose "practice of twenty years . . . qualified her" to deliver the annual address of the Ohio Female Medical Education Society with "thoroughness and ability."[38] The *Daily Ohio State Journal* declared that Hunt "created a very favorable impression" when she recently addressed "a meeting of ladies" in Columbus.[39] In a similar vein, the *Cincinnati Daily Times* described Hunt as "a lady of decided professional ability, . . . sure literary attainments and . . . varied conversational powers."[40] But perhaps it was the Columbus paper, the *Daily Capital City Fact*, which was most supportive of Hunt's agenda when it proclaimed that "there are times when the world is in commotion, and the ladies are determined to have a hand in pushing on the ball of reform. Old Fogyism, and one-eyed Conservatism! Please stand aside and let the ladies pass on!"[41]

The positive press, the packed lecture halls with generally appreciative audiences, the successful campaign on behalf of the Medical Loan Fund Association—these developments heartened Hunt. When she recalled her 1855 tour of Ohio in *Glances and Glimpses*, she praised the western state for being much more responsive to female doctors and woman's rights than was the East. Hunt credited the newness of European American settlement of the West for this progress: "The hardy settlers of a new country, who have to *work* for themselves, are very apt to *think* for themselves also—hence no one who has travelled this region can help being struck with the freedom and boldness of thought which now exists" (353).

Hunt's sojourn in Ohio made her more exasperated than ever with the continued refusal of Harvard and other Massachusetts medical schools to accept women. This reaction shaped her participation in the September 1855 New England Woman's Rights Convention. Held in Boston, the meeting attracted various feminist leaders, including Paulina Wright Davis, Susan B. Anthony, William Lloyd Garrison, and Caroline Severance. Hunt played a particularly prominent role, presiding over the convention and delivering the opening address. She also presented a series of resolutions that reiterated her long-held beliefs: the continued exclusion of women from most medical schools on the grounds of "delicacy" merely showed the "impropriety" of men treating female patients; female doctors were needed to end the "present array of quack nostrums and the utter incompetency" of many male physicians and pharmacists; women doctors were also best suited to attacking their society's "strongholds of vice."

But Hunt's speech also highlighted the impact on her of the Ohio trip. She pointedly praised the medical schools she had recently visited, particularly "Dr. Buchanan's Eclectic Medical School of Cincinnati, the Starling Medical College of Columbus, and the Cleveland College." These schools, she stressed, admitted women. They offered a sharp contrast to the sad state of affairs in Massachusetts where women could not study medicine with men in coeducational institutions.[42]

Despite her prominence and success out west, Hunt remained part of a marginalized minority in Boston. The Boston city directory refused to list women doctors, even those with medical degrees, as regular physicians. The 1855 directory, for example, counted fifteen women as "physicians-female"; four of these were designated as medical doctors, and the others were simply categorized under the heading of "no designation." The fact that the category of "female physicians" also included "clairvoyant," "Indian Doctress," and "electropathist," as well as homeopaths and midwives, served to undermine the credibility of women doctors.[43] Meanwhile, the Massachusetts Medical Society, an organization that initially licensed doctors in the state and remained crucial in legitimizing a physician's professional credentials, refused to admit women, even those who were graduates of accredited medical schools. In frustration, in 1878 twelve Boston area female doctors formed their own medical society.[44]

These facts gnawed at Hunt. Bitterly she noted that despite the "courteous manner" in which many discussed the idea of female physicians, the Boston medical establishment was still dominated by "old established cliques," resistant to "*innovators*." Hunt made it a point of noting that she was not surprised when the Massachusetts Medical Society quickly rejected the application of Dr. Nancy Clarke, a graduate of the Cleveland Medical College. "I was sure," she groused, that "they would not admit her [Clarke], would not have the moral courage to establish such a precedent by welcoming woman as their acknowledged coadjutor" (298). As for herself, Hunt noted that most of Boston's male physicians continued to ostracize her: "I was a traitor, outlaw, felon" (297).

One way that Hunt coped with her outlier status was to welcome women who established a medical practice in Boston, doctors such as Clarke and Martha A. Sawin, a graduate from the Female Medical College of Pennsylvania. Far from viewing them as competitors or rivals, Hunt saw these doctors as fellow pioneers who could help her challenge men's monopoly of medicine. For this reason she asserted that "the establishment of female physicians is one of the delights of my life" (298). The presence of other women doctors also alleviated the guilt Hunt felt when she traveled and left her patients unattended. With obvious relief she noted that because other female doctors could minister to ailing women, she felt "more at liberty to leave home" (297).

Hunt was also an avid supporter of Elizabeth Blackwell. Recall that the latter's admission into the Geneva Medical School in November 1847 encouraged Hunt to apply to attend medical lectures at Harvard. When Blackwell returned from Europe and started practicing in New York City, Hunt stressed that her "soul rejoiced." She also referred several of her patients to Blackwell and wrote her a heartfelt letter: "I poured out my feelings in a letter, and gave her the right hand of fellowship" (284). As noted previously, Hunt also became a fundraiser for Blackwell's project, the New York Infirmary for Women and Children. She and Caroline Severance as well as other feminists were key supporters of this pioneering institution, a fact that Blackwell gratefully noted.[45]

Hunt and Severance also provided critical help to Marie Zakrzewska, who migrated to the United States after politics and gender discrimination thwarted her initially promising career as the head midwife of Berlin's Royal Charité hospital. In the fall of 1854, Zakrzewska attended the Western Reserve College in Cleveland owing to the support of three women: Elizabeth Blackwell intervened to get the German émigré admitted into the college from which her sister had recently graduated. Caroline Severance and Harriot Hunt provided financial support for the impoverished Zakrzewska when they found her funding from several organizations, including the Cleveland Medical Loan Fund Association and the Physiological Society of Cleveland (Severance was then president).

Hunt and Severance also took Zakrzewska under their wing. The young German student was a guest in Severance's home and socialized with her, Hunt, and other women activists. These women's emotional support was probably as important as the financial aid. Zakrzewska was only one of four women out of a class of approximately two hundred students enrolled in the Cleveland Medical College. Her poverty, émigré status, and difficulties with English only served to further marginalize her from most of her classmates.[46]

Hunt's description of meeting Zakrzewska was similar to how she recalled her first encounter with Fredrika Bremer. Hunt felt an immediate kinship with Zakrzewska: "When I met her, an electric communication was instantly established between us. I felt that here was a combination of head and heart, which was as uncommon as it was beautiful. . . . Joy filled my soul that one had come from the old world laden with its experiences and its treasures, to cast her lot in the new" (347).

In her autobiographical reminiscences, Zakrzewska gratefully recollected the support and friendship she received from Hunt and Severance. These women, she stressed, not only helped finance her schooling but also became "kind and intelligent as well as sympathizing friends," ones who took her "under their wings to shelter me and to promote my efforts." Hunt and Severance did not proselytize about woman's rights. Zakrzewska initially rejected feminism, agreeing when a newspaper dismissed feminists as "the hens which want to crow." But she credited her two mentors with furthering her conversion to woman's rights. Hunt and Severance introduced her to many reformers, and she listened intently as they discussed various human rights issues, including feminism. These activists, gratefully recalled Zakrzewska, allowed her to "work out my own salvation and see the righteousness of their demands for a larger sphere for women." That these reformers welcomed and encouraged female doctors made Zakrzewska understand that she and women like her would benefit enormously from feminism. Once she realized that she "had tried to crow as hard as any of these women without realizing it," she became a supporter of woman's rights, including the right to vote.[47]

Hunt and Severance helped Zakrzewska become a doctor and a feminist. They also helped Zakrzewska throughout her medical career. A resident physician of the New York Infirmary for Women and Children from its opening in 1857 until 1859, Zakrzewska recognized that this institution would never have existed had it not been for the network of women activists who backed it, women like Hunt and Severance. When Zakrzewska sought funds to establish the New England Hospital for Women and Children in Boston, she quickly turned to Hunt and also Severance, who by then had relocated to the city. She often stayed with Hunt while in Boston and through her and Severance met not only leading reformers, such as the Welds, Sarah Grimké, and Antoinette Brown Blackwell, but also wealthy, reform-minded people who helped fund her proposed hospital. Hunt also introduced Zakrzewska to women doctors in Boston who could offer needed advice and support, such as Dr. Nancy Clarke, as well as Dr. Henry Bowditch, who soon agreed to be a consulting physician at the new hospital.[48]

Although Zakrzewska and Blackwell appreciated Hunt's support, they had to distance themselves from her. To gain professional credibility and acceptance from their male colleagues, licensed female physicians avoided being too closely identified with women healers who lacked medical degrees and practiced alternative health therapies.[49] Zakrzewska, for example, summarily rejected women who sought to train at the New England Hospital for Women and Children if they espoused hydropathy and homeopathy. She was also dismissive of a "mind-cure" approach to healing and emphasized that the physician's task was to use science to cure the body, not heal the mind or spirit.[50]

Despite Zakrzewska repeatedly asserting that "science has no sex," her approach to medicine was permeated by gender concerns. As her biographer has noted, Zakrzewska believed that a female physician had to reject qualities gendered feminine and embrace "masculine-coded traits," such as scientific expertise and rigorous professional training. Ultimately, Zakrzewska believed that a woman had to become more like a man if she was to succeed in medicine. She boasted that when she studied at one noted Berlin hospital, the male students "never seemed to think that I was not of their sex, but always treated me like one of themselves."[51]

Licensed female physicians did not have to embrace Zakrzewska's efforts to behave like a man to accept her major premise: success in medicine required that they substitute science for sympathy when they treated patients, that they reject therapies premised on the assumption that women were more sympathetic, nurturing, than men. The leading female physician in late nineteenth-century America, Dr. Mary Putnam Jacobi, was a particularly forceful exponent of these beliefs. She declared that a woman could be "a medical expert" only if she was "impassive and directive with patients" and substituted "mastery of physiology and chemistry" for "maternalism."[52] In an 1891 essay surveying the history of women in American medicine, Jacobi credited the pioneers who paved the way for female physicians, including Harriot Hunt, but she also stressed their limitations. Antebellum women healers had exhibited "much zeal but little knowledge" of medicine, and their therapies had long been discredited.⁵³

Unfortunately, there are no extant documents that reveal how Hunt felt when licensed female physicians disparaged her approach to medicine. But Sarah Grimké did voice her concerns to Hunt about these practitioners of medicine. Although she believed that it was "peculiarly" women's "sphere to minister to the sick," Grimké resented the way female doctors increasingly relied on science and neglected to establish a heartfelt, emotional bond with their patients. Her comments warrant extensive quotation since they articulate an ideal of women physicians that Hunt shared: "What an unspeakable blessing it will be to the world, if women of the right stamp, women of strong minds & acquainted ... with the science of medicine are spread ... over the land but in addition to talent & strength there must be *Love[,]*-no woman can justly fulfill her mission as a physician without a love spirit, ... and no woman deserves the name of physician who cannot hold intercourse with the spirits of her patients and minister to the higher nature. Hence I fear nothing more, than that women unblest with this gift and whose highest attainment is a scientific knowledge of medicine should crowd into the profession- I have not yet seen one who has passed through the colleges who comes up to my beau ideal of a physician."⁵⁴

Such comments dovetailed with Hunt's belief that a physician must establish a rapport with her patient's innermost self or soul and listen to the latter's "heart history." Whereas recently trained female doctors sought to emulate their male colleagues by treating the body as scientifically as possible, Hunt's approach to medicine echoed that of Swedenborg—the body was merely a receptacle for the spirit, and if one established harmony between the two, disease would disappear and there would be no need for medicines. For Hunt, the physician's major role was "introducing patients to *themselves*," teaching them to listen to their inner spirit and to follow the supposedly eternal physiological laws prescribed by nature and God (371).

Although a believer in the spiritual world, Hunt never embraced spiritualism, the movement that gained popularity during the 1850s, especially when professed mediums such as the famous Fox sisters conducted séances where they allegedly communicated with the dead. Hunt's failure to join the spiritualist bandwagon was odd since she belonged to the three groups noted for their support of this activity. Spiritualists' claims that a benign God existed, that salvation was open to all, and that there was a harmonious order between the spiritual and material world attracted Universalists and Swedenborgians. Many advocates for woman's rights also espoused spiritualism. They were attracted by spiritualists' commitment to individual rights for all human beings, opposition to patriarchy, support for egalitarian marriages, and acceptance of women in public roles, including as mediums and physicians. Spiritualists also gained the loyalty of many alternative health practitioners, especially women, when they not only welcomed female healers but also proclaimed that listening to one's own spirit cured people from illness.[55]

Although Hunt undoubtedly knew many people who embraced spiritualism, her closest friend did not. In the late 1840s, Sarah Grimké wrote Hunt that she had recently attended a séance where the medium asked her if she wished to convey any message to her beloved mother in the afterlife. Grimké tartly replied that "nothing occurs to me at present. I have constant communication with my mother." Despite her belief in the spirit world, Grimké was skeptical about séances. As she told Hunt: "The danger is that we mistake intercourse with spirits for spirituality, & deem ourselves on the high road to perfection, when we are only adding *ideas* to our stock of knowledge about spiritual things."[56]

Hunt shared Grimké's misgivings about séances. "I believe in spiritual manifestations," she stated, "in those holy unseen influences which arrest us from the within, and the *effect* is seen on the *outer*." Remaining leery about séances and the mediums who conducted them, Hunt stated: "Those nervous twitches speak not of harmony—those morbid feelings tell not of order, those unnatural actions savor not of health. This is the dark side of spiritualism. . . . I am not satisfied of the use of so many hours being given to table-tippings, rappings, twitchings, jerkings, etc. When we are to be arrested, the voice will sound *within*—if not, vain are outward voices" (357).

Hunt's association of spiritualists with disorder and disharmony and her suggestion that these people were charlatans who duped gullible people occurred during a growing backlash against séances. By the early 1850s, prominent Swedenborgians became alarmed at the growing number of their fellow congregants who espoused spiritualism. They denounced this movement for rejecting many of their founder's key religious precepts, including his belief in hell and his advocacy of the Bible as the "most authoritative source of religious truth." But perhaps what most troubled leaders of the New Church was that spiritualists ignored Swedenborg's warnings against trying to contact the dead. Such a practice allegedly transgressed natural and religious proscriptions and failed to recognize that only Swedenborg was privileged to have "exclusive contact with the spirit world."[57]

Leading scientists also offered scathing criticisms of spiritualism and séances. Matters came to a head in 1857 when three of Harvard's most renowned faculty members—zoologist and geologist Louis Agassiz, astronomer Benjamin Peirce, and chemist Eben Norton Horsford—were asked to investigate séances by the *Boston Courier*. After three sessions these men denounced séances as a "stupendous delusion" that "lessen[ed] the truth of man and the purity of woman."[58]

Such a scorching indictment of spiritualism, especially those by Harvard's leading men of science, encouraged Hunt, a woman committed to enhancing her credibility as a respectable, professional physician, to distance herself from this movement. So too did the growing opposition voiced by leaders of her church. Despite continuing to grieve for her departed parents and niece, Hunt doubted that séances could enable her to contact them. She remained focused on trying to improve the lives of people in this world rather than seeking to communicate with the dead.

During the 1850s she sought to support female doctors and promote health reform and woman's rights. In 1856 Hunt attempted to reach a wider audience by publishing her autobiography. *Glances and Glimpses* heightened Hunt's already high public profile and enabled her to focus on grievances to which she had only alluded in her speeches and lectures, such as the cruelty and injustice of conventional marriage for women. It also inadvertently revealed the anguish and loneliness that continued to mar Hunt's life.

Chapter 7

Glances and Glimpses—Harriot Hunt's "Heart History," Jeremiad, and Reform Manifesto

Toward the end of 1854, Sarah Grimké urged Harriot Kezia Hunt to "Write on—Write on" and finish her autobiography.[1] Fortunately, Sarah Grimké and Theodore Weld helped Hunt by editing her narrative.[2] Advanced copies of *Glances and Glimpses*, a richly detailed work of 418 pages, became available in late December 1855.[3] *Glances and Glimpses* was the first autobiography authored by a woman who was prominent in the antebellum feminist movement. Few other woman's rights activists published an autobiography, and those who did waited until the late nineteenth century to do so. Jane Swisshelm's *Half a Century*, for example, appeared in 1880, and Elizabeth Cady Stanton did not publish *Eighty Years and More* until 1898. For reasons soon to be discussed, female autobiographies, especially a full-length life narrative like *Glances and Glimpses*, were highly unusual in the antebellum era.

In the fall of 1855, John P. Jewett and Company, a leading Boston press best known for publishing *Uncle Tom's Cabin* in 1852, began advertising Hunt's life narrative. This press initially trumpeted Hunt's accomplishments as a way to market her book. In December 1855, for example, the publisher used banner headlines to note that the autobiography of an "EXTRAORDINARY WOMAN," that of "DOCTOR HARRIOT K. HUNT," would soon appear.[4] Advertisements in numerous papers promised that Hunt's "remarkable" narrative would recount the "Life Experiences of a Rare Woman." The press highlighted Hunt's medical career: "A professional woman? Yes, reader, a professional woman, . . . one eminent in her profession" and "unafraid to make some professional disclosures . . . the world should know." In the same advertisement the publisher emphasized that "Dr. Harriot K. Hunt" was also the woman who annually issued "able" protests against the "injustice of *taxation without representation.*" Her autobiography, proclaimed Jewett and Company, would be "a volume of *keen satire, genuine wit, capital hits* at the *tom-fooleries* of the age, and [a] book of sterling good sense."[5]

During the first several months of 1856, Jewett and Company began marketing Hunt's book in a new way. Advertisements now stressed that *Glances and Glimpses* was "Emphatically A 'Home Book!' " They featured blurbs from different journals and newspapers praising Hunt's autobiography as a book that offered "a beautiful picture of home," one that was a "testimony to the value of HOME" and conveyed "the earnestness and devotedness of woman." Although extant records do not confirm that these were comments from actual reviews, they were probably paid insertions by the publisher. Their prominent inclusion in advertisements shows that Jewett and Company was increasingly portraying Hunt's text as one offering a paean to traditional domesticity and womanhood.[6]

By April of 1856 another shift was becoming evident in the way Jewett and Company marketed Hunt's book. Gone were the earlier advertisements emphasizing that Hunt was a "professional" and "eminent" woman who annually protested against the "injustice" of taxing women while denying them the right to vote. Instead, the publisher patronized Hunt. Echoing Fredrika Bremer's somewhat condescending depiction of her, advertisements now described Hunt as "The Little Doctor" and then added that she was a "Peculiar One . . . Too." They no longer highlighted Hunt's innovative approach to medicine but emphasized how women patients flocked to her because of her "healthful, joyous, contagious laugh." Advertisements also reiterated that *Glances and Glimpses* was a "genuine 'Home Book,' a book for the fireside, and one which every woman should own and read." Fearing that such a proclamation might not be enough to drum up sales, the publisher declared that it wanted to find "THREE HUNDRED BRIGHT, INTELLIGENT GIRLS, who would like to go from house to house all through New England selling this book." Jewett and Company promised that such girls would get copies of the book on such favorable terms that they would "make money."[7]

Of course, such an offer suggested that *Glances and Glimpses* was not selling well and that the publisher was scrambling to find new ways to peddle the book. Invoking the popular ideology of domesticity to hawk Hunt's narrative also revealed how eager Jewett and Company was to increase flagging sales.

But such a marketing strategy misrepresented *Glances and Glimpses*. This autobiography was a radical text, one that skewered conventional marriage and domesticity. Its author was a pioneering professional woman and feminist who advocated an end to patriarchy and the emancipation of women. Likely realizing that offering a frank, accurate view of Hunt might discourage sales, Jewett and Company increasingly portrayed her in ways that demeaned and trivialized her and obfuscated the subversive nature of her book. To appreciate the boldness of Hunt's autobiography, it is important to situate the book in the context of autobiographical writing in antebellum America.

Life narratives were a popular staple in the highly competitive literary market when *Glances and Glimpses* was published. Autobiographies by self-made men who succeeded in business, politics, reform, and the professions, especially the ministry, regularly appeared. Authors of such works hoped to emulate the phenomenal success of Benjamin Franklin's classic narrative, first published in England in 1793. Although autobiographers were traditionally privileged white men, the antebellum era saw the publication of memoirs by all sorts of people. Former slaves, ex-sailors, soldiers, reformed drunkards, adventurers, frontiersmen, and criminals now told their life stories and thereby asserted a public identity.

As literary scholars and historians have noted, such books did not provide a straightforward account of their authors' lives. Like all autobiographical writing, these antebellum narratives instead illuminated how the authors/subjects remembered and interpreted their lives, how they constructed public self-representations of themselves to burnish their reputations, vent their grievances, settle scores, advocate for various reform agendas, and gain badly needed money. Autobiographies now and then are complex, multivalent texts that can reveal but also obscure or distort crucial aspects of their authors' lives. They also offer a window into the society that produced them.[8]

A Bibliography of American Autobiographies, which lists the life narratives published in the United States until 1945, shows over six hundred antebellum autobiographical works, out a total of 6,377 texts. Yet women wrote only a few over forty of these books.[9] Female autobiographies published before the latter part of the nineteenth century were often more episodic and disjointed than were those produced by men.[10] Initially, they were also briefer, although by the early 1850s female narratives were becoming longer and more detailed.[11] Not surprisingly, many focused on domestic matters. Some were women's plaintive accounts of marriages to drunken or cruel husbands.[12] Other narratives illuminated the lives of antebellum homemakers in the Northeast.[13] Some women also authored accounts describing their lives as western pioneers. One such author was Eliza Wood Burhans Farnham, now best remembered as an innovative penologist and reform-minded matron of female prisoners at Sing Sing.[14] In 1846 she published her memoir *Life in Prairie Land* about her time in Illinois and in 1856 produced her recollections about living in California.[15]

Many antebellum female autobiographies also detailed their authors' lives as Christian missionaries, schoolteachers, preachers, and slaves. In her 1842 memoir, Lucy Richards, for example, described her work as a Methodist missionary and teacher among the Oneida Indians in New York State, while Harriet Livermore's 1826 text recalled her preaching in various New England and New York communities.[16] African American female authors published works describing their lives as Christian missionaries, preachers, or slaves. Jarena Lee and Zilpha Elaw, for instance, authored memoirs that discussed their preaching the gospel, while Harriet Jacobs's *Incidents in the Life of a Slave Girl* offered a searing portrait of what she suffered under slavery and how she escaped.[17]

The existence of women's autobiographies in the antebellum era should not obscure two points. First, most books focused on women's domestic or religious lives, and when they did discuss women's work outside the home, it was usually in their capacity as teachers, missionaries, or preachers. Second, the salient characteristic of female narratives is how few existed prior to the Civil War. The paucity of such books is not surprising. Few women had the literacy, leisure, financial means, or credibility to produce full length narratives.

But perhaps the most important reason why few women authored autobiographies was that this genre of literature privileged the self. Life narratives reflected as well as promoted the notion of the individual as an autonomous being shaping his or her destiny. As George Gusdorf, a leading theoretician of the genre of autobiography, stressed in 1956, "Consciousness of self," the belief that the individual is a "discrete" unit unto him- or herself, is a precondition for the development of autobiography.[18]

But women have long been taught to efface their sense of self and individuality. They have been socialized from an early age to construct a sense of self in relation to others—their parents, siblings, husbands, children, and so forth.[19] Such socialization made it initially very difficult for women to write autobiographies because it required that they focus on their own individual selves. This genre of literature also challenged women to forge a public identity for themselves, one that asserted their right to exercise power in the civic domain, a daunting challenge for most antebellum women, especially when they faced public opprobrium for leaving the private domain of domesticity.[20] To write an autobiography was such an inherently subversive act for women that it is a wonder that any assumed this task in the nineteenth century. According to the noted literary scholar Carolyn Heilbrun, it was not until the advent of the modern feminist movement in the early 1970s that women finally began producing autobiographies that openly asserted their individuality.[21]

But the ground was laid in antebellum America when a minority of women produced full-length autobiographies. Like other non-privileged writers, female autobiographers were likely to be defensive, even apologetic, about writing their life story.[22] They stressed that family or friends had urged them to publish their recollections and also apologized for any errors of grammar and style. Unlike their male counterparts, female autobiographers usually masked their ambition and avoided taking credit for their own accomplishments. Eager to appear self-effacing, most women writers were unable to acknowledge that it was their own ability, grit, and industry that led to their achievements. Instead they credited God, family, or even luck or fate for their alleged good fortune.

They also invoked the discourse of traditional femininity to legitimize their public activism and the publication of their life story. Repeatedly these women portrayed themselves as stereotypical females—they were allegedly nurturing, intuitive, and devoted to selfless service to their families. Female autobiographers who did not marry but became teachers, missionaries, and healers stressed that their careers were a surrogate for marriage and motherhood. Like traditional homemakers, they cared selflessly for others.

Many nineteenth-century female autobiographers also muted their sufferings—they learned to conceal their pain and used their narratives to show how they channeled their sorrows into religious duty and service to humanity. But perhaps most important, these writers rarely expressed anger in their works, lest they would appear shrill and unfeminine. Repeatedly, then, female autobiographers learned to hide their emotions and ambitions in order to establish their legitimacy and gain their readers' sympathy. Female autobiographers were "selves in hiding."[23]

One author who illustrated many of the above characteristics of antebellum female autobiographers was the popular actress and playwright Anna Cora Mowatt.[24] In 1854 she produced a 448-page narrative entitled *Autobiography of an Actress; or, Eight Years on the Stage*.[25] Sarah Grimké and Harriot Hunt were Mowatt's friends as well as fans, and both read her life story. After telling Hunt how much she had enjoyed Mowatt's autobiography, Grimké added in a bantering tone: "I guess when your autobiography comes out I shall be quite cured of my abhorrence of 'Memoirs written by herself.' Anna Cora gave me the first curative dose and I think you will finish the work."[26]

Since Mowatt was already a celebrity and had a ready audience for her book, one would expect that she would be a confident autobiographer, yet this was not the case. Like so many other nineteenth-century women who assumed a public role, Mowatt was defensive about both her career and narrative. She started her autobiography with an apology—the only reason she was publishing her text, she claimed, was because her dearly beloved husband, now dead, had urged her to do so.[27] She remained defensive throughout her autobiography. She insisted that it was only with great reluctance that she overcame her repugnance to engage in what was then a risqué profession. Invoking the rhetoric of domesticity, she claimed that "the idea of becoming a professional actress was revolting," but she did this to protect her gravely ill husband from destitution and "preserve [their] home."[28]

The rhetoric of prescribed femininity was so powerful in the nineteenth century that both Elizabeth Blackwell and Elizabeth Cady Stanton appropriated it in their respective autobiographies. Blackwell portrayed herself as selflessly dedicated to the welfare of not only her patients but also humanity. She repeatedly de-emphasized her ambition and humbly described herself as one who followed God's plan for her.[29] Blackwell also muted expressions of anguish and anger, even when she recounted suffering tragedies and abuse. She did not dwell, for example, on the sorrow she experienced when an eye infection blinded her in one eye and ended her dream of becoming a surgeon. She also avoided discussing her private life other than to note her adoption of an orphaned Irish child when her loneliness became "intolerable."[30]

Afraid of undercutting the major purpose of her autobiography, advancing public support for female physicians, Blackwell carefully avoided any expression of anger against men who opposed her medical practice. The doctors who refused to help or recognize her as a colleague, the men who harassed her when she went out on night calls, those who sent her nasty anonymous letters—Blackwell briefly noted this but checked any expressions of bitterness. Rather, she blandly declared that "with common sense, self-reliance, and attention to work in hand," women could pursue medical careers.[31] Blackwell also pointedly noted that she rejected participating in the first woman's rights convention held in Worcester, Massachusetts, because she feared it smacked of antimale bias.[32]

Although Stanton was not as self-effacing as Blackwell, she too invoked the mantle of traditional femininity in *Eighty Years and More*. In her preface she stressed that she would focus mainly on her "private life as the wife of an earnest reformer, as an enthusiastic housekeeper, proud of my skill in every department of domestic economy, and as the mother of seven children."[33] Throughout her narrative Stanton avoided appearing as the committed radical that she was and instead presented herself as "largely harmless, benign and motherly."[34] Stanton also carefully excised expressions of anger or resentment about patriarchal power from her autobiography for fear of alienating her audience and omitted discussing any disappointments or conflicts in her personal life, such as her troubled marriage.[35]

Eighty Years and More is a deceptive book. Despite her claims that she would focus on her private life, most of Stanton's narrative discusses not only her personal struggle but also those of all women for basic rights and freedoms. Stanton appropriated popular notions of domesticity to promote her feminist agenda and make it palatable to her readers in the late nineteenth century. The fact that the founding mother of American feminism felt the need to adopt this strategy in the 1890s underscores how difficult it was for nineteenth-century women to openly demand their rights.

Hunt's autobiography simultaneously appropriated and defied the rhetorical strategies prescribed for such works. Ostensibly, Hunt followed the script of many other nineteenth-century female memoirists. She was at times self-effacing and defensive, even apologetic, about writing a life narrative. Even the title, *Glances and Glimpses*, deprecates the seriousness of her text. The length of her book, the obvious care with which she detailed her story, belied her claim that she was merely providing her "kind reader" with only "glimpses of a life" (ix). Her subtitle, *Fifty Years Social, Including Twenty Years of Professional Life*, provided a more accurate description of the ambitious scope of Hunt's book.

In her preface Hunt readily conceded that "*critics*" and "*satirists*" would find much to criticize in *Glances and Glimpses*. There are, she asserted, "plenty of *defects*, plenty of rough *granite* for your *hard* natures to hammer upon; an overflow of *enthusiasm* for you to brand as mere *impulse*." She pleaded with both critics and readers to "be kind in your severity, charitable in your criticisms," and to "find the 'stand-point' of the *writer*" before they held a "microscope" to her work and saw its many "flaws" (xi–xii). Hunt therefore assumed the pose expected of women writers in the mid-nineteenth century when she made such comments—she appeared humble and apologetic. But she also shrewdly tried to preempt condemnation of her work by suggesting that critics were carping and unkind.

Like other antebellum women authors, Hunt idealized, indeed sacralized, domesticity. Repeatedly she stressed how her family nurtured and anchored her. She trumpeted her devotion to her parents by telling her readers that they would find in her book "a lamp lighted at the sacred *altar* of home, and fed by oil pure and fresh from the cruise of parental influence" (ix). Similar to other unmarried career women of the nineteenth century, Hunt also asserted that her profession became a surrogate for marriage and motherhood. She was "wedded to Humanity," channeled her "maternal nature" into her "*profession*," which "seemed hallowed to me; my patients were my family" (214, v).

Hunt seemed to deprecate her abilities in describing what enabled her to write her life story. She presented herself as a passive figure rather than as the driven, creative woman she actually was. Echoing Harriet Beecher Stowe's famous claim that God actually wrote *Uncle Tom's Cabin* and she was merely his instrument, Hunt asserted that she "heard a voice" telling her to write. "In simplicity I have obeyed, doing what my hands found to do; I feel a debt has been paid to humanity, a burden rolled off my heart, and a recognition of my home responsibilities publicly expressed" (417).

Hunt's autobiography shows that she carefully used her text to forge public personas that fit the prescribed views of femininity in antebellum America. As the preceding chapters have shown, Hunt repeatedly presented herself as a loving, dutiful daughter and sister—she started her own school to help her financially distressed parents; became a doctor to cure her grievously ill sister; and built up her practice to support her impoverished, widowed mother. Of course another public persona Hunt presented in her autobiography was that of the selfless healer and reformer, committed to the welfare of others. She emphasized that what drove her activism was dedication to the cause of "human rights" (214, 224, 249).

One need not doubt the sincerity of Hunt's professed love for family or commitment to serving humanity to recognize that she presented herself in ways that burnished her reputation and also masked her ambition and radicalism. As Patricia Spacks has argued, one must view all autobiography as a "theatrical performance of the self" in which authors artfully craft public identities for themselves.[36] As noted earlier, when women did this they often hid how they sought success and independence. Prescribed views of femininity made it necessary for female authors to obscure how committed they were to empowering not only themselves but women in general. This was the case with Harriot Hunt. She invoked traditional feminine discourse, including tributes to conventional domesticity and selfless, nurturing women, for the same reason that Stanton did in her autobiography. Both women hoped that using the ideology of domesticity to present feminist arguments would help gain badly needed public support for the woman's rights movement.

Ostensibly *Glances and Glimpses* straddled conflicting models of femininity. This was evident in Hunt's dual dedication to both her sister and Sarah Grimké. The first dedication not only highlighted Hunt's love for her "only sister" but also paid homage to the path Sarah chose after she left the Hunt medical practice to become a wife and mother. Harriot praised her sister's decision to embrace traditional domesticity. Sarah's "high and holy marriage" had enabled her to become a mother. Hunt suggested that she experienced vicariously the happiness of motherhood through her sister. The children Sarah bore "gladden[ed] with joy" her own life and Harriot felt she "shared that relation" of motherhood, at least "in part" (v).

But this dedication smacked of sentimentality. Hunt's paeans to her sister's "high and holy marriage" and blessed maternity bordered on the fulsome. By contrast, the second dedication to Grimké, one of the pioneers of American feminism, was more brief and direct. Hunt praised Grimké as a woman of "high-toned principles" and "moral courage" who had "elevated, deepened, and brightened" her "public life" and taught her to "apply the touchstone of truth to every subject." Hunt also credited Grimké with being an inspiration and model for all women committed to improving the world. Directly addressing her friend, Hunt gratefully declared: "As a woman, rare and true, you have done much for me, and also for every woman engaged in the reforms of the day" (vii). This encomium highlighted Hunt's allegiance to the feminism that Grimké embodied. Although she loved her sister dearly, Hunt acknowledged that in the end it was Grimké who offered her a model of womanhood that was more relevant to the kind of life she led.

Hunt was unable to retain the mask of demure, passive, and self-effacing femininity throughout her text. Even her reminiscences of an idyllic childhood home inadvertently undercut her professed homage to domesticity. Such reminiscences became a mantra, a trope, and the more they were repeated the more one wondered how accurately they described the actual reality of Hunt's early life. As Carol Heilbrun has observed, nostalgia for childhood in women's memoirs often masked "unrecognized anger."[37] Such nostalgia also implicitly rebuked the adult world in which female memoirists lived. The reason why so many of these authors had fond memories of their childhood was because that was the one time in their lives when they enjoyed relative freedom, it was a time before they had to assume the circumscribed lives of women.[38]

Glances and Glimpses challenged traditional feminine discourse when Hunt detailed how she rose from poverty to become a successful, independent woman. Her pride was evident in recounting her many achievements— establishment of a school; success as a doctor, despite staunch male opposition; and a career as a noted health reformer and woman's rights activist. Hunt made it a point to note that it was her hard-earned success that enabled her to pay off the mortgage on the family home and provide comfortably for her widowed mother and herself. When Hunt recalled hobnobbing with nationally recognized reformers and political leaders such as Gerrit Smith, Lucretia Mott, and Elizabeth Cady Stanton, she advertised her own growing prominence. In short, Hunt's autobiography was that of a woman who was anything but self-effacing. Hunt often dropped the mask of prescribed feminine passivity to reveal her ambition, tenacity, grit, and accomplishments.

Glances and Glimpses was also a subversive text because Hunt did not hide the enormous personal price she paid for her maverick career and reform activism. She stressed her loneliness, the keen sense of loss and abandonment experienced when her parents died. Hunt's accounts of suffering breakdowns after the death of loved ones and her yearning to regress to childlike dependency underscore her periodic bouts of depression and desperation (225–26). Her sister Sarah's marriage also left her bereft, evidenced when Hunt admitted that Sarah's marriage was a "great loss" for her and created a "widowed feeling" that "never wholly left" her (165, 166). Hunt reprised these views at the end of her narrative when she declared that Sarah's "marriage ... left me alone.... The departure of my mother to the spirit land ... left me *alone* in our home [and] ... a lonely orphanage was added to the solitary duties ... of my professional life" (416). As these comments reveal, themes of loneliness and abandonment haunt *Glances and Glimpses*. However unintentional on Hunt's part, *Glances and Glimpses* became her "heart history," a text where she confessed her struggles and the anguish she periodically experienced.

But if she revealed certain parts of her personal life, Hunt was circumspect about others. She ultimately played what one scholar has described as a "peekaboo" game with her readers, revealing just enough about her life to snag her audience's interest but not anything that would damage her reputation or violate her privacy.[39] Like any wise autobiographer, Hunt walked a fine line between concealment and confession. At the end of her narrative Hunt stressed how she hid important aspects of herself. In doing this, she highlighted how deceptive the genre of autobiography is, how it is ultimately a public performance that obscures as much as it reveals about its subject/narrator. In a boasting tone Hunt told her readers: "I have only shown you the *outside* of [my] life, and . . . you will see nothing, *know* nothing of my *interior* self. The *I* is still concealed behind this *paper tapestry*—still inshrined [sic] within a holy of holies, into which human eye has *never* looked–where human foot has never trod. Even now I stand in *conscious hiddenness*. True, you see *some* of the things I have done—*some* of the trials, sorrows, and joys of a happy life. But these are no more ME than the physique that my spirit wears" (416). Hunt's view of the narrative she constructed as nothing more than a "paper tapestry" that concealed her "interior self" suggests that she felt a certain contempt for the text she created and its readers. She implied that she was playing with her audience. Her book offered a kind of psychological striptease where readers could get merely "glances" and "glimpses" of her life but not view the inner core of Hunt's identity.

But Hunt's comments might have been a stratagem to challenge her readers. She was deliberately provocative when she bragged about standing before the public in "conscious hiddenness." Her words encouraged readers to peruse her narrative as a kind of puzzle, one that required them to decipher what lay hidden behind its author's public personas and protestations. Ultimately, *Glances and Glimpses* did reveal something fundamental about Hunt's identity for readers who probed beneath the surface of the text. Hunt lived a woman-centered life, one where her closest friends, associates, and patients were other women.

Her autobiography also hinted that she was romantically attracted to other women. Her recollection as a young girl of having "many love attachments" with some of her schoolmates suggested this (21). So too did her depiction of her friendship with Fredrika Bremer, a woman for whom she felt intense feelings that "electrify the soul" (235–37). As discussed earlier, Hunt's correspondence with Sarah Grimké hinted at a romantic attraction between these two women, but her autobiography skirted this issue, merely noting a deep friendship between them. Hunt evaded any open discussion of romantic feelings in her text, especially if they were for other women; such an admission would have made her a pariah in the homophobic society in which she lived. That Hunt might have harbored such feelings, however, made her remark that she stood in "conscious hiddenness" before her readers all the more poignant.

Glances and Glimpses revealed not only a complicated narrator but also a conflicted one. Hunt repeatedly undercut her own arguments and rhetorical strategies, which was evident when she contradicted her portrayal of herself as a demure woman by highlighting her considerable abilities, initiative, and determination. Even as she ostensibly invoked prescribed views of femininity and domesticity, she showed how she defied these strictures to succeed in a male-dominated profession and challenge women's exclusion from power.

But perhaps the autobiography is most conflicted when Hunt quickly shifts gears after defiantly asserting that her "interior self" remained hidden. Such remarks highlighted the importance Hunt placed on protecting not only her privacy but also her individuality, her sense of self, from her readers' prying eyes and censure. As soon as she made these comments, however, Hunt then appeared ready to erase any notion of self at all. She urged her readers to regard her life and autobiography as no more than a conduit for promulgating the welfare of humanity. Just as a statue is of "*no account*, save as it unfolds and impresses" upon viewers the "laws of grace and proportion," she emphasized, "*so am I nothing*." Her only desire, she continued, was that people read her book to recognize the "harmonious laws of our humanity" and address women's "*unsatisfied* aspirations after knowledge, independence, and enlarged usefulness"(416–17).

Once again Hunt presented herself as a passive figure lacking agency or individuality. She highlighted this point by comparing herself to a statue whose purpose was to lead the viewer to focus on important issues beyond itself. At times Harriot Hunt was willing to efface herself if that meant gaining her audience's support for her reform agenda, especially the cause of woman's rights. But, paradoxically, she also insisted on readers recognizing her as the ambitious, successful, and determined woman she was. Even as she urged readers to look beyond her particular self and focus on the cause of human rights, Hunt also asserted her importance as an individual worthy of attention and respect.

Glances and Glimpses utilized a grab bag of rhetorical strategies to attract readers and gain support for its author's views. But Hunt took a bold risk when she did something that few women autobiographers did in the nineteenth century—she used her book to articulate her anger against patriarchal power. Although antebellum feminist leaders used various kinds of texts, including essays, lectures, novels, and speeches, to protest male domination, Hunt's life narrative was the only antebellum American autobiography authored by a woman to offer a detailed exposé of patriarchal power in its myriad forms. This author/activist weaponized the genre of autobiography to show how this power oppressed women. What made Hunt's analysis so compelling was that she grounded her denunciation of patriarchy in her own life experiences and those of the women she doctored and befriended. More than a century before feminists proclaimed that "the personal is political," Hunt vividly described how the injustices she, friends, and patients endured reflected women's oppression in a misogynistic society.

When she described the "heart histories" of individual women, Hunt neither sensationalized their sufferings nor presented them in a maudlin fashion. As Cynthia Davis has cogently noted, Hunt's carefully selected excerpts of female suffering enabled her to simultaneously convey the anguish many women experienced and establish a critical distance from their plight.[40] Hunt had to do both if she was to accomplish two crucial goals. She wanted to gain the reader's sympathy for individual women who were abused. But Hunt's case studies of female suffering were also designed to provoke anger at what women in general endured because of patriarchal oppression. Ultimately, therefore, Hunt's accounts of female "heart histories," including her own, were a way to mobilize support for a more gender-equal society. As she stated early on in her text, "heart histories" not only "appeal powerfully to our sympathies" but "rouse our indignation at the degradation and uselessness of our sex" (50). Detailed analysis of *Glances and Glimpses* and its use of women's "heart histories" illustrate Hunt's larger political agenda.

Throughout her narrative Hunt surveyed how men wielded power to illustrate a crucial point: male domination of key institutions not only oppressed women but also betrayed America's democratic principles and ensured its moral decline. As discussed earlier, Hunt was contemptuous of most politicians, including northern ones who truckled under to the "Slave Power." But for Hunt such actions were symptomatic of a much larger betrayal. In a particularly heartfelt lamentation she asked: "Where is freedom in 1855? Where is principle? Where is public virtue [?] . . . What have we done with the antique jewels, bought at great price by our fathers, for the brow of a people? They are gone. We have sold them for luxury, wealth, and power" (42).

Hunt was not alone in her nostalgia for an earlier, supposedly more virtuous and noble America. Nor was she unusual in thinking that the United States was in moral decline and had abandoned the heroic sacrifices of the revolutionary generation. Proclaiming these sentiments became a popular staple of countless literary works, sermons, and lectures.[41] Like other nineteenth-century female activists, Hunt looked to women, with their allegedly pious, nurturing, and selfless natures, to regenerate the nation: "Will it not be through woman, as the moral elevator of the race, that deliverance will again come?" (317).

But *Glances and Glimpses* did not merely issue platitudes about female moral responsibility. It excoriated women's growing marginalization from politics. While recollecting her mother's avid interest in politics, Hunt pointedly declared that in the early Republic women "were not stigmatized for having an interest in the National housekeeping, as well as the domestic!" (4). But as she surveyed mid-nineteenth-century America, she found that women were increasingly forbidden any role in politics. Their voices were silenced, and when they tried to express a political opinion, men peremptorily told them to stay in their private world of domesticity. "The chain has been tightened," Hunt groused. Her anger, frustration, and sense of betrayal at women's exclusion from politics was particularly evident when she wistfully recalled a more gender-inclusive politics in earlier decades: "Parlors in my childhood were used for caucuses, and women were not excluded. Men did not then leave their families, evening after evening, for political headquarters; but Home was made the place for high-toned conversation on the movements of the day, and the feminine element was felt in the discussion. . . . Now, men hire rooms to discuss political questions in, and we are told to keep our 'sphere'! We are not even supposed to have an *interest* in the very laws under which we live—which control our destinies, and shape our lives—by which we are tried, judged, and condemned, and which we are taxed to support!" (44–45).

Anger at women's exclusion from political power led Hunt to risk public opprobrium by criticizing the founding fathers and the American Revolution. "Our forefathers," she asserted, were "selfish" because the "*white* man's freedom was all that they claimed" (265). Hunt's bitterness at the failed promise of the American Revolution was also apparent when she reproachfully stated that "Faneuil Hall was not *our* Cradle of Liberty. We had no hand in the rocking. If we *had* had, perhaps the child would have turned out better. But *men* rocked *that* cradle!" (44).

Despite these comments, Hunt recalled "feeling a glow of pride" when in the fall of 1840 the women of Boston held a "great fair at Faneuil Hall" to gain funds to complete the building of the "Bunker Hill Monument," an edifice she lauded as an "enduring memorial of liberty and patriotism." But Hunt complained that it was "half a monument" because it recognized only the sacrifices and freedoms of men. Americans at this point, she added, had merely "half a freedom." Women were needed to complete "the temple of freedom," to make American "freedom entire and beautiful." But for this to occur, proclaimed Hunt, her countrymen needed to broaden their conceptions of liberty and citizenship: "Civil liberty now is a monopoly. It belongs to one sex, though it was secured by the blood and prayer and toil of generations of both sexes. Now its blessings are sexual! It is for John and Peter, not Mary and Deborah. But it will not be always so" (163).

Hunt's conviction that the American Revolution was incomplete because it liberated only men while bypassing women underscored her anger against male rule. This anger also stoked her criticism of mainstream churches. Like Sarah Grimké, Hunt accused ministers of hijacking the Christian message so as to gain power over others, especially women. She developed this charge by pointedly noting women's pivotal role in establishing the early church. It was they, she stressed, who "were last at the cross, and first at the resurrection, proclaiming the sad and the joyful in the Christian ministry." Yet Hunt claimed that ministers of all the leading "denominations" had wrongly shunted women aside and usurped their rightful roles in the church. Men, she fumed, "had taken upon themselves to become *mothers*, and provide for the spiritual household." The all-male clerical establishment now "preached, regulated, counselled, and decided upon every church measure—whilst the true representative of the church—the bride, or female element, was an automaton responding yes, amen." Hunt excoriated this development as a "sad perversion" of genuine Christianity (201–2).

But Hunt did not merely rail against the clergy's arrogation of power. Her autobiography espoused an androgynous view of God and quoted biblical passages to support her argument. She also gendered the church as feminine. "The church, our mother," she boldly declared, "recognizes 'neither male nor female'—she prepares not one kind of food for my brother and another for my sister, 'for they are all *one* in Christ Jesus.'" It was therefore "unholy" and "unrighteous" to oppose women's ordination as ministers. Hunt also proclaimed that the church could never fulfill her Christian mission as long as "narrow minds" constructed "boundary lines" of male and female spheres and excluded women from the ministry (202). Such an unnatural "sexuality" in the church thwarted her "high and holy mission." Only "a *union* of the two elements, male and female, in spiritual ministrations," she proclaimed, could achieve a genuine Christianity (204).

Glances and Glimpses was a jeremiad against male doctors as well as ministers and politicians. The text expanded on the litany of grievances against the American medical establishment that Hunt first made in her speeches and lectures. She denounced male physicians' use of harsh or "quack" medicines, their physical examinations that often shamed and humiliated women, their unwillingness to listen to their female patients, their failure to practice preventive medicine, and their opposition to female colleagues.⁴² Of course, Hunt's autobiography recounted her failed efforts to study at Harvard's medical school and also lambasted the faculty and students who opposed her (217–19; 265–71).

Male domination of the nation's economy also galled Hunt. She lashed out at the men who ran Wall Street and the leading mercantile houses, railroads, and banks. They were "performers," she sneered, who dealt in "gold and silver, in dollar and cents," and enacted a tawdry and selfish play lacking in any morality or decency (331–32). Hunt expanded on this theme by surveying the poverty in antebellum America. Bitterly, she described how impoverished children scrambled into abandoned buildings "eager to snatch some of the rubbish" to provide badly needed fuel to warm their families on cold winter nights. "Visit the wharves," Hunt admonished her readers, and see "the fruit children, organ players, strolling vagrant girls," desperate to earn money (366).

Glances and Glimpses was especially hard hitting when Hunt discussed how economic and gender discrimination worked hand in hand to oppress countless women. She used her own life story to convey how difficult it was for women to earn decent wages in antebellum America. Recalling her struggles to find work to help her impoverished family, Hunt wondered why "healthful, remunerative employment" was not available to women as well as to men (49). Although she had fond memories of running her school, Hunt recognized what a grueling, demeaning, and low-paying job teaching was for women. Her narrative reproached her society for not treating female schoolteachers better. The "miserable remuneration," she stressed, not only "sadly crippl[ed]" a teacher's "usefulness" but also sapped her "self-respect" (102). It also undermined her status in society. A female educator suffered the "stigma" of being derided as "only a teacher" and therefore unworthy of respect. Hunt noted that many young female teachers, out of desperation and poverty, often married men they neither liked nor respected. Who could blame such women for "marrying an imbecile," asked Hunt, when a female teacher was "underrated" and "underpaid" and "her self-respect" was gone and she became an "underling—pinched, degraded, contemned ... weary, and miserable" (103–4).

Hunt's autobiography also publicized the desperate circumstances of women who worked in the needle trades. She noted the "heart histories" of her patients, the dressmakers and seamstresses who complained about the grueling labor, little money, and poor health they endured, to show the difficult lives of working-class women (133–34). Although she understood how tough life could get for laboring men, Hunt recognized that for women the struggle to survive on their own was especially grueling. She decried the fact that women faced gender discrimination in the marketplace, consistently earning less than men for the same or comparable work. Why, Hunt wondered, was it possible for a man who practiced "industry and frugality" to get a "home and a competence as his reward," whereas such remained an elusive dream for most working women? "What does the laboring woman get for *her* years of toil, industry, and frugality," she bitterly asked, but poverty, illness, and the contempt of others (133).

Women's economic disempowerment, their subordination in churches, their exclusion from politics and medicine—Hunt's autobiography discussed these injustices to expose how patriarchal power oppressed women. "My sex," she fumed, "have been duped, overreached, ridiculed, and slandered." Hunt said this in the context of denouncing male itinerant lecturers on physiology whose addresses were a "decoy" to sell quack remedies to naïve women (283). But she could just as easily have been excoriating other groups of men who duped and betrayed women. There were all sorts of men, she repeatedly exclaimed, who abused their power to hurt women in need of their help and protection.

Glances and Glimpses particularly dramatized this issue when it addressed how men sexually exploited women. Hunt's angry diatribes against slaveholders who impregnated and then abandoned their female slaves and of adulterous husbands who caused her women patients so much anguish illustrated this point. Such comments were part of a larger feminist discourse against predatory male sexuality. By the mid-1850s, the image of the lustful slaveholder who raped his female slaves and then sold them was a trope in abolitionist literature. When feminists at woman's rights conventions tackled the issue of prostitution, they did so not only to gain sympathy for "fallen women" but also to publicize and condemn male sexual privilege. Female moral reformers also did this when they exposed men who visited brothels and denounced those who seduced and then deserted their female lovers.[43]

Glances and Glimpses featured several poignant accounts of seduction. Hunt recalled how one of her young students, a "beautiful, gifted child, from Maine," allegedly "as ignorant at sixteen, as my girls of six or eight years," had her "mind and soul" destroyed when seduced and then abandoned by a youth (107, 108). Another "wretched victim of *seduction*" was "in deepest agony," filled with "shame," when her lover not only seduced her but also defrauded her of her hard-earned money, funds that her father needed "to save his little homestead." But as Hunt bitterly stated, the young woman had "*no* redress" and suffered "shame" and "ruin" while her lover escaped punishment (385).

But the case of seduction that most angered Harriot was that of a young girl who lived in the Hunt home after her family had abandoned her. She was seduced and impregnated by a clerk who refused to marry her. With grim satisfaction Hunt noted that she confronted this "wretch," got him expelled from his lodgings, and exposed his misbehavior to the young woman he was courting. Although the seduced girl was able to rebuild her life after her out-of-wedlock baby died, this story haunted Hunt. She used it to dramatize how men's lechery marred women's lives (145–48).

For as upset as Hunt was at the seducer of her ward she reserved her greatest anger not at particular men but rather at the entrenched practices and institutions that ensured women's continued subordination. *Glances and Glimpses* is at its most scathing when it censured the institution most Americans regarded as sacred and at the foundation of any civilized society—marriage. Hunt's comments occurred in the context of a growing feminist criticism of patriarchal power within matrimony. This discourse merits discussion because it shaped Hunt's autobiography and gave her the courage to express her anger at the subjugation of wives.

During the antebellum era, a minority of woman's rights advocates portrayed patriarchal marriage as an unjust and humiliating institution. Sarah Grimké pioneered in this criticism when she declared in her *Letters on the Equality of the Sexes* that woman "generally loses her individuality, her independent character, her moral being" when she married. Increasingly, she became no more than a "cipher," completely "absorbed into him [her husband]." After discussing how the law of coverture legalized this process by denying wives any kind of independent legal or political existence, Grimké concluded that a woman who married was no better than a slave.[44]

Other antebellum feminists also targeted the institution of marriage as the major source of female oppression. Criticism of men's marital tyranny over their wives became a staple of the speeches given at the annual woman's rights conventions in which Hunt regularly participated. This criticism was particularly pronounced at the 1851 convention, where Hunt delivered a major speech on the need for women doctors. She likely heard leading feminists deliver denunciations of marriage. Lucy Stone, for example, declared that wives were often "a ceaseless drudge or a blank" in their own homes and "a starved and dependent outcast before the law." Ernestine Rose bemoaned the fact that when women married, they lost their "entire identity" and were taught that "blind submission" to their husbands was a "virtue."[45]

Condemnation of conventional marriage and domesticity also appeared in various feminist periodicals that emerged during the early to mid-1850s. Articles published in journals such as the *Lily* and the *Una* portrayed marriage as "the slavery of woman" and wives as "household chattels." Authors derided as "twaddle" the prescribed view that wives had a duty to submit to their husbands and asserted that the image of the home as a "sanctuary" all too often masked the rule of men who were "cruel and suspicious tyrant[s]."[46]

Elizabeth Oakes Smith, a popular lecturer and reformer, expressed similar views when she published a series of articles in the *New York Tribune* that appeared in book form in 1851 as *Woman and Her Needs*. Wives, she bitterly opined, were "a sort of puppet, to be placed, like Tom Thumb, upon a giant's palm," while men regarded them with a "tolerating, half-amused indulgence" (35).[47] She also rebuked her society for allowing men to exercise "a savage lordliness" where they "usurp all the privileges of freedom" and then "dole out bits of freedom" to women as they would "atoms of food to half-starved wretches" (19, 36). Smith also denounced the practice of young women marrying much older, affluent men, a situation that happened to her when she was only sixteen. Such "baby wives," she fumed, were "defrauded" of the opportunity to "grow and blossom" into full womanhood (42). Smith ultimately portrayed marriage as a kind of living death or an entombment for women. Once a woman married, she bristled, she had to "merge her being, be absorbed and annihilated in marriage—be an extinct world, a gone-out soul" (43).

Perhaps the most radical denunciation of marriage in antebellum America came from Mary Gove Nichols, the initially popular lecturer on women's health and prominent water-cure advocate. When she began espousing free-love doctrines in the 1840s, Nichols became "radioactive" for woman's rights advocates, committed to protecting their movement from any hint of sexual impropriety.[48] Harriot Hunt was one of Nichols's critics. In *Glances and Glimpses* she recalled that during her regular visits to Lynn, Massachusetts, in 1838, she boarded several days a month with the then Mary Gove. Although Hunt praised Gove's lectures on health reform and physiology, she condemned her free-love doctrines: "I shudder at their character, and would remove myself from *every influence* tending to favor them. My sympathies are with their deluded followers, many of whom know misery as the result of their conversion" (139–40).

In 1854, Mary Gove Nichols copublished with her second husband, Thomas Low Nichols, an antimarriage diatribe. The middle third of *Marriage*, written by Mary, offered numerous case studies of wives who suffered at the hands of abusive, adulterous, and neglectful husbands. The Nicholses used the testimony of unhappy wives to condemn matrimony as an inherently oppressive institution and to proselytize their free-love doctrines.[49]

The following year Mary Gove Nichols published *Mary Lyndon*, a "thinly fictionalized autobiography."[50] In many respects *Mary Lyndon* was also a captivity narrative. It detailed how miserable Nichols was in her first marriage to a dour, domineering Quaker. Lyndon/Nichols was trapped in a marriage that was destroying her spirit, intellect, and freedom. Nichols used her book to justify her divorce and happy remarriage to her second husband as well as to advocate for free-love principles.

But even someone as radical as Mary Gove Nichols felt that she could reveal the pain of her first marriage only by using the novelistic form, by creating fictional personas for herself and the primary people who shaped her life. Although quickly identified as the author of *Mary Lyndon*, Nichols did not list her name on the title page when her text was first published, feeling the need to use the cover of fiction to reveal her marital troubles.[51] Perhaps this strategy enabled her to distance herself emotionally from the anguish and humiliation she endured while married to her first husband. But Nichols's appropriation of fictional techniques to reveal her life story was also a way to make more palatable her bold demands for liberating women from despotic husbands at a time when matrimony was widely viewed as sacrosanct.

To criticize the institution of marriage was a radical, subversive act in mid-1850s America. But this is what Harriot Hunt did in *Glances and Glimpses* when she discussed how conventional marriage and domesticity subjugated women. She did so in a forthright manner, unafraid to express anger at what wives suffered. She must have realized that her actions risked alienating the public and hurting her medical practice, but Hunt was nothing if not a risk taker.

When she explored how the home could become a kind of tomb or prison for women, Hunt drew on the testimony offered by her numerous female patients. She had both the privilege and the burden to listen to these women as they confessed to her their unhappiness as wives. In *Glances and Glimpses* Hunt bore witness to what these women suffered; she testified on their behalf when most were too timid, too intimidated, or too resigned to give testimony on their own. She declared that "many a woman in gentle love and humble cheerfulness, cover[s] up the cancerous sores and corruption of *private* life." But Hunt asserted that women needed to reveal what lay hidden behind a healthy or beautiful exterior. It was necessary, she firmly declared, to confront unpleasant facts about the home just as one must recognize that the "beautiful pond lily floats on stagnant waters, concealing the filthy scum which covers them" (200).

Like all good writers, Hunt recognized that an anecdote about a particular person often drove home a point much more than abstract analyses of institutions. By recounting the confessions of wealthy wives who felt bored, lonely, and dissatisfied, Hunt highlighted how a web of money and fashion often entrapped women. The "fashionable class" of women, she asserted, "fritter away their time in elegant stores, in millinery shops, and at mantuamakers [sic]" (412). According to Hunt, a woman who lived this kind of life was often "melancholy" and "loathe[d] herself." The fashion she craved ironically became her downfall: "her soul is imprisoned in whalebone as well as her body" (278).

Glances and Glimpses also narrated the "heart histories" of middle-income homemakers to illustrate how marriage and domesticity became a trap for women, one that made them ill and prematurely old. As Hunt grimly asserted: "I have seen parched, shriveled, half-baked women . . . their skins crying aloud for moisture, and certainly a very peculiar drought rests upon such. Well, this drought was not entirely physical; it was felt in the *soul*" (408). Hunt fumed with anger at the many homemakers she treated whose lives had been destroyed by the rigors of household drudgery and too many children. The "dignity" of their "womanhood" had "sunk" in the "drudgery" of the kitchen and nursery (408). In an effort to take care of her husband and children, a woman, lamented Hunt, often became "a broken down invalid, with overworked, overanxious, crippled energies, and withered mind inscribed upon her wrinkled, somber face" (409).

She counterposed the homemaker's decline with the husband's growth. Because the man was working outside the home, engaged in business and other public activities, he had been "developing *mentally*." Regularly in contact with "*minds* full of energy, thought, and emulation . . . *he* is wide awake, he attends lectures, he goes to the club, to the political meeting" (409). Predictably, his wife soon bored him. Her "*unfed mind* and overworked body" made her a "cipher in the world of intelligence—an invalid—and sometimes a burden, not a blessing to her family—loved with the love of pity, rather than that of reverence, served from duty rather than deep filial affection" (410). In short, the self-sacrificing wife and mother became a pitiful, stunted figure while her husband remained mentally alert and physically rigorous.

Hunt stressed that such a decline was the result of the prescribed views of femininity that society imposed on women and that they internalized with tragic consequences for themselves and their families: "Is she [the homemaker] to blame? No, she has only lived out *her* ideal—*this era's* ideal of woman's sphere—she has offered herself up a willing sacrifice upon the altar of domestic duty." Hunt stressed that homemakers were routinely sacrificed because of society's misguided belief that women had to care selflessly for their families and ignore their own development. Such women were "mentally and bodily immolated," she exclaimed, and then wondered why people condemned the "Hindoo widow who burn[ed] herself upon the funeral pyre" but ignored the "Christian wife who starve[d] her *mind* to death, and move[d] about her house a living corpse" (409).

The grim lives that countless women endured as wives made it imperative that girls be educated so as to avoid marrying other than for love. Hunt made clear what the end purpose of education was for women—not only to hone their intellectual abilities but also to rely on themselves. Young women who were educated, she stressed, learned "self-reliance" and could be "trained to some healthful, remunerative employment" (49). But education, she believed, protected and empowered women in other ways. Educated women would not be so easily duped or exploited by predatory men. Women knowledgeable about their own bodies would be less likely to be hoodwinked by male doctors who sold them quack remedies and subjected them to harsh, invasive treatments. Widows who educated themselves about their husbands' financial affairs and rejected the canard that "to meddle with business . . . was the sphere of *man*" would not be swindled of their life savings and property (372). Girls who were not naïve and ignorant would be less likely to be seduced.

Glances and Glimpses was bitter about society's failure to adequately educate its female children. Like other antebellum feminist critics, Hunt censured parents who neglected their daughters' education and focused only on their marriage prospects: "Girls are educated—for what? They are sedulously trained—for what? For nothing but marriage! They are early taught to consider what are their chances and attractions for the market!" (48). Hunt emphasized that she deliberately used the word "market" because she felt that young girls were groomed for a kind of prostitution when they were taught that their paramount goal was to snag an affluent husband who would take care of them. In a comparison that she must have known would upset many of her readers, Hunt claimed that young females in the United States were no better than those in "a Turkish harem." American women, like their counterparts in an Eastern harem, were allegedly trained to be "dependent," "weak," "silly" women, so "degraded" that they viewed as "honorable" their "future sale for wealth [and] social position" (49). Hunt's anger was palpable as she described how "young, bright, promising school-girls" were "dwarfed into young ladies" in their obsessive quest for a suitable husband. They became "silly, coquettish, overdressed [and] fashionable" in a desperate effort to "be sold to the highest bidder!" (50).

Hunt also excoriated parents for ignoring the individuality of their children by trying to fit them into uniform patterns of behavior, ones where prescribed gender divisions were rigidly enforced. She declared: "Parents, in the development of your children, it is for you to beautify *all* uses, not to sexualize them; giving to a feminine boy, manhood; and to a masculine girl, womanhood" (101–2). Not surprisingly, Hunt advocated a more gender-neutral approach to childrearing. Boys, she said, should learn "every pleasant kind of handiwork that girls are [taught]." Girls should engage in activities traditionally reserved for boys. They should be able "to run, and walk, and play with hoop, and ball, and kite out of doors" (101). Through such advice Hunt sought to free not only children but also adults from the "treadmill routine" of regimentation that stifled their individuality and thwarted their full development as human beings (99).

Hunt's words and ideas resonated with those of the prominent Transcendentalist and feminist thinker Margaret Fuller. Like Fuller, Hunt recognized how fluid the notion of gender was and condemned society's efforts to pigeonhole the sexes into separate spheres and rigid roles. Her recognition that there were "feminine boys" and "masculine girls" echoed Fuller's assertion that "there is no wholly masculine man, no purely feminine woman" but that "male and female . . . are perpetually passing into one another."[52] Hunt's declaration that "*both* the male and female element" was "essential" to achieve "the wholeness," "the completeness," of Christianity (206) echoed Fuller's beliefs that "a ravishing harmony" of male and female spheres would create a transcendent unity and enable "divine energy" to "pervade nature."[53]

Hunt used *Glances and Glimpses* to articulate her ideas about how to create a more humane and just world, one where human beings were not forced into constricted gender roles and where women were treated as men's equals. This text also conveyed its author's tremendous sadness at living in a world permeated by patriarchal oppression. Even when her autobiography became a diatribe against male misogyny, Hunt poignantly revealed the pain she suffered when men denigrated, ostracized, and vilified her, which was evident when she declared that most Boston physicians regarded her as a "traitor, outlaw, [and] felon" (297). It was also apparent when she detailed her failed efforts to attend lectures at Harvard. "Shall I ever forgive the Harvard Medical College," she lamented, "for depriving me of a thorough knowledge of that science [of anatomy]" (122).

Glances and Glimpses also conveyed Hunt's fervent desire for a home. Throughout her narrative she repeatedly, indeed almost obsessively, discussed how she sought to preserve her family home, especially when her father's death, poverty, and Sarah's illness hindered her efforts. Hunt's pain was obvious when she recounted her family having to leave their home and rent it out. Her efforts to regain the house in the North End and her establishment of a home for herself and her mother and sister in another part of Boston feature prominently in Hunt's life story. For Hunt, owning her own home validated her identity as an independent and successful professional woman as well as a dutiful daughter and sister. It also nurtured her emotionally, fulfilling what Susan B. Anthony, another unmarried feminist, called the "home instinct" or the deeply felt need for a single woman to live in her own household, beholden to no one.[54]

The idea of home had a metaphoric as well as literal meaning for Hunt. She looked forward to the day when women, including herself, would finally be welcomed as equal family members in the home known as the United States of America. Ultimately, her autobiography was not merely a rant against the oppression she and her sex faced but also a heartfelt call to make her country more welcoming to all citizens, to make those traditionally marginalized, especially women, feel as if they were now part of the American family.

Glances and Glimpses was a complicated text. It told the story of an individual's upward mobility and success despite difficult struggles. But it was also a denunciation of patriarchy, highlighting the discrimination and abuse countless women suffered, including its author. Not surprisingly, Hunt's narrative garnered mostly negative reviews. The *Boston Daily Atlas*, for example, condemned Hunt's "extreme views" regarding the "social and political wrongs of womankind" and bemoaned that "so much . . . rhetorical power [and] . . . valuable efforts" were "wasted upon a meaningless and empty abstraction."[55] Another paper declared that the author of *Glances and Glimpses* was merely supporting "the hobbies of the day" when she promulgated "peculiar notions" regarding "the sphere and rights of woman."[56]

Predictably, publications noted for their commitment to prescribed gender roles or political and religious conservatism were notably hostile to Hunt's autobiography.[57] Their condemnation of Hunt's religious unorthodoxy as well as commitment to woman's rights showed that reviewers recognized how the two were inextricably linked—how adherence to liberal sects promoted feminist activism. The *Happy Home and Parlor Magazine*, for example, denounced the alleged "egotism" of *Glances and Glimpses* with its "needless commendation of Universalism" and "Swedenborgianism" as well as its "extreme woman's-rights-doctrine."[58] Although grudgingly admitting that *Glances and Glimpses* provided some "valuable" medical advice, the *New Englander* declared that Hunt's religious views did "not strike us very favorably." As for Hunt's advocacy of woman's rights, this periodical conceded that Hunt had "'rights' growing out of her intellectual and professional character." But the journal quickly added that hers was an unusual case because these rights "cannot be claimed by all her sex."[59] The *Country Gentleman* was even more critical of Hunt's text, claiming that it espoused religious views characteristic of "radical progressionists." Hunt's "eclectic" mixture of Universalist and Swedenborgian doctrines, coupled with her "reformatory schemes," asserted this journal, undermined the merits of *Glances and Glimpses*. This text was "ultra in theory and tendency" and "vain" in its "independence of all common-place ideas" and confidence in "its general superiority."[60]

When reviewers condemned *Glances and Glimpses* as "vain" and "egotistical," when they disparaged its woman's rights doctrines as an "ultra," "extreme" cause or as a mere hobby, they revealed a common strategy—use gendered language to discredit the text and demean its author. One Washington, D.C., newspaper merely noted the book's publication and then snidely remarked that at least Hunt did not wear "Bloomers."[61] A Massachusetts paper linked Hunt to "Lucy Stone, Antoinette Brown, Lucretia Mott, and other strong-mindeds" who "brazenly" advocated for the "'Woman's Rights movement.'"[62] Meanwhile the *New Englander* disparaged Hunt as "too *mannish*."[63]

Even publications that ostensibly praised Hunt often peppered their comments with condescending remarks about her character or personal appearance. The *New Hampshire Patriot and State Gazette*, for example, praised Hunt as "the little doctor" who wrote in "so pleasant a style as to entertain and charm the reader."[64] The *New York Daily Times* commented on Hunt's age and looks, admiring her for admitting to being "a fair half century" old, even though she looked younger by "a good half dozen years."[65] Another paper demeaned Hunt by portraying her as a Pollyanna. It described "Miss Hunt" as "one of those genial, hopeful, mirth-inspiring souls that almost compel you to look through their own bright spectacles."[66]

Reviewers occasionally chided Hunt for marring an otherwise excellent autobiography by raising controversial issues such as woman's rights. The *Christian Examiner and Religious Miscellany*, for example, claimed that the first three quarters of *Glances and Glimpses* offered "pleasant" descriptions of Hunt's "happy family life" in Boston's North End and praised her "healing mission" to help ailing women. But the reviewer groused that Hunt spoiled her book when she embraced "the questionable views of the Woman's Rights party." This author hoped that Hunt's "own clear, good sense, and her excellent judgment and practical wisdom, will sooner or later draw her off from the fellowship of those females who would amount to a sore nuisance if there were not, happily, so few of them."[67]

In a similar vein, the *New York Daily Times* lauded *Glances and Glimpses* for its recollections of Hunt's early life and struggles to establish her career. Such accounts were "highly interesting" and "the best part of the book." But Hunt's advocacy for woman's rights alienated the reviewer. Although conceding that Hunt made a "plain, forcible argument" for enfranchising women, the writer complained that she was a "strong-minded woman" whose narrative lost momentum when it focused on gender issues: "The latter half of her story . . . is nearly swamped by . . . assertions respecting the rights and wrongs of women [and] is rather heavy reading."[68]

Such comments underscore a crucial fact: many reviewers did not understand how committed Hunt was to promoting gender equality and to restructuring her society. The most positive reviews of *Glances and Glimpses* in the mainstream press were those which claimed that Hunt's autobiography promulgated orthodox Christian values and the joys and sacredness of domesticity. Such reviews either minimized if they did not omit altogether Hunt's discussion of the need for a thorough reformation of gender relations. The author of the first review of *Glances and Glimpses* for the *Boston Evening Transcript*, identified as "A Grandmother," expressed her gratitude to the "gifted authoress" for writing a book that conveyed the "beautifully finished picture of *home* in all its relations" and offered parents a "faithful delineation of family discipline."[69] A later reviewer declared that nothing could be "more heart-cheering" than "Dr. Hunt's description of her early life," with its detailed descriptions of how her parents, "so full of love and care," nurtured and guided their children.[70] Both reviewers omitted any mention of Hunt's advocacy of woman's rights and other unorthodox views. So too did the *New Hampshire Patriot and State Gazette*. It described *Glances and Glimpses* as a "well written and interesting narrative," designed "to entertain and charm the reader." The paper stressed that "Miss Hunt" offered "a great deal of sound advice in respect to the physical and mental training of children" and also praised "her strong common sense and her brave, cheerful Christian spirit."[71]

Other reviewers buried critical references to Hunt's feminist beliefs toward the end of their comments while highlighting her book's alleged paeans to domesticity. The *California Farmer and Journal of Useful Sciences*, for example, asserted that *Glances and Glimpses* was valuable because Hunt taught how a good home instilled "sweet lessons" that enabled adults to "overthrow all obstacles" they encountered or "endure with more patience and resignation the world's sneer." It particularly recommended Hunt's narrative to "*mothers*" and "young persons" just beginning to travel "the troubled sea of life." Although the reviewer acknowledged that "Dr. Hunt [was] a strong advocate for *Woman's Rights*" and wanted women to become "lawyers, doctors, and ministers," he wondered if she would "ever be able to have it her way." Rather than elaborate on this comment, the writer quickly shifted gears by arguing that there was no "space to go into the full merits of [Hunt's] work at this time." He ended his commentary by recommending *Glances and Glimpses* for its "deep moral tone."[72]

Probably the most important analysis of *Glances and Glimpses* occurred in the *North American Review*, the premier journal for the nation's educated citizenry. Once again the unnamed reviewer ignored or missed the radical message Hunt articulated in her book. Rather, he praised the "domestic sketches" she offered of her childhood in the North End when this area still had "an air of comfort" and "quaint respectability." He also admired Hunt's portrait of her parents. Her recollections of their industry, "sound sense," and "sturdy integrity" created a "charming picture of independence, modest refinement, . . . and mutual helpfulness." This writer also lauded Hunt's "good service in her calling" and added that there was "a portion of the physician's functions" which could be "delegated to women properly trained for the office." But the reviewer also qualified this support by noting his "strong preference" for "the regular school of medicine." He admired Hunt's "honesty and zeal, her kindly temper and gentle spirit"; he described her narrative as "both pleasant and suggestive."[73] But in the end the reviewer could not see how angry and subversive Hunt was in her autobiography. Even the foremost periodical in antebellum America missed what Hunt's autobiography was about: a scathing indictment of her society and a call to transform its most basic institutions, including that of marriage.

Ironically, the few journals that supported Hunt's beliefs, the *Liberator* and the *Universalist Quarterly and General Review*, often minimized the radical content of her book by portraying it in ways that reinforced prescribed views of domesticity and gender. An author identified only as "H. B." began a review in the *Liberator* by praising Hunt's book as "a genuine *live* book." But then the writer stressed that what was most important about *Glances and Glimpses* was that Hunt praised the home as the incubator of a person's future moral character. "H. B." also excoriated "the soulless, aimless lives of two-thirds of American women, whose God is fashion; whose idol is the insipid novel; who are ever ready to ridicule and slander every true woman" such as Hunt. There was no mention, however, of how *Glances and Glimpses* examined the role patriarchy played in making women frivolous and ignorant.[74]

The *Universalist Quarterly* also echoed the gendered stereotypes that Hunt sought to discredit in her autobiography. The reviewer portrayed her as an author characterized by emotion, enthusiasm, and piety, but not analytic reasoning. In other words, Hunt was depicted as the stereotypical female writer, which was evident when the reviewer lauded *Glances and Glimpses* for its "gushes of heart-feeling . . . and sincerity of religious expression" and for offering "all the external stimulant of an exciting novel." Claiming that the book "boils and foams with vitality," the writer opined that "Miss Hunt writes not from her mind, but from her feelings and soul." The review ended by stressing that Hunt's text warranted a wide audience since it "preach[ed] the unspeakable worth and sacredness of home."[75]

The inability or refusal of many reviewers to grapple with the radical content of *Glances and Glimpses* showcased their entrenched conservatism. Many such writers did not know what to make of a text that challenged established gender roles and institutions even as it appeared to be a "pleasant" book, redolent with nostalgic tales of happy domesticity in the early Republic. Several critics described *Glances and Glimpses* as a "curious book" or "one of the curiosities of literature."[76]

As critical or patronizing reviews of *Glances and Glimpses* appeared, friends tried to soften whatever disappointment Hunt felt. Angelina Grimké, for example, urged Hunt not to be "troubled" by such negative comments. "If it [the book] does good, that is the great thing," asserted Grimké. She added that Hunt was "so extensively & personally known" that she did not have to feel "anxiety" about people criticizing her narrative.[77] Sarah Grimké also wrote Hunt an encouraging letter. She told her that Gerrit Smith had liked *Glances and Glimpses* "very much" and urged Hunt to send a copy of the book to her friend Sarah Mapps Douglass, the noted African American abolitionist and educator.[78]

Predictably, people who were religious liberals and active in Boston's reform circles were those who bought and sympathetically read Hunt's autobiography. Daniel Child was one such man. He and his wife, Mary, were middle-class Bostonians, Unitarians, reform activists, and friends with Hunt. As he noted in his diary, Daniel enjoyed reading *Glances and Glimpses* after receiving it as a Christmas gift from his sister-in-law.[79] But such readers as Daniel Child were not enough to ensure the commercial success of *Glances and Glimpses*. The book met the fate that the majority of texts produced in the competitive antebellum marketplace did, quickly disappearing from public view.[80]

Hunt never responded publicly to reviews of *Glances and Glimpses*. Nor did she leave any record about how she felt when her autobiography failed to attract many readers. Instead, Hunt did what she always did when faced with hostility, disparagement, and indifference—she soldiered on. During the latter half of the 1850s she remained active in reform and also tended to her patients. The last fifteen years of Hunt's life, from 1860 to 1875, were difficult, even painful, ones for her. The Civil War and the Reconstruction era, as well as the bitter divisions that roiled the postwar woman's rights movement, upended her world while illness marred her final years.

Chapter 8

Confronting War, Old Age, and Other Challenges

On June 27 and 28, 1860, approximately fifteen hundred of Harriot Hunt's friends, patients, and relatives visited her home to celebrate her twenty-five-year career in medicine. Various reports described this occasion as her "silver wedding" anniversary. As the *Liberator* noted in its detailed coverage of the event, people had gathered to celebrate the "25th anniversary of the union of Miss Harriot K. Hunt and Harriot K. Hunt, M.D." Hunt's home was garlanded with flowers and mementos from her past, including sketches of her childhood home and the Bible she had received from her beloved childhood pastor, the Reverend John Murray. Twelve young women dressed in white and representing the months of the year preceded Hunt into her crowded parlor. She then entered the room accompanied by her sister. Both had wreaths on their heads. Encomiums lauding her medical work and woman's rights activities were offered by various people, including Caroline Severance, Dr. Marie Zakrzewska, and the noted sculptor Harriet Hosmer. The tributes of prominent feminists who could not attend, such as Lucretia Mott and Frances D. Gage, were read. So too were the congratulatory messages of other notable people, including Drs. Elizabeth and Emily Blackwell. One of the highpoints of the celebration was when the managers of the Hospital for Women and Children presented Hunt with a gold ring. The following day representatives from the Physiological Institutes of Woburn and Charlestown and other organizations called on Hunt to pay their respects. That evening, festivities continued with a "bridal cake" and other refreshments.[1]

The June 1860 celebration highlights how Hunt's career became a surrogate for marriage. The authors of the *History of Woman Suffrage* declared that it was fitting to offer Hunt "many bridal offerings" because, as she herself often stated, "her love element had all centered in her profession."[2] In a similar vein, Hunt's friend, the philanthropist and reformer Ednah Dow Cheney, stressed that the "pure gold ring" Hunt received was a way "to consecrate the marriage to her profession."[3] But there were some who thought Hunt's celebration was inappropriate. Woman's rights advocate Martha C. Wright complained to Elizabeth Cady Stanton that her sister Lucretia Mott had received one of Hunt's "bridal cards" inviting her to her anniversary party and asking for "a sentiment" or written tribute. Wright then snidely commented: "I wondered whether if some Boston Adonis of mature age should be accepted someday, it [would] be considered bigamy and whether succeeding patients [would] be less legitimate than previous ones—There is a 'sentiment,' but probably not the one prayerfully suggested to my sister."[4]

Hunt's request showed that she carefully planned her silver anniversary. In late May of 1860 she wrote to her friend Anna Parsons, noting preparations for her "festival" and asking her to contribute a "sentiment." Although she was temporarily confined to her home due to a recent leg injury, Hunt was in good spirits. The prospect of being feted by family, patients, and friends heartened her, and she declared that Parsons would be there in spirit if not in person at her celebration. "The soul has feelers," happily proclaimed Hunt, and joined people together even when they were physically apart.[5]

Practicing medicine anchored Hunt's life. She continued to see patients until at least several years before her death. She bonded with them, and they with her. Physician and reformer Mary Safford Blake stressed these points when she interviewed Hunt on her sixty-sixth birthday.[6] Blake noted that Hunt still had "a large consultation practice." Toward the end of her life, many of the women Hunt treated sought to help her when she became sickly. As she told Blake: "I can't begin to tell you how my patients vie with each other in bringing me fruit and flower offerings, and every delicacy, and come to proffer aid when I am ill." Hunt also stressed how being a doctor gave her life joy and meaning: "I have been so happy in my work; every moment occupied; how I long to whisper it in the ear of every listless woman, 'do something, if you would be happy.'"[7]

Hunt followed her own advice. Until felled by illness and old age, she always sought to "do something." She not only practiced medicine but engaged in a swirl of reform activism. This chapter will explore Hunt's myriad endeavors during the approximately last twenty years of her life. It will especially examine her leadership in the Ladies' Physiological Institute, her preaching in various churches during the latter 1850s, her ambivalent reactions to the Civil War and Reconstruction, and her persistent campaigns on behalf of woman's rights, especially the right to vote. Hunt's deepening relationships with the Wright family, Sarah Grimké, and other female reformers also merit discussion, as does Hunt's use of her last will and testament to shape her legacy.

In the early spring of 1856, members of the Ladies' Physiological Institute elected Hunt president and soon purchased a copy of *Glances and Glimpses* for their organization's library. These actions and Hunt's re-election in 1857 highlighted the institute's high regard for her.[8] Her presidency was an eventful one. She played a pivotal role in getting the institute to offer needed financial help to establish the New York Infirmary for Women and Children; Marie Zakrzewska addressed the institute during the fall of 1856, and the organization soon responded to her request for money by donating materials valued at $300 to a fund-raising fair for the planned infirmary.[9] Hunt also served on the committee that revised the institute's constitution and bylaws.[10] During her tenure as president, the Ladies' Physiological Institute decided to rescind their initial resolution thanking Mary Gove Nichols for "spreading a knowledge of physiology."[11] No doubt the latter's free-love principles had led institute members to reconsider. In 1857 Sarah Grimké congratulated Hunt on her reelection as institute president and praised her for getting the society to remove its "endorsement" of the "preeminently repulsive" Nichols.[12]

Hunt had many irons in the fire during the latter half of the 1850s. One of her most crucial activities remained fighting for woman's suffrage. She continued issuing her annual declarations to Boston officials, protesting her having to pay taxes while being denied the right to vote. But the growing sectional crisis over slavery added a new dimension to Hunt's campaign. John Brown's recent execution after his failed raid on Harper's Ferry, Virginia, in 1859 to liberate slaves, for example, exacerbated Hunt's anger at women's persistent disenfranchisement. "Now, at this period of conflict between liberty and oppression, this month of human sacrifice," she bitterly noted, "the taxpaying woman, ignored in representation," was still forced to support a government which "sustain[s] laws" that "violate her perceptions of justice."[13]

By the late 1850s, a growing minority of women were not only formally protesting the injustice of disenfranchisement but refusing to pay their taxes despite facing jail, confiscation of their property, and ostracism. Lucy Stone, who had urged women to take such action at the 1852 woman's rights convention, decided to practice what she preached. In January 1858, she informed the tax collector of Orange, New Jersey, that she would no longer pay taxes since she could not vote. Town officials seized some of her household goods, including engraved portraits of such prominent reformers as William Lloyd Garrison, and sold them at public auction. Fortunately for Stone and her family, a supportive neighbor bought the items and she was able to purchase them from him. The *New York Times* condemned Stone's actions as a "sham," especially because she had prearranged with her neighbor to purchase what had been confiscated. Although Stone defiantly vowed to repeat her act of civil disobedience, no evidence exists that she did so. Yet her action dramatized the increasing determination of suffragists.[14]

Other women also braved public condemnation when they refused to pay their taxes in the late 1850s. In the fall of 1858 in Worcester, Massachusetts, Sarah Wall invoked the Declaration of Independence and the United States Constitution to justify her decision to "henceforth pay no taxes until the word *male* is stricken from the voting clauses of the Constitution of Massachusetts." Wall quickly faced prosecution from the city collector and lost her case in the courts in 1863.[15] In Claremont, New Hampshire, during the years 1857–59, Mary L. Livermore was forced to work on the public road when she refused to pay her taxes.[16] In 1859 in Upstate New York, Lydia Sayer Hasbrouck had many of her possessions confiscated by the tax collector and advertised for sale after she refused to pay her taxes. Like Livermore, she was forced to work on the public roads. But Hasbrouck struck back—she excoriated such actions in the *Sibyl*, a feminist paper that she edited. As she noted in one 1862 article, "Uncle Sam's legal thief" made his "yearly visit" to her home to "see what he could grab from our household goods."[17] Theft—that is what Hasbrouck and other suffragists believed was occurring when officials took their property after they refused to pay their taxes to a government that denied them a basic right of citizenship in a democracy, the right to vote.

As the struggle for female suffrage intensified during the late 1850s, Hunt and other activists renewed their efforts to convince the Massachusetts State Legislature to enfranchise women. Passage in 1855 of a law granting married women rights over property they brought to the marriage or acquired afterward through inheritance, gift, or bequest undoubtedly gave hope to suffragists that the state legislature would support their arguments.[18] In March 1857 Lucy Stone and other noted supporters of woman's rights, including Wendell Phillips and

Unitarian minister James Freeman Clarke, addressed the legislature's Judiciary Committee. The galleries filled quickly as people jockeyed for seats to hear these reformers assert how unjust it was to deny "self-government" and "equal rights" to female citizens. In his address Clarke echoed Hunt's longtime argument when he noted that to deny taxpaying women the vote was akin to the injustice American men had suffered at the hands of the British Parliament.[19]

In February of 1858 suffragists tried again to sway the Massachusetts Legislature by addressing the Joint Special Committee on the Qualifications of Voters. Hunt was one of the featured speakers. She pointed out the injustice of denying "intelligent women" the vote while granting it to all male citizens, some of whom were "apologies for men." Hunt added that woman "would never take her true place in this Republic until she is recognized at the ballot-box." She also asserted that women should be able to "hold office, and sit side by side with the male Representatives in the Legislature."[20] Hunt also gave legislators a "piece of her mind" when she condemned the practice of sending "silly boys to College" while "sensible girls fold[ed] their hands in despair at home." When the chairman of the committee asked Hunt why few women demanded the suffrage, she tartly responded: "If women who were choked could be expected to breathe?"[21]

Lucy Stone, Wendell Phillips, Sarah Wall, and other suffragists also sought to convince the Judiciary Committee to delete the word "male" as a qualification for voting in the state of Massachusetts.[22] Suffragists enjoyed the support of the noted Massachusetts philanthropist, reformer, and legislator Samuel E. Sewall. A staunch advocate for woman's rights, he played a major role in Massachusetts granting property rights to wives.[23] In 1858 Sewall addressed the Massachusetts Legislature's Judiciary Committee. He urged legislators to live up to the ideals of the Declaration of Independence and the principles of natural rights it enshrined by enfranchising female citizens. Sewall singled out Hunt's annual protests for praise and looked forward to her address. Like Hunt, Sewall invoked the "great war-cry of the Revolution . . . that taxation without representation is tyranny."[24]

But the Judiciary Committee refused to budge. Massachusetts would not grant its female citizens the right to vote until 1920 with passage of the Nineteenth Amendment. In the 1850s most state legislators remained skeptical about the need to enfranchise women. This doubt was evident when one representative asked Hunt why a majority of women seemed to be satisfied with the status quo. She retorted by asking why slaves in the South seemed "so happy and contented."[25]

Hunt's frustration and bitterness at women's disenfranchisement was evident in a letter she wrote to Sewall several months before her address to the Judiciary Committee. She noted that she had paid her taxes that morning but then promptly gave yet another one of her annual protests to Boston authorities. Despite having a friend look "aghast" at her, Hunt was not dissuaded from protesting. "My plan was laid for doing something. The naturalization of that ignorant Irish boy was not lost upon me," she firmly declared. Hunt's words underscored how it continued to rankle her that she, a knowledgeable, native-born Bostonian, was denied the vote while allegedly ignorant male immigrants quickly gained this right once they became naturalized citizens. She told Sewall that she would soon make fifty copies of her protest and send it to leading feminists such as Lucretia Mott and Sarah Grimké as well as to him. She also urged Sewall to give her protest a "conspicuous mention" in the state legislature and preface it with his own remarks in support of suffrage.[26]

As she noted in her letter to Sewall, Hunt was "a working bee" in the latter half of the 1850s. There is no evidence that she was slowing down, even though she occasionally had bouts of illness, suffered accidents, and was over fifty years old. Her work on behalf of woman's rights energized her. It also meant that she remained in the crosshairs of those who opposed equal rights for women. Shortly after Hunt addressed the Massachusetts Judiciary Committee, the *New York Times* used satire to discredit her. The editors claimed that Hunt was "one of the dozen women in the United States who pine because Nature did not make them men." Like Lucy Stone and the "other small band of female reformers" who demanded the suffrage, Hunt, argued the *Times*, would not rest until the following resolution was passed: "*Be it enacted*, That all women shall become men; this act to take effect immediately." But in a bantering tone the paper stated that it would not support this measure because "we do not wish to see women abolished. We would rather not do without them." The editors quickly added, however, that if women were "all like Dr. Hunt and Lucy Stone we might think differently." Entitled "Abolishing Women," the editorial concluded by urging the Massachusetts Legislature "to exercise a judicious conservatism" and reject the move to enfranchise women.[27]

But not all mainstream newspapers were hostile to Hunt's efforts on behalf of suffrage. In fact, her persistent protests won grudging admiration even from some papers that ostensibly rejected her arguments. After declaring that suffrage was "by no means universal" among men, editors of a Boston newspaper conceded that Hunt's arguments had merit: "We admire the spirit with which [Hunt] maintains what she regards as her rights. It must be confessed that it is far easier to laugh at her argument than to answer it; for women, it must be admitted, are represented in our Legislature very much in the same way that our ancestors were in the British Parliament."[28] The last sentence was particularly revealing. The editors' "confession" that they agreed with the gist of Hunt's arguments suggests that her annual protests were garnering growing public respect if not support.

In 1859 Hunt ratcheted up her activism. She played a prominent role in the woman's rights convention held that May in Boston. By that time, bitter sectional divisions between the North and the South roiled the nation, and secession and civil war loomed. In the midst of these alarming developments, the *Liberator* heralded the gathering of feminists in the city. Editor William Lloyd Garrison noted that "rumors of wars abroad" and "the arrogant claims of the slave power at home" discouraged hopes for the "progress of reformatory ideas." It seemed, lamented Garrison, that "no advance has been made" in the struggle for justice and equality. Yet those who spoke at the woman's rights convention, including Hunt, encouraged Garrison. Their comments, he declared, reminded Americans that "the world moves still," that God wanted the world to "advance."[29]

Unfortunately, Hunt's speech to the convention has not survived. But the *Liberator* noted that she spoke in "a very earnest and forcible manner" about the need for female suffrage. The official report of the meeting described Hunt's address as "acute and pointed" and regretted that there was "no worthy report" of it.[30] But once again Hunt and other feminist advocates provoked controversy. The *Boston Post* was particularly scathing and sarcastic in its coverage of the convention: "The women's rights women,—the strong minded women,—the shrill voiced women, and women of sharp features,—the women who prefer cowhide boots to Cinderilla [sic] slippers, and woolen socks to silken hose,—the women in favor of the free and independent use of pitchforks, razors, butcher knives and broom handles,—the women of voluble speech and elongated tongues, held a Convention.... Every seat was occupied by the women and a few of the 'weaker sex' were sprinkled around the *out-skirts*, like thistles in a bed of roses, or thorns in a thistle bed." The paper singled out Hunt for particular criticism. It portrayed her as a defiant, radical woman who offered simplistic solutions to complicated issues. Hunt, stressed the editorial, demanded "the equality of husband and wife," "denounced the narrow views in relation to women," and believed that the "only hope of remedy" was to have women attend "Harvard and other colleges." The *Boston Post* also disapprovingly noted that Hunt adamantly opposed taxing women who could not vote. Ignoring the fact that Hunt annually paid her taxes even as she lawfully protested her disenfranchisement, the paper depicted her as a rabble-rouser. Hunt allegedly urged women to defy the law by refusing to pay their taxes and boasted of doing this herself: "As long as women are not represented in Government she would not have them pay taxes. Let them be taxed and let them refuse to pay.... She closed by predicting that there was a good time coming."[31] Such comments made it seem as if Hunt relished defying the government and even sought its overthrow.

Hunt obviously remained a controversial figure in the late 1850s. But she was also a woman who attracted many supportive reformers and friends. When the latter arranged a "soiree" in 1857 to honor Hunt, Sarah Grimké admiringly wrote: "You have the most choice & loving circles of friends of any woman I know."[32] During the latter part of the 1850s, two noted reformers, Caroline Severance and Caroline Dall, worked with Hunt on a number of issues.[33] Their lives repeatedly intersected, and they became friends. As noted previously, Severance and Hunt met during the 1852 woman's rights convention in Syracuse, New York, and in the mid-1850s they toured Ohio together, campaigning on behalf of woman's rights.

Dall knew Hunt as early as 1851. They and other reformers attended a discussion of Margaret Fuller at Bronson Alcott's home.[34] Dall also socialized at Hunt's home, especially during the September 1855 woman's rights convention in Boston.[35] By that time the two women were friendly enough that Hunt could tease Dall when the latter objected to Elizabeth Oakes Smith addressing the meeting in overly fancy dress. Dall fumed at what she described as Smith's "opera costume." But she also appreciated how "Garrison & H. K. Hunt" told her that the "greatest fun of the whole Convention" was watching her face register "various expressions of regret, disgust, & annoyance" as Smith talked. Dall jested in return that next time she would wear a "black veil" to conceal her expressions.[36]

Dall, Severance, and Hunt belonged to many of the same organizations and shared a common reform agenda during the latter part of the 1850s. Severance and Dall, for example, were influential members of the Ladies' Physiological Institute and worked with Hunt on the committee to revise the organization's constitution and bylaws.[37] They also shared Hunt's commitment to promoting women in medicine. As noted earlier, Severance was a major benefactor of Marie Zakrzewska.[38] As for Dall, she publicly advocated for women doctors.[39] She also befriended Zakrzewska and edited and partly wrote her autobiographical sketch entitled *A Practical Illustration of "Woman's Right to Labor"* (1860).[40]

Dall and Severance also played prominent roles in the woman's rights conventions in which Hunt participated. Severance, for example, was president of the 1859 meeting in Boston and did such an able job that even the hostile *Boston Post* had to admit that she "filled the chair in a perfectly satisfactory manner."[41] Dall called the meeting to order and was a featured speaker. Her talk included a survey of the increasing numbers of women in various trades and occupations, and she also addressed the Massachusetts State Legislature's Judiciary Committee, urging woman's suffrage, shortly after Hunt did the same.[42]

Public lectures that Dall delivered from the late 1850s to the mid-1860s highlight how closely her ideas dovetailed with those of Hunt. Like Hunt, Dall demanded that medical schools admit women since they were allegedly best suited to treat female patients. She also urged the formation of a female medical society to increase the number of women physicians. After noting the broad range of wage-earning jobs that women did, Dall condemned their low pay. She also predicted that as women became more economically independent, they would demand political rights. But the issue that most galvanized Dall was that of woman suffrage. Like Hunt and other antebellum suffragists, Dall viewed the movement to enfranchise women as part of a wider struggle to advance the cause of democracy and human rights. "'Woman's rights' are identical with 'human rights,'" she proclaimed, and any government that ignored this fact was "tyrannical."[43]

In one 1860 lecture, Dall praised Hunt's work on behalf of female suffrage: "Dr. Harriot K. Hunt had done well in entering her protest, year by year, against the tax which was levied upon her while her right of voting was denied."[44] But in a later lecture Dall mildly rebuked Hunt, even as she called her "our sturdy friend." She wished that Hunt would have had "the heart" to refuse to pay her taxes and let the city government take her property for "non-payment of taxes." Hunt's annual protests, she feared, had little effect: "The City government sits as serene and patient under her inflictions as if she had never spoken. Her protests probably got back to the pulp of the paper-mill; and, but for the newspaper, we should never know that they were written."[45]

As her comments suggest, Dall came to view Hunt's annual protests as too timid and ineffective. Although she admired Hunt as a feminist pioneer, she also felt that women had to be more confrontational in demanding their rights. Like Lucy Stone, Dall urged women to defy the law and refuse to pay their taxes. She also exhorted "five thousand female property-holders" to protest by "calling their own caucus, and storming the City Hall with well-concerted words." Only such combative actions, Dall asserted, would "compel" the government to finally take women's grievances seriously.

Despite disagreements about how best to wage the suffrage struggle, Dall and Hunt remained colleagues and friends. Hunt had a knack for bringing together different groups of people. Like other female activists, such as the prominent abolitionists the Weston sisters, Hunt used her home as a place where reformers could meet and discuss mutual interests, plan future activities, and forge friendships.[46] In short, Hunt's Boston home nurtured a wide reform network. Recall that it was there that Marie Zakrzewska, just starting her medical practice, met Sarah Grimké, the Welds, and other noted Boston reformers and female physicians who later helped her professionally.

The abolitionist and woman's rights advocate Sallie Hollie fondly remembered visiting Hunt's home for teas and parties in the mid-1850s. Hunt, she said, was a "round and short and merry woman" and also a "lively and entertaining" one, who regaled her guests with funny stories about her life. But what Hollie most treasured about her times at the Hunt home were the people she met. She seemed a bit celebrity struck when she described visiting Hunt's home after the September 1855 woman's rights meeting and being introduced to such feminist luminaries as Sarah Grimké, Paulina Wright Davis, and Caroline Severance. The most impressive person to Hollie, however, was Caroline Dall, who at the convention delivered a report surveying Massachusetts laws regarding married women. Hollie gushed that Dall was a "person of culture and genius," someone who reminded her of Margaret Fuller. Dall also had fond memories of that evening in Hunt's home. In her diary she happily noted that Hunt and many of her guests, including Severance and Hollie, warmly praised her presentation.[47]

At times Hunt brought together two friends who ended up helping each other during difficult periods in their respective lives. Ednah Dow Cheney gratefully recollected how Hunt helped her cope with the sorrow she felt after her husband's death: "My friend . . . would not let me rest in the indolence and selfishness of grief." Instead, Hunt sent Marie Zakrzewska to talk to Cheney about her plans for the New York Infirmary for Women and Children. Cheney not only became one of the hospital's benefactors but also resumed her life of philanthropy and reform.[48]

Zakrzewska also regarded Harriot Hunt as a kind of lifesaver. Shortly after the hospital opened in May 1857, she wrote Hunt about how grateful she was for the help she received from her and Severance. Addressing Hunt as "my dear friend," she stressed that she was "homesick" for her. As for herself, Zakrzewska declared that she felt "alive, happy, healthy & highly spirited." She had finally established a community, a niche, for herself and it exhilarated her: "I feel the first time myself since my life in New York, I wish to embrace the whole world for gratitude of this feeling, . . . and all this together makes me thanking God, that I live, lived & will live to be useful to my contemporaries & perhaps even to posterity."[49] Such testimony highlights how Hunt nurtured her friends and did so in ways that promoted the two causes closest to her heart, women's health and women's rights.

For as many friends and colleagues as Hunt had, however, her closest ties remained with her sister's family. The diary of Hunt's nephew Edmund Wentworth Wright, which he kept from his twelfth year in 1856 to his nineteenth in 1863, shows that his family and "Aunty" Harriot regularly visited each other, spent holidays together, and at times traveled together.[50] When Hunt visited the Wright home, she often brought guests. Edmund recalled, for example, that when his aunt spent a Sunday afternoon with them in early April 1857, Mr. and Mrs. Severance, Dr. Marie Zakrzewska, and Bronson Alcott accompanied her. In June 1858 Harriot Hunt and fellow feminist Frances D. Gage visited the Wright home. The Wrights also went with Hunt to visit the Shakers. In early August 1858, for example, Edmund wrote in his journal that he and his family were on their way to "spend a week with Aunty" at the Shaker community in Harvard.

Harriot Hunt and the Wrights also came together to share momentous political events that roiled their community. In one December 1859 diary entry, Edmund stated that his family and aunt attended a "very large meeting" at Tremont Temple in Boston to protest the hanging of John Brown. The Wrights were also present at major milestones in Hunt's life. Edmund proudly noted, for example, how he and his mother attended the Ladies' Physiological Institute when his aunt was elected "President by a large majority" in May 1857. He also recorded in his diary his aunt's celebration of her twenty-five years in medicine in June 1860.

The closeness between Harriot Hunt and her sister's family grew deeper when the Wrights moved from nearby Dorchester, Massachusetts, to Boston in April 1862. Edmund stated in his diary that part of what made the Wrights' move to Boston so "pleasant" was that "Aunt Harriot live[d] almost opposite" his new home and was able to visit "almost every day." Other diary entries noted that Hunt regularly had tea or meals with the Wrights. Edmund also gratefully acknowledged the generous gifts his aunt gave him and his family. When he and his brother Theodore were admitted into Harvard College in July 1862, he recalled that Hunt gave each of them an engraved "splendid seal ring." In an October journal entry Edmund was particularly appreciative of his aunt's latest act of generosity—she had pledged to give her nephews a "very bountiful" gift of $1,000 apiece when they graduated.

During the late 1850s and 1860s Hunt drew closer not only to the Wright family but also to Sarah Grimké. In 1859 Grimké reminded Hunt that they were kindred spirits who had shared much over the years: "*We dear sister have had an ample share of the joys of life with enough of its sorrows, its trials, its perplexities to impose upon us a salutary discipline, to give us rich & varied experiences.*"[51] Hunt continued to confide in Grimké. In 1857, for example, she told Grimké that she was planning to add yet another role to her already full life, that of preacher. Grimké wondered if her friend was "really studying theology." As for herself, Grimké stressed that she could "not enjoy the drilling through the musty volumes of theological dogmas" required to "get ordained." But Grimké admitted that she would "enjoy" the "preaching part." She urged Hunt to let her know when she would make her "debut as a minister" and promised that she would be there.[52]

Although Hunt was never ordained a minister, she did preach in various churches from 1859 to at least the early 1860s. Various newspapers in 1859 reported her preaching at different Universalist churches in New England. In April, for example, the *New York Times* noted that Hunt had "commenced preaching the Gospel" in Athol, Stoneham, and other Massachusetts towns, while in September the *Boston Traveler* declared that she had preached in sixteen Universalist churches in Maine earlier that summer.[53] Unfortunately, none of Hunt's sermons have survived, but several papers praised her preaching. The *Boston Evening Transcript*, for example, stated: "Her manner was reverential and pleasing. Her discourse was characterized by earnestness and deep religious feeling, and an instinctive appreciation of her subject; and was listened to with much satisfaction by an attentive audience."[54]

One detailed and very positive account of Hunt's sojourn in Maine appeared in the *Liberator* in the fall of 1859. Identified only as "A. B.," the author declared that Hunt had spoken "about twenty times in ten or twelve towns" during her tour of Maine, which lasted from late June to early September. According to this writer, Hunt combined lecturing with preaching. She not only spoke on matters related to "her profession" and woman's rights but also "preached" in "pulpits." Hunt therefore "united the offices of physician and spiritual leader." The anonymous author admiringly stated that Hunt had attracted people in "large numbers—radicals and conservatives—and [they] had their minds instructed, their consciences aroused, and their hearts softened." Hunt's "missionary tour to Maine" had been "a grand success."[55]

Hunt's family often listened to her preach. Edmund Wright described how he and his parents "heard Aunty preach" in different Boston churches, including a Methodist one, during the spring and summer of 1861. When Hunt "preached all day" in Boston's Music Hall one Sunday in April 1861, for example, the Wright family attended the morning session. Then seventeen-year-old Edmund admiringly recorded in his diary that Hunt "preached very well I thought for a lady." Later journal entries showed his growing admiration for Hunt's preaching and pride in the accolades she received: "Aunty preached this morning to a very fine congregation. . . . It was liked by all whose opinion was worth anything. . . . Aunty is very well liked as a preacher." The next month he wrote, "We all went to meeting and heard Aunty preach. It was quite a good sermon and all seemed very much pleased."[56]

Harriot Hunt defied society's strictures when she boldly ascended a pulpit and assumed a role traditionally reserved for men. She put into practice what a number of feminists, including she and Grimké, had long urged—challenge men's power in the churches by having women preach and even become ministers. One of the reasons why "A. B." admired Hunt was that she "had not stopped to argue abstractly whether woman may speak in public" but instead asked both "men and women to come and hear her lecture and preach." In other words, Hunt had appropriated public spaces like the lecture hall and church pulpit, showing that women had as much right as men to speak there.

Hunt joined a small band of women when she became a female preacher. During the approximate period from the 1740s to the 1840s, over one hundred women preached in evangelical sects such as the Baptists, the Christian Connection, and the Methodists. A motley group, they included African American women, such as the former slave-turned-abolitionist and woman's rights advocate Sojourner Truth, and Harriet Livermore, the daughter of a prominent congressman and jurist from New Hampshire, who preached several times before Congress. The majority of female preachers, however, came from impoverished backgrounds and were generally uneducated, even illiterate. Many women preachers were "biblical feminists." Unlike Sojourner Truth, they espoused only a spiritual equality between the sexes and urged women's continued subordination to men in temporal matters.[57]

But there were religious sects that not only accepted women preachers but also urged greater temporal as well as spiritual equality between the sexes. These included the sects Hunt gravitated toward, the Shakers and Quakers. The Universalists and Unitarians also tended to be more welcoming to women preachers than were mainline churches. As noted earlier, the Universalist Church, to which the Hunt family belonged, was among the earliest to ordain women, including those who became major woman's rights activists after the Civil War, such as Olympia Brown.⁵⁸ The Unitarians also accepted women preachers and ministers. One of their female congregants who began preaching shortly after Hunt was Caroline Healey Dall. She noted that in the 1860s she was preaching in "regular Unitarian churches" throughout Boston and surrounding areas.⁵⁹

But women preachers were always a controversial minority and became more so during the antebellum era. As evangelical sects transformed themselves into more affluent and respectable denominations, they began to ostracize these women during the 1830s and erase any institutional records about them. Ministers who earlier had valued female preachers now sought to silence them. As they were shunted aside and criticized, women evangelists declined in numbers by the end of the 1830s.⁶⁰ During the early 1840s, the Millerites, a sect proclaiming the imminent end of the world and the Second Coming of Christ, welcomed female preachers, but the failure of the apocalypse to arrive soon discredited this group and its proselytizers.⁶¹

The women preachers who emerged in later decades often sought to distance themselves from their forebears, if they even knew about them at all. Women who began preaching in the 1850s were more educated and emotionally restrained than their earlier female counterparts. This later generation often felt embarrassed by the emotional intensity and illiteracy of previous women evangelists. They also frequently used the pulpit to preach abolitionism and woman's rights and to denounce patriarchal power in its various guises.⁶² Hunt and Dall exemplified such female preachers.

Irrespective of the differences among women evangelists in nineteenth-century America, many of their contemporaries, especially the mainstream clergy, regarded them as "unnatural," "unfeminine," and "disorderly." It is therefore surprising that New England newspapers did not denounce Hunt's preaching and that several even commended her performance in the pulpit. This response suggested that a growing minority of Americans had begun to accept the notion of female preachers, just as they did female doctors. By the late 1850s, a woman who was educated and preached the gospel message effectively seemed neither unnatural nor irreverent to many reform-minded Americans. This was particularly the case in Boston, the epicenter of reform activism. And given that Hunt preached mostly in Universalist churches, her way was smoothed as this denomination had long supported rights for women as well as their religious activism. It also probably helped that, by the time she began preaching, Hunt was a well-known, middle-aged physician and woman of property who counted as among her friends some of Boston's leading citizens.

The favorable coverage she received when she preached and lectured in 1859 likely heartened Hunt. But there were professional reversals as well as successes in her life. One of Hunt's bitter disappointments was the closing in 1860 of the New England School of Design. Established in November 1851 with fifty-seven students enrolled, the school was part of a network of institutes, including those in Philadelphia and New York, that taught women about the theory and practice of industrial design. Female students learned such subjects as wood engraving, drawing, fabric design, anatomy, and lithography. The goal was not only to educate women in the industrial arts but also to make them employable. Although several female graduates forged successful careers as artists, the majority of them ended up teaching design themselves.[63]

Hunt and her friends Ednah Dow Cheney and Dr. Josiah Flagg played a pivotal role in establishing the New England School of Design. After visiting Philadelphia and seeing the Franklin Institute School, Cheney and Flagg committed themselves to establishing a sister school in Boston. They received the enthusiastic support of Hunt.[64] Twenty-seven people met at Hunt's home to discuss initial plans for the New England School of Design (274–75). In an early January 1854 letter to Anna Parsons, Hunt noted how pleased she was with the school and hoped for its success.[65]

Yet by the late 1850s, various factors, including the fallout from the economic depression of 1857, the decision of Massachusetts to end its state subsidy, and the dwindling number of students, doomed the New England School of Design.[66] Hunt was both sad and angry about the school's failure. As she told Anna Parsons, the "Death warrant" the "Executive Society of the School of Design" issued was "a great wrong" and an "outrage" to currently enrolled students. It also had a "lamentable" impact on "Woman," grumbled Hunt.[67] But ultimately there was nothing either she or other supporters could do to save the school.

Whatever professional and personal disappointments Hunt experienced in the late 1850s paled in comparison with the unprecedented crisis that she and her generation faced when the Union foundered and the Civil War began in April 1861. The four years of fighting, the horrific casualties, and the myriad political and social changes the nation experienced transformed Hunt's world. Women throughout the North mobilized on behalf of the Union cause. They nursed wounded soldiers and participated in various fund-raising projects and relief work. They also formed organizations to facilitate the war effort. The United States Sanitary Commission and its various chapters, such as the New England Women's Auxiliary Association, solicited and coordinated war relief and played a crucial role in supplying Union hospitals and camps. The Woman's National Loyal League also supported the war effort and campaigned for abolitionism.[68]

The war had a profound impact on the leaders of the woman's rights movement. When the conflict began, Elizabeth Cady Stanton stated that it was "music" to her "ears" because it personified "a simultaneous chorus for freedom," one that would abolish slavery and further the cause of woman's rights.[69] This belief led Stanton and other leading feminists to assume a prominent role in the above-noted organizations. Stanton and Susan B. Anthony organized the Woman's National Loyal League.[70] At this organization's first meeting in New York City in the spring of 1863, they were joined by other prominent feminists, such as Lucy Stone, Angelina Grimké Weld, and Ernestine Rose.[71] League women soon gathered thousands of petitions to pressure the Lincoln administration to abolish the institution of slavery. By February of 1864, they had sent more than 12,000 such petitions with over 100,000 signatures.[72]

And what of Harriot Hunt? Curiously, her name did not appear in the Woman's National Loyal League roster of officers or speakers featured at its opening meeting. Nor did she seem to be active in other civic organizations that mobilized women in support of the Union cause, such as the New England Women's Auxiliary Association of the U.S. Sanitary Commission. Why not? The paucity of primary documents for this period in Hunt's life makes it difficult to investigate this question. Perhaps Hunt was ill or she was stretched thin with her many responsibilities and therefore unable to participate as fully as she would have liked in the war effort. When the war began in April 1861, Hunt was fifty-five years old and probably needed to conserve her energies if she was to continue her medical practice and the reform activities that most mattered to her. In a January 1860 letter to Sarah Grimké, Hunt mentioned that she had been unable to visit dear friends during the recent Christmas holidays because of her demanding medical practice: "My cases are so imperative I cannot leave. My winter has been very busy and my success startles even HKH."[73]

Hunt now had a woman who lived with her and took care of her home and needs. In 1857 Sarah Grimké told Hunt how glad she was that a "kind companion" was "ministering" to her "daily wants."[74] The companion's name was Rachael Babcock; the 1860 federal census identified her as a thirty-nine-year-old "mulatto" "servant."[75] By now, Hunt was a woman who could easily afford to hire a housekeeper and companion. As noted earlier, the census of 1860 showed that she had real estate appraised at $24,000 and a personal estate valued at $12,000.[76] By the early 1860s, newspapers stressed that she owned "valuable property in Boston."[77] In 1864 Hunt reported an annual income of over $2,300 after deducting numerous expenses, including her payment of over $600 in national, state, and local taxes.[78] When one considers that in 1870 the annual earnings of nonfarm employees in the United States was only $489, Hunt was obviously one of the city's most affluent residents.⁷⁹

But the war took its toll on her, just as it did on poorer citizens. Hunt's annual protests against "taxation without representation" showed that she ultimately had very ambivalent feelings about the conflict. This was evident in her 1861 annual protest. Like Stanton and other reformers, Hunt hoped that the Civil War would initiate "a struggle for a higher perception of freedom . . . when bondage after bondage is being removed." She looked forward to the day when the freedom promised in the Declaration of Independence would no longer be limited only to white males. The "national eagle," she fervently hoped, was "spreading her wings over those hitherto only nominally protected, *woman is beginning to take courage, and is willing to bide her time, till man shall be morally strong enough* to recognize her rights as *citizen* in a republic."⁸⁰

But Hunt voiced her bitterness and sorrow as well as hope about the war. She saw slavery, the leading cause of the war, as a direct consequence of men's stranglehold on political power. "*Woman, in her womanhood,*" she emphatically declared, "*could never have permitted slavery*, an institution which blights every thing she holds sacred, through her conjugal and maternal nature." White males, she stressed, because of their "ignorance, love of power and selfhood," and commitment to "crushing the colored race," were to blame for the Civil War. Hunt was under no illusions about how bitter, hard-fought, and bloody this conflict would be. The fact that women were denied any right to voice their views about a war that grievously hurt them and their families galled her: "Now, she [woman] is to be taxed to bear her part in a civil war which she has had nothing to do in creating; family ties have been and are still to be ruptured by deaths the most aggravating; widows and fatherless children are to be thrown upon the world. *Man*, through taxation, is to devise and control the means to meet these exigencies, while *woman* is passively to submit to *his* decisions, though it reduce her property to a minimum of its former value; so '*taxation without representation*' assumes a deeper significance than ever before in the history of our country."

Such comments offer another vantage point from which to view Hunt's failure to join female wartime organizations. Even though she hoped the war would ultimately inaugurate an era of freedom, Hunt realized this conflict would cost the nation much blood and treasure. The fact that women were expected to sacrifice their families and property and "passively submit" to men who caused this terrible tragedy made Hunt leery of actively supporting the war.

Nevertheless, she did display her patriotism in one important way. In 1866 the government of Massachusetts gratefully acknowledged that almost six hundred of its prominent citizens during the war paid "representative recruits" to fight on behalf of the Union even though they themselves were not subject to the draft. The list included some of the state's most notable citizens, including Edward Everett, George B. Emerson, Richard Henry Dana, Henry Wadsworth Longfellow, and James Russell Lowell. Out of the seventy-nine "ladies" who hired a recruit, the government report singled out only one woman for her contribution—"Harriot K. Hunt."[81]

Hunt's actions showed that she supported the Union struggle. But her decision to hire a recruit to fight was also a way for her to pursue woman's rights. Because she was a woman, Hunt was not liable to the draft and therefore had no need to hire a substitute to fight in her stead. But she asserted a crucial right of citizenship when she did hire a young man to fight—Hunt "claimed the right of being represented on the battle-field by an able-bodied substitute." As a writer in the popular magazine the *Ladies Repository* admiringly noted in 1870, Hunt's actions "proved her fidelity to her own principles."[82]

Whatever bitterness and misgivings Hunt may have felt initially about the war seemed to dissipate toward the end of this conflict. Now Hunt stressed that the war would advance the cause of freedom for women as well as African Americans. No doubt major Northern victories as well as Lincoln's Emancipation Proclamation issued in January 1863 contributed to her optimism. Her annual protest for 1864 linked the struggle for black rights with that for women. Hunt hailed not only the Union's impending victory but also the coming end of slavery: "The question of freedom in a free country is, in a most wonderful manner, becoming developed, through the fulfillment of our obligations to the colored race. Nobleness of soul has burst forth through conventionalism, customs and habits. Latent principles, embodied in the Declaration of Independence, are now demanding thought and practical application."[83]

Hunt then quickly segued to the issue of suffrage. According to her, the nation was at a crossroads. "The question of suffrage now stands before the country as a gigantic subject," she declared, and Americans wrestled with the issue of "by whom, for whom, and to whom this right belongs." Hunt expressed confidence that the historic events unfolding in the nation would result not only in the full "emancipation" of people of color but also cause Americans to grant the vote to women. Her optimistic tone was evident when she declared toward the end of her protest: "So, cheerfully, hopefully, and trustingly, I enter again my protest against *taxation without representation* . . . and the present method of suffrage will follow slavery in due time."

But Hunt's optimism, like that of other suffragists, was short lived. By the late 1860s the woman's rights movement had splintered; some feminists, such as Lucy Stone, supported Frederick Douglass's contention that Americans must concentrate on granting black men the suffrage, whereas Stanton, Anthony, and others demanded that women as well as men of color be enfranchised. The latter group of suffragists became especially embittered when the Fourteenth and Fifteenth Amendments to the Constitution were adopted in 1868 and 1870, respectively. The former amendment declared that states would lose representation in Congress if they denied the "right to vote" to "male inhabitants" who were citizens and at least twenty-one years old. The Fifteenth Amendment declared that no citizens could be denied the franchise due to "race, color, or previous condition of servitude." In effect, this latter amendment enfranchised formerly enslaved African American men but not women.[84]

Like Stanton, Anthony, and other notable feminists, Hunt feared that triumphant Republican politicians would soon betray the cause of female suffrage. This worry tempered the joy she expressed for the political rights gained by African American men. "I am proud of my city," she proclaimed in her 1866 annual protest, because "color is to be ignored in our halls of legislation." Yet Hunt also noted with disgust how politics was becoming an increasingly corrupt, raucous process, one that continued to exclude female citizens. "All kinds of party machinery" and "demagogues," she complained, resorted to "frenzied activity" to gain "male votes" for their respective candidates. These "party zealots," angrily added Hunt, courted "drunkards," "libertines," and "raw, green emigrants" while refusing to enfranchise "millions of intelligent, virtuous, native-born citizens" who were women.[85] Hunt's protest resonated throughout the suffrage movement during the late nineteenth and early twentieth centuries, highlighting how growing numbers of suffragists resorted to nativist and class arguments and invoking the idea that women deserved the vote because they were allegedly more moral than men.

Hunt's persistent demands for the franchise attracted the ridicule of the editor of the *Springfield Republican*. In November 1863, shortly after Hunt had issued her annual protest, the paper offered a sarcastic, insulting view of her. It misstated both her name and marital status and ignored that Hunt was a well-known physician. "Mrs. Harriot Rosia Hunt, a Boston woman of pantaloon proclivities," sneeringly declared the editor, "pays her taxes under protest, and sighs for the day when women as well as men will have the privileges of paying poll taxes and depositing votes."[86] Hunt's annual protest for 1864 also attracted the contempt of the *Springfield Republican*. Although this time the paper called her "Dr. Harriot K. Hunt," it still deprecated her views by declaring that "the natural right of woman to be man is as clear as the right of a hen to crow—there's no use arguing the case."[87]

But Hunt had her defenders. The *Liberator* rebutted the editorial comments of the *Springfield Republican* by resorting to ridicule and sarcasm: "The natural right of an editor . . . to make a donkey of himself is as clear as any other right—there's no use arguing the case."[88] The following month the *Liberator* issued another volley against the editor of the *Springfield Republican* when it accused him of "persistently treat[ing] the friends of emancipation with whom he differs, with contempt and ridicule." The *Liberator* took particular exception to the "low fling" hurled against "Dr. Harriot K. Hunt." But in the end the paper was confident that the editor of the *Springfield Republican* and his supporters were on the wrong side of history. Sooner or later, predicted the *Liberator*, "the laws of nature and an enlightened public opinion" would force them to "yield . . . on the question of Woman's freedom and her enfranchisement."[89]

And how did Hunt respond to attacks against her? She seemed to relish the controversy she provoked and persisted in advocating for a woman's right to vote. Shortly after the Civil War ended, Elizabeth Blackwell wrote to her adopted daughter that she had recently visited Harriot Hunt in Boston. Hunt had read her latest annual protest and declared "with peals of laughter" that she planned to sue the city of Boston for "taxing her without representation." According to Blackwell, Hunt remained as "jolly as ever" but also determined to prosecute the cause of female suffrage.[90]

By the mid-1860s, however, Hunt had begun to slow down. She no longer seemed to travel on lecture tours or preach in different churches.[91] Although she still saw patients at her home, she stopped making house calls.[92] The resumption of the annual woman's rights conventions, which had been temporarily suspended during the war, predictably attracted Hunt's support. She served as one of the vice presidents of the 1868 convention, together with William Lloyd Garrison and other stalwarts of the feminist cause.[93] But Hunt did not seem to have delivered a major address there. There is no record of her attending any other postwar woman's rights conventions.

But in 1868 Hunt did help to establish the New England Women's Club, which became a template for the many women's clubs that emerged in the United States during the latter half of the nineteenth century. Composed primarily of middle- and upper-class women, these clubs promoted their members' involvement in various philanthropic and reform activities. They politically mobilized countless women and nurtured their sense of sisterhood and empowerment. Not surprisingly, club women often became suffragists.[94]

The first several meetings of the New England Women's Club were held in Hunt's home. Although men could join this organization, the founders stressed that it was "to be officered and controlled by women." Members also emphatically declared that "the club was to be no lounging-place for the drones" but instead offer "a broader home for those who love and labor for the great human family."[95] As such comments suggest, the New England Women's Club rejected the idea of being just a social club. Rather, it tackled major political and economic issues. This organization developed various proposals to help working-class women, such as establishing a loan fund for the impoverished and a public employment registry. Club members also provided major funding to help the New England Hospital for Women and Children. Not surprisingly, Dr. Marie Zakrzewska was a featured speaker as well as one of its members. The club's various charitable and philanthropic activities also included aid to immigrants, prison reform, and the establishment of kindergartens for impoverished children.

But the club was particularly concerned with promoting the education and political rights of women. Members helped establish various education classes and funded scholarships to women's colleges. To prepare women for college, the club worked to establish the Girls' Latin School in Boston. It also played a pivotal role in campaigning for woman's right to vote and serve on school boards in Massachusetts. Finally, its members heard lectures on the need to allow women to vote in all elections.[96]

The activities sponsored by the New England Women's Club and its campaigns for reform were causes long dear to Hunt. Her friends Caroline Severance and Ednah Dow Cheney were fellow club organizers, and the former served as the first president of the organization. In short, the New England Women's Club was an organization that seemed tailor made for Hunt. But although her home was where the club began, her name does not appear on the list of officers or speakers. Neither the club's records nor its official history make any further mention of Hunt after noting her presence at its founding.

Hunt was probably unable to participate in the New England Women's Club owing to illness. When she died on January 2, 1875, several months after her sixty-ninth birthday, her death certificate stated the causes as uremia and Bright's disease, ailments both indicative of kidney failure.[97] Obituaries noted that she had been ill for quite a while and her death was long expected.[98] The last several years must have been difficult for Hunt. The loss of those dearest to her as well as debilitating disease marred her final years. In July 1867 Sarah Hunt Wright died at the age of fifty-eight.[99] Sarah Grimké died in December

1873 when she was eighty-one.[100] The deaths of her beloved sister and dear friend undoubtedly anguished Hunt. But she continued to try to be productive. She still consulted with some patients and tried to write a sequel to her autobiography.

In October of 1871, Harriot Hunt also made her will.[101] It is a meticulously detailed document that reflects how careful Hunt was to dispose of her considerable estate. Area newspapers ran articles discussing the will, approvingly noting how Hunt sought to provide for her patients as well as family and friends and also used her wealth to fund various charities.[102] Hunt's will stipulated that her patients' confidentiality was to be ensured by destroying their records. This information included what patients owed her. Hunt also instructed that no bills were to be sent to any of her patients. Instead, she left it "to their discretion" to pay to her estate "any amount for which they may feel indebted."

Hunt's cash bequests totaled $12,200. Not surprisingly, she left the bulk of her estate to her sister's five children. Each of them received $1,000 from their aunt's estate, and three of the four nephews received an additional $300 "in recognition of their family names and in harmony with my love of pedigree."[103] Hunt also made cash bequests to other relatives and friends. Roxalana Grosvenor, for example, received $100. Hunt also left money to support various philanthropic projects. She bequeathed $1,000 each, for example, to help Boston's poor and to aid "sick nurses." She also gave $1,000 to the "Home for aged colored women." Predictably Hunt also used her wealth to promote the medical education of women. She bequeathed $1,000 to the "Homeopathic Hospital." She also instructed Angelina Grimké Weld and several other friends to invest the sum of $1,000 and use the income for the "purchase of medical text books for women students within the New England States."

Hunt was especially particular about how she disposed of the real estate she had amassed. Her will shows that she remained deeply attached to her current home on Green Street and also to her childhood residence on Fleet Street in Boston's North End. She sought to preserve intact these properties and the adjoining houses that she also owned. Hunt was emphatic that the Fleet Street property should be retained in the family for as long as possible because it was "a place ever sacred through memories and fraught with intense associations, having formed a nucleus for my prosperity—never having lost its life power."

Hunt placed various restrictions on how her heirs, the Wright children and their progeny, could dispose of her estate. She stipulated, for example, that the income from the Fleet Street properties was to "accumulate for the term of ten (10) years as a fund for future improvement, only placing such repairs as are necessary." Only after ten years' time could the Wrights sell the property. But even then Hunt imposed restrictions—monies gained from such a sale were to be invested in real estate, and if her heirs tried to circumvent the terms of the will, they would forfeit their portion of the inheritance. Leaving nothing to chance, Hunt stipulated that if her sister's children did not leave heirs, the money from the Fleet Street properties was to go to the "Boston Provident Association," which would provide extra coal and flannels for "poor widows and unmarried women of American birth."

Regarding her current house on Green Street, Hunt instructed her heirs to keep it open one to three months during the year so that her friends and patients "may find still an open door to enter a home that they have consecrated by their blessings." Hunt also stipulated that there be "fragrant flowers freely distributed" throughout her home. This house and the one adjoining it, she instructed, were to be "kept as united property." Undoubtedly recognizing that at some point the Wright children or their progeny might rent or even sell her beloved home, Hunt specified that her residence was "never to be let, leased[,] or used for the sale of anything deteriorating or physically enervating, [such] as gambling, intemperance[,] tobacco[,] social perversions[,] or anything which tends to separate the soul from its source." This was "my home," emphatically declared Hunt, "the result of my professional life," and she clearly was committed to protecting it even after her death.

Hunt's will honored the memory of her beloved eldest niece and namesake, Harriot Augusta Wright, the child whose early death devastated her. When Hunt bequeathed the Fleet Street properties to her sister's five surviving children, she made it a point of dividing their shares six ways. Her remaining niece was to receive a double portion, her own as well as that of her older, deceased sister. Harriot Augusta, Hunt stressed, was "the first born" and although "transferred . . . early to another world" deserved "a continued place in the family."

Hunt also used her will to try to preserve her written work and to advance the suffrage cause. She stipulated that the plates of her now-out-of-print autobiography, *Glances and Glimpses*, as well as the second "unfinished" volume of her narrative be given to the New England Women's Club. Hunt urged club members to consult her friends and "steadfast reformers," such as Angelina Grimké Weld, Samuel Sewall, and Caroline Severance, regarding how best to dispose of these materials. Hoping that all her writings would be published, including her annual protests against "taxation without representation," Hunt specified how the profits from their sale should be used—tracts "on the suffrage question" should be bought and distributed to Boston area libraries.

Harriot Hunt's detailed instructions about how to dispose of her estate showed her determination to promote her legacy, protect her homes, honor her beloved dead niece, and support the reform causes nearest to her heart. But in the end, the passage of time took its toll—Hunt's properties were eventually sold, the plates to *Glances and Glimpses* have disappeared, as has the unfinished manuscript of the second volume of her autobiography, and its author is largely forgotten in contemporary times. But one can still visit Hunt's gravesite found in the Mount Auburn Cemetery in Cambridge, Massachusetts. A marble statue of Hygeia, the ancient Greek goddess of good health, which Hunt commissioned from the African American sculptor Edmonia Lewis, adorns her grave.[104]

In her 1902 reminiscences, Ednah Dow Cheney offered a tribute to Hunt. She portrayed her friend as "a rare type of woman in whom heart and intellect, fancy and sound common-sense were all mingled in strange profusion." Cheney also claimed that Hunt was "among the most remarkable" of "the pioneers of women physicians." Although denied the "advantages of a college education," Hunt "made a path for women on which many a noble successor has followed." Besides these accolades, Cheney emphasized what so many others noted about Hunt—her "joyous laugh," one that was "contagious" and helped those around her, including her patients.[105]

But perhaps what was best about Cheney's recollection was an anecdote she told about Hunt. Once when Hunt had to visit the Boston courthouse, she protested against chains at the building's entrance. These had been erected to deter crowds from rescuing fugitive slaves. Hunt, asserted Cheney, "would not stoop under a chain" and insisted it be taken down.[106] This was a fitting story to tell about a woman who devoted her life to tearing down barriers that denied women their opportunities and rights

Note on Digitized Nineteenth-Century Newspapers and Journals

Newspaper articles cited in this book can be accessed from numerous databases, but especially GenealogyBank.com, America's Historical Newspapers, 19th Century U.S. Newspapers, Chronicling America: Historic American Newspapers, American Periodical Series and ProQuest Historical Newspapers: *The New York Times* (1851–2010) with Index (1851–1993). American Periodical Series Online provided me with articles from nineteenth-century periodicals and journals.

Notes

Abbreviations

Countway Library: Francis A. Countway Library of Medicine, Harvard Medical Library, Boston, MA.
HUA: Harvard University Archives, Cambridge, MA.
MJA: Massachusetts Judicial Archives, Boston, MA.
Schlesinger Library: The Arthur and Elizabeth Schlesinger Library on the History of Women in America, Radcliffe Institute for Advanced Study, Harvard University, Cambridge, MA.
Weld-Grimké Family Papers: William L. Clements Library, University of Michigan, Ann Arbor, MI.
WRHS: Western Reserve Historical Society, Cleveland, Ohio.

Introduction

1. "Obituary [of Harriot Kezia Hunt]," *Boston Daily Advertiser*, January 5, 1875. See also the obituaries in the *Boston Morning Journal*, January 5, 1875; the *Salem Register*, January 7, 1875; the *Boston Traveler*, January 9, 1875; and the *Lowell Daily Citizen and News*, February 25, 1875.
2. These remarks appear in Elizabeth Cady Stanton, Susan B. Anthony, and Matilda Joslyn Gage, eds., *History of Woman Suffrage*, 3 vols. (1881; repr., New York: Arno and New York Times, 1969), 2:582–83.
3. See the dedication page of ibid., vol. 1.
4. Mary Roth Walsh, *"Doctors Wanted: No Women Need Apply": Sexual Barriers in the Medical Profession, 1835–1975* (New Haven, CT: Yale University Press, 1977), xiv, 1.
5. Susan Wells, *Out of the Dead House: Nineteenth-Century Women Physicians and the Writing of Medicine* (Madison: University of Wisconsin Press, 2001), 28–30.
6. Nora N. Nercessian, *"Worthy of the Honor": A Brief History of Women at Harvard Medical School* (Boston: Prepared for the Committee on the Celebration of 50 Years of Women at Harvard Medical School, 1995), 10–20.
7. Harriet H. Robinson, *Massachusetts in the Woman Suffrage Movement: A General, Political, Legal and Legislative History from 1774 to 1881* (1881; repr., Forgotten Books, 2012), 22; Stanton, Anthony, and Gage, *History of Woman Suffrage*, 1:259–60, reprints Hunt's first protest in 1852.
8. See, for example, "Speech of Harriot K. Hunt to the 1851 Women's Rights Convention, Assembled in Worcester, MA," in the *Proceedings of the Woman's Rights Convention, Held at Worcester, October 15th and 16th, 1851. . . .* (New York: Fowler and Wells, 1852), 59–62, accessed from *Women and Social Movements in the United States, 1600–2000: Scholar's Edition*, ed. Kathryn Kish Sklar and Thomas Dublin, http://asp6new.alexanderstreet.com.

9. Martha H. Verbrugge, *Able-Bodied Womanhood: Personal Health and Social Change in Nineteenth-Century Boston* (New York: Oxford University Press, 1988), 49–80.
10. Julia A. Sprague, *History of the New England Women's Club from 1868 to 1893* (Boston: Lee and Shepard Publishers, 1894); Karen J. Blair, *The Clubwoman as Feminist: True Womanhood Redefined, 1868-1914* (New York: Holmes & Meier Publishers, 1980), 31–38.
11. Arlene Marcia Tuchman, *Science Has No Sex: The Life of Marie Zakrzewska, M.D.* (Chapel Hill: University of North Carolina Press, 2006), 66–67, 68, 75, 171; Walsh, "Doctors Wanted," 82–89; Virginia G. Drachman, *Hospital with a Heart: Women Doctors and the Paradox of Separatism at the New England Hospital, 1862–1969* (Ithaca, NY: Cornell University Press, 1984), 35.
12. Stanton, Anthony, and Gage, *History of Woman Suffrage*, 3:299; Robinson, *Massachusetts in the Woman Suffrage Movement*, 135.
13. Caroline Skinner, *Women Physicians and Professional Ethos in Nineteenth-Century America* (Carbondale: Southern Illinois University Press, 2014), esp. 7–8, 13, 49, 64–65; Lamar Riley Murphy, *Enter the Physician: The Transformation of Domestic Medicine, 1760-1860* (Tuscaloosa: University of Alabama Press,1991), 213–18; Regina Markell Morantz-Sanchez, *Sympathy and Science: Women Physicians in American Medicine* (1985; repr., Chapel Hill: University of North Carolina Press, 2000), esp. 35, 57; Regina Markell Morantz, "The Perils of Feminist History," *Journal of Interdisciplinary History* 4, no.4 (Spring 1974): 655–60; Walsh, "Doctors Wanted," esp. 20–34. See also Dorothy Eleanor Battenfeld, "'She hath done what she could': Three Women in the Popular Health Movement: Harriot Kezia Hunt, Mary Gove Nichols, and Paulina Wright Davis" (master's thesis, George Washington University, 1985), esp. 37–42, 62–73, and Janet Karen Henderson, "Four Nineteenth-Century Professional Women" (EdD diss., Graduate School of Education of Rutgers, State University of New Jersey, 1982), ProQuest (UMI 821823), 45–48, 68–112.
14. Wells, *Out of the Dead House*, 29–30; Nina Baym, *American Women of Letters and the Nineteenth-Century Sciences: Styles of Affiliation* (New Brunswick, NJ: Rutgers University Press, 2002), 177–180; Cynthia J. Davis, *Bodily and Narrative Forms: The Influence of Medicine on American Literature, 1845-1915* (Stanford, CA: Stanford University Press, 2000), 63–72; Joan Burbick, *Healing the Republic: The Language of Health and the Culture of Nationalism in Nineteenth-Century America* (New York: Cambridge University Press, 1994), 220–21, 331–32, and 182–90. See also Caroline Skinner, "Delicate Authority: Ethos in the Public Rhetoric of Nineteenth-Century American Women Physicians" (PhD diss., University of Louisville, 2006), ProQuest (UMI 3228056), 98–131.
15. Sally G. McMillen, *Lucy Stone: An Unapologetic Life* (New York: Oxford University Press, 2013); Carla Bittel, *Mary Putnam Jacobi and the Politics of Medicine in Nineteenth-Century America* (Chapel Hill: University of North Carolina Press, 2009); Tuchman, *Science Has No Sex*.

Chapter 1: The Making of a Maverick

1. Kezia Wentworth was born on November 5, 1770, and Joab Hunt on November 7, 1769; they were married on November 6, 1791, in Boston. Their marriage record appears in the *Boston, Massachusetts Marriages, 1700-1809*, from ancestry.com. The notice of Harriot Hunt's birth appears in *Massachusetts, Town and Vital Records, 1620-1988*, ibid. Boston city directories in the late eighteenth and first two decades of the nineteenth centuries identify Joab Hunt's occupation. See, for example, the *Boston Directories* for 1796 and 1805, *U.K. and U.S. Directories, 1680-1830*, ibid.
2. Although no birth record has been found for Harriot's sister, the *Massachusetts, Town and Vital Records, 1620-1988*, noted the death of Sarah Hunt Wright on July 8, 1867, and gave her birth year as "about 1809," from ancestry.com.
3. Alex R. Goldfeld, *The North End: A Brief History of Boston's Oldest Neighborhood* (Charlestown, SC: History Press, 2009), 11–110; Paula J. Todisco, *Boston's First Neighborhood: The North End* (Boston: Trustees of the Public Library of the City of Boston, 1976), esp.19–21; Peter R. Knights, *The Plain People of Boston, 1830-1860: A Study in City Growth* (New York: Oxford University Press, 1971), 13.
4. The *Boston Directories* for 1806 and 1807 confirm that the Hunts moved from Lynn Street to Fleet Street.

5. Goldfeld, *North End*, 96; Todisco, *Boston's First Neighborhood*, 20–21.
6. *Abstract of the Repairs and Expenditures on the French corvette* Le Berceau, *by order of the Secretary of the Navy, under date April 2, 1801 . . .*, reprinted in the *Telescope*, May 6, 1802.
7. Donald R. Hickey, *The War of 1812: A Forgotten Conflict* (Champaign: University of Illinois Press, 2012), 7.
8. *Boston Directory*, 1806.
9. Hunt's advertisement appeared in *True American*, May 30, 1803.
10. *Boston Directory*, 1789; "Vote Distributors," *Boston Commercial Gazette*, April 1, 1816, and "Faneuil Hall Caucus," *Boston Daily Advertiser*, April 1, 1816.
11. "An Act to Incorporate the Associated Housewrights in Boston" appears in multiple New England newspapers, including the *Essex Register*, July 3, 1822; the *Salem Gazette*, July 9, 1822; and the *Christian Register*, August 9, 1822.
12. Noted in "Mechanic Association," *New England Galaxy &Masonic Magazine*, December 18, 1818, and "Mechanick Festival," *Columbian Centinel*, December 9, 1818; Gary J. Kornblith, "Self-Made Men: The Development of Middling-Class Consciousness in New England," *Massachusetts Review* 26, no. 2/3 (Summer–Autumn, 1985): 462–63.
13. Steven C. Bullock, *Revolutionary Brotherhood: Freemasonry and the Transformation of the American Social Order, 1730–1840* (Chapel Hill: University of North Carolina Press, 1996), 137–273.
14. *Massachusetts, Mason Membership Cards, 1733–1990*, no. 634, "Hunt, Job [Joab]," from ancestry.com
15. Bullock, *Revolutionary Brotherhood*, 91–98, 209–11. For reminiscences of St. Andrew's Lodge and its early nineteenth-century members, including Joab Hunt, see R. W. Moore, *A Memorial of the Half-Century Membership of R. W. Charles W. Moore* (Cambridge, MA: Printed at the Riverside Press, 1873); Moore noted that most of the lodge members in the early 1820s were "'North End Mechanics'" (25).
16. Bullock, *Revolutionary Brotherhood*, 139.
17. Ibid., esp. 138,184–86, 198–206; Paul Goodman, *Towards a Christian Republic: Antimasonry and the Great Transition in New England, 1826–1836* (New York: Oxford University Press, 1988), 12, 40–42.
18. Donald R. Hickey, *Don't Give Up the Ship! Myths of the War of 1812* (Champaign: University of Illinois Press, 2006), 98.
19. Hickey, *War of 1812*, 238–39.
20. Samuel Eliot Morison, *The Maritime History of Massachusetts, 1783–1860* (1921; repr., Boston: Houghton Mifflin, 1961), 213.
21. Benjamin W. Labaree, "The Making of an Empire: Boston and Essex County, 1790–1850," in *Entrepreneurs: The Boston Business Community, 1700–1850*, ed. Conrad Edick Wright and Katheryn P. Viens (Boston: Massachusetts Historical Society, 1997; distributed by Northeastern University Press), 345, 351–52, 355–56, 358.
22. Charles Sellers, *The Market Revolution: Jacksonian America, 1815–1846* (New York: Oxford University Press, 1991), and Douglass C. North, *The Economic Growth of the United States, 1790–1860* (New York: W. W. Norton, 1966), survey these developments.
23. Standard histories of this development include Bruce Laurie, *Artisans into Workers: Labor in Nineteenth-Century America* (New York: Hill & Wang, 1989), and Sean Wilentz, *Chants Democratic: New York City and the Rise of the American Working Class, 1788–1850*, 1984 ed. (New York: Oxford University Press, 1986).
24. Morison, *Maritime History of Massachusetts*, 214.
25. Scott Reynolds Nelson, *A Nation of Deadbeats: An Uncommon History of America's Financial Disasters* (New York: Alfred A. Knopf, 2012), 66–79; Sellers, *Market Revolution*, 103–71.
26. Sellers, *Market Revolution*, 87.
27. Daniel Peart, *Era of Experimentation: American Political Practices in the Early Republic* (Charlottesville: University of Virginia Press, 2015), 15–46; Gary J. Kornblith, "Becoming Joseph T. Buckingham: The Artisanal Struggle for Independence in Early-Nineteenth-Century Boston," in *American Artisans: Crafting Social Identity, 1750–1850*, ed. Howard B. Rock, Paul A. Gilje, and Robert Asher (Baltimore, MD: Johns Hopkins University Press, 1995): 123–34; Andrew

R. L. Cayton, "The Fragmentation of a 'Great Family': The Panic of 1819 and the Rise of the Middling Interest in Boston, 1818–1822," *Journal of the Early Republic* 2, no.2 (Summer 1982): 143–67.
28. Ronald P. Formisano, "Boston, 1800–1840: From Deferential-Participant to Party Politics" in *Boston, 1700–1980: The Evolution of Urban Politics*, ed. Ronald P. Formisano and Constance K. Burns (Westport, CT: Greenwood Press, 1984), 29–57.
29. Oscar Handlin, *Boston's Immigrants: A Study in Acculturation*, rev. and enlarged ed. (Cambridge, MA: Belknap Press of Harvard University Press, 1959), 239.
30. Robert A. McCaughey, "From Town to City: Boston in the 1820s," *Political Science Quarterly* 88, no. 2 (June 1973): 191–213.
31. Thomas H. O'Connor, *The Athens of America* (Amherst: University of Massachusetts Press, 2006), 37.
32. Goodman, *Towards a Christian Republic*, 69.
33. "Massachusetts Charitable Mechanic Association," *Boston Courier*, November 22, 1830, and December 27, 1830, listed Buckingham as a member of the committee that organized forthcoming lectures at the association.
34. Moore, *Memorial of the Half-Century Membership*, 22.
35. Ann Lee Bressler, *The Universalist Movement in America, 1770–1880* (New York: Oxford University Press, 2001), and Russell E. Miller, *The Larger Hope: The First Century of the Universalist Church in America, 1770–1870*, 2 vols. (Boston: Unitarian Universalist Association, 1979). Miller cites the growing numbers of Universalist societies by 1820 (*Larger Hope*, 1:161).
36. Charles A. Howe, "How Human an Enterprise: The Story of the First Universal Society in Boston during John Murray's Ministry," *Proceedings of the Unitarian Universalist Historical Society* 22 (1990–91): 19–34.
37. Bressler, *Universalist Movement in America*, 80–85; Miller, *Larger Hope*, 1:487–533.
38. Bressler, *Universalist Movement in America*, 85–88.
39. Ronald Schultz, *The Republic of Labor: Philadelphia Artisans and the Politics of Class, 1720–1830* (New York: Oxford University Press, 1993), 131–32, 225–26; Bruce Laurie, *Working People of Philadelphia, 1800–1850* (Philadelphia: Temple University Press, 1980), 69–76.
40. Bullock, *Revolutionary Brotherhood*, 176; Bressler, *Universalist Movement in America*, 77–80; *American National Biography Online*, s.v. "Ballou, Hosea," http://www.anb.org/articles/08/08-00080.html.
41. Linda Kerber, *Women of the Republic: Intellect and Ideology in Revolutionary America* (1980; repr., New York: W. W. Norton,1986), 189–93; Mary Beth Norton, *Liberty's Daughters: The Revolutionary Experience of American Women, 1750–1800* (1980; repr., Ithaca, NY: Cornell University Press, 1996), 263–67.
42. Lucia McMahon, *Mere Equals: The Paradox of Educated Women in the Early American Republic* (Ithaca, NY: Cornell University Press, 2012), offers a more recent discussion of this development. See also Kerber, *Women of the Republic*, 189–264, and Norton, *Liberty's Daughters*, 256–94.
43. Mary Kelley, *Learning to Stand and Speak: Women, Education, and Public Life in America's Republic* (Chapel Hill: University of North Carolina Press, 2006), 66–111.
44. For an introduction to Murray's life and writings, see Sheila L. Skemp, ed., *Judith Sargent Murray: A Brief Biography with Documents* (Boston: Bedford/St. Martin's Press, 1998).
45. Ibid., 26, 28.
46. Bressler, *Universalist Movement in America*, 88–96; Miller, *Larger Hope*, 1:534–73; and Blanche Glassman Hersh, *The Slavery of Sex: Feminist-Abolitionists in America* (Champaign: University of Illinois Press, 1978), 141, 143, 151.
47. *American National Biography Online*, s.v. "Brown, Olympia," http://www.anb.org/articles/15/15-00097.html; *Notable American Women: 1607–1950*, s.v. "Chapin, Augusta Jane" and "Hanaford, Phebe Ann Coffin," http:search.credoreference.com.; see also Bressler, *Universalist Movement in America*, 90–91, 94, and Miller, *Larger Hope*, 1:564–73.
48. Kelley, *Learning to Stand and Speak*, esp. 16–33; see also Mary Kelley, "Reading Women/

Women Reading: The Making of Learned Women in Antebellum America," *Journal of American History* 83, no. 2 (September 1996): 401-24.

49. Hamilton Andrews Hill, "Trade, Commerce, and Navigation," in *Professional and Industrial History of Suffolk County, Massachusetts*, ed. William T. Davis, 3 vols. (Boston: Boston History Company, 1894), 2:122.
50. "B," "From the *Boston Courier*," *Boston Daily Advertiser*, September 19, 1827.
51. Several Boston newspapers advertised this protest meeting. See, for example, the *Boston Daily Advertiser*, October 8, 1827.
52. Hill, "Trade, Commerce, and Navigation," 2:122, noted that by the time this repeal occurred, the Canton trade was based in New York and never returned to Boston.
53. Thomas Woody, *A History of Women's Education in the United States*, 2 vols. (New York: Octagon Books, 1974), 1:489.
54. Jo Anne Preston, "Domestic Ideology, School Reformers, and Female Teachers: Schoolteaching Becomes Women's Work in Nineteenth-Century New England," *New England Quarterly* 66, no. 4 (December 1993): 531-51; see 531 for the statistic. See also Geraldine J. Clifford, *Those Good Gertrudes: A Social History of Women Teachers in America* (Baltimore, MD: Johns Hopkins University Press, 2014), 25-27, 33-35; James M. Wallace, "The Feminization of Teaching in Massachusetts: A Reconsideration," in *Women of the Commonwealth: Work, Family, and Social Change in Nineteenth-Century Massachusetts*, ed. Susan L. Porter (Amherst: University of Massachusetts Press, 1996), 43-61; and Richard M. Bernard and Maris A. Vinovskis, "The Female Teacher in Ante-Bellum Massachusetts," *Journal of Social History* 10, no. 3 (Spring 1977): 332-45.
55. Woody, *History of Women's Education in the United States*, 1:491. Preston, "Domestic Ideology, School Reformers, and Female Teachers," 536, notes that in the early 1870s female teachers in Massachusetts earned less than 40 percent of male ones.
56. Quoted in Woody, *History of Women's Education in the United States*, 1:490. For the original source see H. Augusta Dodge, ed., *Gail Hamilton's Life in Letters*, 2 vols. (Boston: Lee & Shepard, 1901), 1:79-80, 112-13.
57. For discussions of these developments in different institutions, see Michael Meranze, *Laboratories of Virtue: Punishment, Revolution, and Authority in Philadelphia, 1760-1835* (Chapel Hill: University of North Carolina, 1996); Louis P. Masur, *Rites of Execution: Capital Punishment and the Transformation of American Culture, 1776-1865* (New York: Oxford University Press, 1989); and Myra C. Glenn, *Campaigns against Corporal Punishment: Prisoners, Sailors, Women, and Children in Antebellum America* (Albany: State University of New York Press, 1984).
58. Michel Foucault, *Discipline and Punish: The Birth of the Prison*, trans. Alan Sheridan (New York: Pantheon Books, 1977), pioneered in arguing this perspective.
59. Catherine Kelly, "Gender and Class Formations in the Antebellum North," in *A Companion to American Women's History*, ed. Nancy A. Hewitt (Malden, MA: Blackwell Press, 2002), 104, especially stresses this point.
60. Moore, *Memorial of the Half-Century Membership*, 22.
61. Ibid., 22-23.
62. Accounts of Joab Hunt's death appeared in various newspapers such as the *Newburyport Herald*, November 20, 1827; the *Salem Gazette*, November 20, 1827; and the *Masonic Mirror: and Mechanics' Intelligencer*, November 24, 1827. See also Moore, *Memorial of the Half-Century Membership*, 23.
63. *Newburyport Herald*, November 20, 1827, and the *Masonic Mirror: and Mechanics' Intelligencer*, November 24, 1827. Moore, *Memorial of the Half-Century Membership*, 22, echoed these comments when he praised Hunt for his "energetic vigor, honest industry, and inventive genius."
64. Goodman, *Towards a Christian Republic*, analyzes different aspects of the Antimasonic crusade. See also Bullock, *Revolutionary Brotherhood*, 277-307.
65. Moore, *Memorial of the Half-Century Membership*, 23; Bullock, *Revolutionary Brotherhood*, 284.

66. "Joab Hunter [sic]," *North Star* (Danville, VT), June 16, 1829; the *Jamestown (NY) Journal*, June 10, 1829, and July 1, 1829. See also Goodman, *Towards a Christian Republic*, 6.
67. Moore, *Memorial of the Half-Century Membership*, 23.
68. "Joab Hunt Estate Inventory," *Probate Records*, no. 28510, vol. 126, Part 1,1828, 156–57, Suffolk County, Massachusetts, MJA.
69. See *Probate Records*, no. 28510, vol. 342, 1818–39, 116, ibid.
70. This notice appeared in the *Boston Commercial Gazette*, December 20, 1827.
71. Robert D. Richardson Jr., *Emerson: The Mind on Fire* (Berkeley: University of California Press, 1995), esp.79–80, 86–91, 97–98, 288–92, 538.
72. Miller, *Larger Hope*, 1:98.
73. Ralph Waldo Emerson, "Self-Reliance," in *Ralph Waldo Emerson: Selected Essays*, ed. Larzer Ziff (1982; repr., New York: Penguin Classics, 1985), 177.

Chapter 2: Establishing a Medical Career

1. William G. Rothstein, *American Physicians in the Nineteenth Century: From Sects to Science* (Baltimore, MD: Johns Hopkins University Press, 1985); Paul Starr, *The Social Transformation of American Medicine* (New York: Basic Books, 1982), esp. 30–78; Joseph F. Kett, *The Formation of the American Medical Profession: The Role of Institutions, 1780–1860* (New Haven, CT: Yale University Press, 1968), esp.181–83.
2. Catherine L. Thompson, *Patient Expectations: How Economics, Religion, and Malpractice Shaped Therapeutics in Early America* (Amherst: University of Massachusetts Press, 2015), esp. 1–48; John Harley Warner, *The Therapeutic Perspective: Medical Practice, Knowledge, and Identity in America, 1820–1885* (1986; repr., Princeton, NJ: Princeton University Press, 1997), esp. 22–23, 29, 93–95; Rothstein, *American Physicians in the Nineteenth Century*, 41–53; James C. Whorton, *Crusaders for Fitness: The History of American Health Reformers* (Princeton, NJ: Princeton University Press, 1982), 13–37.
3. Elaine G. Breslaw, *Lotions, Potions, Pills, and Magic: Health Care in Early America* (New York: New York University Press, 2012), 153–59; James C. Whorton, *Nature Cures: The History of Alternative Medicine in America* (New York: Oxford University Press, 2002), 3–130; John S. Haller Jr., *Medical Protestants: The Eclectics in American Medicine, 1825–1939* (Carbondale: Southern Illinois University Press, 1994), 37–93; Lamar Riley Murphy, *Enter the Physician: The Transformation of Domestic Medicine, 1760–1860* (Tuscaloosa: University of Alabama Press, 1991), 70–100; Rothstein, *American Physicians in the Nineteenth Century*, 55–61; Susan E. Cayleff, *Wash and Be Healed: The Water-Cure Movement and Women's Health* (Philadelphia, PA: Temple University Press, 1987); Jane B. Donegan, *"Hydropathic Highway to Health": Women and Water-Cure in Antebellum America* (New York: Greenwood Press, 1986).
4. John L. Thomas, "Romantic Reform in America, 1815–1865," *American Quarterly* 17 (Winter 1965): 656–81; Rothstein, *American Physicians in the Nineteenth Century*, 55–61.
5. Haller, *Medical Protestants*, 48, 101, 96.
6. Kett, *Formation of the American Medical Profession*, vii, 31; Rothstein, *American Physicians in the Nineteenth Century*, 145.
7. Regina Markell Morantz-Sanchez, *Sympathy and Science: Women Physicians in American Medicine* (1985; repr., Chapel Hill: University of North Carolina Press, 2000), 31–32; Cayleff, *Wash and Be Healed*, 68–73, 93; Donegan, *"Hydropathic Highway to Health,"* 38–49.
8. Ellen S. More, *Restoring the Balance: Women Physicians and the Profession of Medicine, 1850–1995* (Cambridge, MA: Harvard University Press, 1999), 19.
9. Thomas Neville Bonner, *To the Ends of the Earth: Women's Search for Education in Medicine* (Cambridge, MA: Harvard University Press, 1992), 6, 172n2.
10. Arlene Marcia Tuchman, *Science Has No Sex: The Life of Marie Zakrzewska, M.D.* (Chapel Hill: University of North Carolina Press, 2006), 137–55, and Mary Roth Walsh, *"Doctors Wanted: No Women Need Apply": Sexual Barriers in the Medical Profession, 1835–1975* (New Haven, CT: Yale University Press, 1977), 35–75, offer particularly detailed discussions of this school and Gregory. Walsh lists the women's medical colleges established during the nineteenth century (180).
11. Steven J. Peitzman, *A New and Untried Course: Woman's Medical College and Medical College of Pennsylvania, 1850–1998* (New Brunswick, NJ: Rutgers University Press, 2000), 1–44.

12. Edward C. Water, *Women Medical Doctors in the United States before the Civil War: A Biographical Dictionary* (Rochester, NY: University of Rochester Press, 2016), 329–44, lists the names and schools of these female doctors. See 355–56 for a list of Boston's women physicians.
13. See, for example, Breslaw, *Lotions, Potions, Pills, and Magic*, 113–33; Ellen S. More, Elizabeth Fee, and Manon Parry, eds., *Women Physicians and the Cultures of Medicine* (Baltimore, MD: Johns Hopkins University Press, 2009), esp. 2–3; Bonner, *To the Ends of the Earth*, 6–12; Morantz-Sanchez, *Sympathy and Science*, 51–56; Walsh, "Doctors Wanted," esp. xii, 15, 106–46.
14. Robert A. Nye develops this argument in "The Legacy of Masculine Codes of Honor and the Admission of Women in the Medical Profession in the Nineteenth Century," in More, Fee, and Parry, *Women Physicians and the Cultures of Medicine*, 141–59.
15. Peitzman, *New and Untried Course*, 6.
16. Ibid., 5–8, 9–11; More, *Restoring the Balance*, 17–19.
17. Tuchman, *Science Has No Sex*, 156, 168, 172–73; Virginia G. Drachman, *Hospital with a Heart: Women Doctors and the Paradox of Separatism at the New England Hospital, 1862–1969* (Ithaca, NY: Cornell University Press, 1984), 53; Walsh, "Doctors Wanted," 85, 86, 93, 117,149, 157; Agnes C. Vietor, ed., *A Woman's Quest: The Life of Marie E. Zakrzewska, M.D.* (New York: Arno Press, 1972), 336.
18. Peitzman, *New and Untried Course*, 32.
19. Elizabeth Mott, *The Ladies' Medical Oracle: Or, Mrs. Mott's Advice to Young Females, Wives, and Mothers. . . .* (Boston: Printed and published for the authoress, 1834), 216, noted this as did the Mott's newspaper advertisements. See, for example, "Patent for the U.States," *Salem Gazette*, September 5, 1834, and January 20, 1835. See also Susan L. Porter, "Mrs. Mott: 'The Celebrated Female Physician,'" *Historic New England Magazine* (Winter/Spring 2005), 11, http://www.historicnewengland.org/NEHM/2005WinterSpringPage11.htm.2.
20. "Patent for the U.States."
21. Mott, *Ladies' Medical Oracle*, esp. 10, 17–18, 215.
22. Mott touted the curative powers of her "Life Elixir" throughout her book. See, for example, ibid., 20, 39–40, 82, 95, 150, 165–66.
23. Ibid., 5, 14.
24. Ibid., 6, 9, 14.
25. Porter, "Mrs. Mott."
26. For a record of Mott's death, see *Massachusetts Town and Vital Records, 1620–1988*, from, ancestry.com. His obituary appears in the *Boston Traveler*, September 25, 1835.
27. See, for example, "To the Ladies," *Boston Traveler*, March 29, 1836, and October 14, 1836.
28. See, for example, "To the Ladies," *Boston Post*, November 25, 1836. See also "To the Ladies!," *Boston Traveler*, in the following issues: December 9, 1836; December 20, 1836; and February 24, 1837. Mott advertised in other newspapers as well. See, for example, "Mrs. Mott, the Celebrated Female Physician," in the *Lowell (MA) Patriot*, March 30, 1837, and April 6, 1837.
29. Noted in many of the advertisements cited in the previous note. See also "To Invalids," *Boston Daily Evening Transcript*, June 24, 1837, and July 1, 1837.
30. See, for example "The Misses Hunt, Female Physicians," in the following issues of the *Boston Traveler:* May 7, 1839; August 27, 1839; October 25, 1839; and May 1, 1840.
31. See, for example, the advertisement "To the Ladies" in the following issues of the *Gloucester (MA) Telegraph*: June 1, 1839; August 3, 1839; November 2, 1839; and May 2, 1840, and "To Invalids," *Newburyport (MA) Herald*, August 17, 1838.
32. Porter, "Mrs. Mott."
33. See, for example, the advertisements in the *New-Hampshire Patriot and State Gazette*: "Female Physician, Mrs. Mott," March 30, 1843, and "Female Physician," November 23, 1843. See also Mott's advertisement in the *Boston Courier*, July 14, 1842.
34. No documents have been found to show what the fees were.
35. Will of Harriot K. Hunt, Suffolk Probate File Papers, Docket no. 56530, MJA. A photocopy of this document is found in the Harriot Kezia Hunt Papers, Schlesinger Library.
36. David Stack, *Queen Victoria's Skull: George Combe and the Mid-Victorian Mind* (New York: Hambledon Continuum, 2008), esp. 33–93, 125–41.
37. Ibid., 90.

38. Ibid., 80.
39. Robert C. Fuller, *Alternative Medicine and American Religious Life* (New York: Oxford University Press, 1989), 38–65.
40. Ibid.; John S. Haller Jr., *Swedenborg, Mesmer, and the Mind/Body Connection: The Roots of Complementary Medicine* (West Chester, PA: Swedenborg Foundation, 2010), 68–91, 131–38, 158–71; Anne Harrington, *The Cure Within: A History of Mind-Body Medicine* (New York: W. W. Norton, 2008), 39–53, 111–19; Whorton, *Nature Cures*, 103–30. Chapter 3 discusses Hunt's conversion to the ideas of Emanuel Swedenborg, a thinker who also promoted a spiritual approach to healing.
41. Susan Wells, *Out of the Dead House: Nineteenth-Century Women Physicians and the Writing of Medicine* (Madison: University of Wisconsin Press, 2001), esp. 13, 16, 19, 28–38.
42. Regina Markell Morantz-Sanchez, "Gendering of Empathic Expertise: How Women Physicians Became More Empathic than Men," in *The Empathic Practitioner: Empathy, Gender, and Medicine*, ed. Ellen Singer More and Maureen Milligan (New Brunswick, NJ: Rutgers University Press, 1994), 42–43; Morantz-Sanchez, *Sympathy and Science*, 188–91.
43. Ann Douglas Wood, "'The Fashionable Diseases': Women's Complaints and Their Treatment in Nineteenth-Century America," *Journal of Interdisciplinary History* 4, no. 1 (Summer 1973): 40–45.

Chapter 3: Coping with Family Tragedy and Professional Rejection during the 1840s

1. Their marriage announcement appears in the *New-Hampshire Sentinel*, October 7, 1840, and the *Christian Watchman*, October 9, 1840.
2. *Massachusetts, Town and Vital Records, 1620–1988*, from ancestry.com.
3. C. Dallett Hemphill, *Siblings: Brothers and Sisters in American History* (New York: Oxford University Press, 2011), 153–85; Lee Virginia Chambers-Schiller, *Liberty, a Better Husband: Single Women in America: The Generations of 1780–1840* (New Haven, CT: Yale University Press, 1984), 127–48. Leonore Davidoff, *Thicker than Water: Siblings and Their Relations, 1780–1920* (New York: Oxford University Press, 2012), 136–37, 140–47, notes a similar dynamic among sisters in Victorian Britain.
4. Martha H. Verbrugge, *Able-Bodied Womanhood: Personal Health and Social Change in Nineteenth-Century Boston* (New York: Oxford University Press, 1988), 51–52, 78.
5. See ibid., 49–80. Many of the records of this institute are found in the Schlesinger Library. Box 1, vols. 1–4, contain the institute's minutes and annual reports for the 1850s, years in which Hunt was particularly active in the organization.
6. Verbrugge, *Able-Bodied Womanhood*, 55.
7. *Massachusetts, Town and Vital Record, 1620–1988*, from ancestry.com. Harriot Wright's death notice appeared in the *Boston Emancipator*, October 15, 1845.
8. For a more recent, incisive introduction to Swedenborg's life and ideas, see John S. Haller Jr., *Swedenborg, Mesmer, and the Mind/Body Connection: The Roots of Complementary Medicine* (West Chester, PA: Swedenborg Foundation, 2010), 1–67.
9. Richard Silver, "The Spiritual Kingdom in America: The Influence of Emanuel Swedenborg on American Society and Culture: 1815–1860" (PhD diss., Stanford University, 1983), ProQuest (UMI 8329776).
10. Marguerite Beck Block, *The New Church in the New World: A Study of Swedenborgianism in America* (1932; repr., New York: Octagon Books, 1968), 100–111.
11. Ibid., 134, 296–97; Haller, *Swedenborg, Mesmer, and the Mind/Body Connection*, 134–35.
12. George Trobridge, *Swedenborg: Life and Teaching* (1935; repr., New York: Swedenborg Foundation, 1962), 162–63.
13. Silver, "The Spiritual Kingdom in America," 210–36, 229 for quotation; Haller, *Swedenborg, Mesmer, and the Mind/Body Connection*, esp. 127, 133, 136–37, 160, 164–65, 172–73, 181–82, 198–210; Robert C. Fuller, *Alternative Medicine and American Religious Life* (New York: Oxford University Press, 1989), 53–58.
14. *Massachusetts, Town and Vital Records, 1620–1988*, from ancestry.com.

15. Stanton's speech is reprinted in *Elizabeth Cady Stanton, Susan B. Anthony: Correspondence, Writings, Speeches*, ed. Ellen Carol DuBois (New York: Schocken Books, 1981), 246–54.
16. Chambers-Schiller, *Liberty, a Better Husband*, 211.
17. Zsuzsa Berend, "'The Best or None!' Spinsterhood in Nineteenth-Century New England," *Journal of Social History* 33, no. 4 (Summer 2004), esp. 942–46; Chambers-Schiller, *Liberty, a Better Husband*, 21, 27, 66; Chambers-Schiller, "The Single Woman: Family and Vocation among Nineteenth-Century Reformers," in *Woman's Being, Woman's Place: Female Identity and Vocation in American History*, ed. Mary Kelley (Boston: G. K. Hall,1979), 338. On British spinsters' commitment to helping others, see Martha Vicinus, *Independent Women: Work and Community for Single Women, 1850–1920* (Chicago: University of Chicago Press, 1985).
18. Harriot K. Hunt to Dr. O. W. Holmes, December 12, 1847, Harvard College Papers, 2nd ser., 15:240–41, HUA. *Glances and Glimpses*, 217–19, discusses Hunt's first application to Harvard and reprints the letters she sent to and received from the school. See also Nora N. Nercessian, *"Worthy of the Honor": A Brief History of Women at Harvard Medical School* (Boston: Prepared for the Committee on the Celebration of 50 Years of Women at Harvard Medical School, 1995), 10–14.
19. O. W. Holmes to Edward Everett, December 11, 1847, Harvard College Papers, 2nd ser., 15:239, HUA. It is curious that Holmes's letter was dated one day *before* Hunt's petition to him. Perhaps Holmes anticipated Hunt's request and drafted his letter to Harvard before he received Hunt's missive. Another possibility is that either Holmes or Hunt misdated their respective letters.
20. Minutes of the Meetings of the President and Fellows of Harvard College, December 27, 1847, UAI 5.130, box 5, Harvard University Corporation Papers, 2nd ser., HUA. The Countway Library also has a digitized copy of these minutes. See Harvard Medical School, Office of the Dean, Records, 1828–1904 (inclusive), 1869–1874 (bulk), RG M-DE01, series 00266, box C: Medical Education, 1828–1878, "Harvard Medical School Papers re admission of women," box 4, folder 5, http://nrs.harvard.edu/urn-3:HMS.Count:med00110.
21. Stephen J. Stein, *The Shaker Experience in America: A History of the United Society of Believers* (New Haven, CT: Yale University Press, 1992), 203, 114.
22. The following works have shaped my discussion of the Shakers: ibid., esp. 2–237; Glendyne R. Wergland, *Sisters in the Faith: Shaker Women and Equality of the Sexes* (Amherst: University of Massachusetts Press, 2011); Brian L. Bixby, "Seeking Shakers: Two Centuries of Visitors to Shaker Villages" (PhD diss., University of Massachusetts, Amherst, 2010), ProQuest (UMI 3397685); Suzanne R. Thurman, *"O Sisters Ain't You Happy?": Gender, Family, and Community among the Harvard and Shirley Shakers, 1781–1918* (Syracuse, NY: Syracuse University Press, 2002), 1–158; and Lawrence Foster, *Religion and Sexuality: Three American Communal Experiments of the Nineteenth Century* (New York: Oxford University Press, 1981), 21–71.
23. Stein, *Shaker Experience*, 133–48; Thurman, *"O Sisters Ain't You Happy?,"* 138–42.
24. Bixby, "Seeking Shakers," 54–139; Stein, *Shaker Experience*, 215–22; Thurman, *"O Sisters Ain't You Happy?,"* 129–33. See also Glendyne R. Wergland, ed., *Visiting the Shakers, 1850–1899: Watervliet, Hancock, Tyringham, New Lebanon* (Clinton, NY: Richard W. Couper Pr., 2010).
25. "Shirley, Massachusetts: 'Day Book No. 3,'" September 1, 1849, vol. 217, reel 39, Hamilton College Microfilm of the Shaker Manuscript Collection, 1723–1952, Rare Books, Communal Society, BX9771, S 42 1976, Clinton, NY. The original manuscript is found in the WRHS.
26. See, for example, the following entries in ibid.: September 3, 5, 9, and 10, 1849; June 3 and 4,1850; July 1,1850; August 30 and 31, 1850; April 10 and 11, 1851; September 8, 1851; and October 18 and 19, 1851. See also "Shirley, Massachusetts: Journal of the Activities of the Ministry at both Shirley and Harvard, 1851–1854," September 25, 1852, vol. 218, reel 39, and "Harvard, Massachusetts: Daily Record of Activities at Both Harvard and Shirley, Massachusetts, 1856–1859," February 15, 1856; April 11, 1858; August 6, 1858; and May 1, 1859, vol. 54, reel 31.
27. Marianne Finch, *An Englishwoman's Experience in America* (1853; repr., New York: Negro Universities Press, 1969), 139–50 (quotations on 148 and 142). The Shakers noted that Hunt and her companion, an "English lady," visited them on April 10, 1851, "Day Book No 3," vol. 217, reel 39, Shaker Manuscript Collection, Hamilton College Microfilm.
28. The Shakers also noted Hunt treating ailing female elders. See, for example, "Harvard,

Massachusetts: Daily Record of Activities at Both Harvard and Shirley, Massachusetts, 1856–1859," May 1, 1859, vol. 54, reel 31, Shaker Manuscript Collection, Hamilton College Microfilm.
29. Finch, *An Englishwoman's Experience in America*, 139.
30. The following entries in the Shaker Manuscript Collection, Hamilton College Microfilm, describe these visits: "Day Book No. 3," September 8–10, 1851, vol. 217, reel 39; "Shirley, Massachusetts: Journal of the Activities of the Ministry at Both Shirley and Harvard, 1851–1854," May 19–22, 1852, vol. 218, reel 39; "Harvard, Massachusetts: Daily Record of Activities at Both Harvard and Shirley, Massachusetts, 1856–1859," May 4, 1856, and June 24 and June 25, 1857, vol. 54, reel 31.
31. Shaker records noted this. See, for example, "Harvard, Massachusetts: Daily Record of Activities at Both Harvard and Shirley, Massachusetts, 1856–1859," April 11, 1858, and May 1, 1859, vol. 54, reel 31, in ibid. See also Finch, *An Englishwoman's Experience in America*, 142.
32. Ibid., June 26 and February 15, 1856.
33. Thurman, *"O Sisters Ain't You Happy?,"* 149–58; see also Thurman, "Shaker Women and Sexual Power: Heresy and Orthodoxy in the Shaker Village of Harvard, Massachusetts," *Journal of Women's History* 10, No. 1 (Spring 1998): 70–87.
34. Finch, *An Englishwoman's Experience in America*, 152–53, recalled meeting a Shaker mother and daughter at Hunt's home who told her a similar tale and praised the Shakers for offering them sanctuary.
35. Ibid., 148–49.
36. "Journal of a trip from Enfield, Connecticut, to Shaker Communities in Maine, New Hampshire, and Massachusetts . . . , August 30, 1850, Edward Deming Andrews Memorial Shaker Collection, Winterthur Library, Winterthur, DE.
37. Regina Markell Morantz-Sanchez, *Sympathy and Science: Women Physicians in American Medicine* (1985; repr., Chapel Hill: University of North Carolina Press, 2000), 35, 151; Morantz, "Making Women Modern: Middle-Class Women and Health Reform in Nineteenth-Century America," *Journal of Social History* 10, no. 4 (Summer 1977): 490–507.
38. Dorothy Eleanor Battenfeld, "'She hath done what she could': Three Women in the Popular Health Movement: Harriot Kezia Hunt, Mary Gove Nichols, and Paulina Wright Davis" (master's thesis, George Washington University, 1985).
39. Sally Gregory Kohlstedt, "Physiological Lectures for Women: Sarah Coates in Ohio, 1850," *Journal of the History of Medicine and Allied Sciences* 33, no.1 (January 1978): 75–81. All quotations in this and the next paragraph are taken from two letters Coates sent to Darlington, dated March 31 and October 4, 1850, reprinted on 79–81.
40. Chapter 4 will discuss Hunt's growing prosperity during the latter 1840s and 1850s.
41. Susan E. Cayleff, *Wash and Be Healed: The Water-Cure Movement and Women's Health* (Philadelphia: Temple University Press, 1987), 141–58, and Jane B. Donegan, *"Hydropathic Highway to Health": Women and Water-Cure in Antebellum America* (New York: Greenwood Press, 1986), esp. 187–90.
42. On Bremer, see Bonnie S. Anderson, *Joyous Greetings: The First International Women's Movement, 1830–1860* (New York: Oxford University Press, 2000), 19–20,182–85, and Brita K. Stendahl, *The Education of a Self-Made Woman: Fredrika Bremer, 1801–1865* (Lewiston, NY: Edward Mellon Pr., 1994). See pp. 85–101 for discussion of Bremer's trip to America. See also Margaret H. McFadden, *Golden Cables of Sympathy: The Transatlantic Sources of Nineteenth-Century Feminism* (Lexington: University Press of Kentucky, 1999), 154–61, and Signe Alice Rooth, *Seeress of the Northland: Fredrika Bremer's American Journey, 1849–1851* (Philadelphia: American Swedish Historical Foundation, 1955).
43. Fredrika Bremer, *The Homes of the New World; Impressions of America*, trans. Mary Howitt, 2 vols. (New York: Harper & Brothers, 1853), 1:142–45.
44. Ibid.
45. Ibid., 145.
46. Ibid., 144.
47. Rooth, *Seeress of the Northland*, xiii, stressed this point.
48. Fredrika Bremer, *Hertha*, trans. Mary Howitt (New York: G. P. Putnam, 1856).

49. Bremer's 1856 letter to Hunt quoted in Rooth, *Seeress of the Northland*, 135–36.
50. Judith M. Bennett, "'Lesbian-Like' and the Social History of Lesbianisms," *Journal of the History of Sexuality* 9, no. 1/2 (January–April 2000), esp. 14–17, 21–24; Martha Vicinus, *Intimate Friends: Women Who Loved Women, 1778–1928* (Chicago: University of Chicago Press, 2004), xxi, xxiv.
51. Besides Bennett, "'Lesbian-Like,'" and Vicinus, *Intimate Friends*, see Rachel Hope Cleaves, "Beyond the Binaries in Early America: Special Issue Introduction," *Early American Studies* (Fall 2014): 459–68; Sharon Marcus, *Between Women: Friendship, Desire, and Marriage in Victorian England* (Princeton, NJ: Princeton University Press, 2007), 1–72; and Carroll Smith-Rosenberg, "The Female World of Love and Ritual: Relations between Women in Nineteenth-Century America," *Signs* 1, No. 1 (Autumn 1975): 1–29.
52. The standard biography on Sarah and her younger sister, Angelina remains Gerda Lerner, *The Grimké Sisters from South Carolina: Pioneers for Women's Rights and Abolition*, 2nd rev. (1967; repr., Chapel Hill: University of North Carolina Press, 2004). See also Lerner, ed., *The Feminist Thought of Sarah Grimké* (New York: Oxford University Press, 1998).
53. Sarah Moore Grimké to Harriot Kezia Hunt, n.d., Weld-Grimké Family Papers.
54. Quoted in Lerner, *Grimké Sisters from South Carolina*, 132. For the original document, see Elizabeth Cady Stanton, Susan B. Anthony, and Matilda Joslyn Gage, eds., *History of Woman Suffrage*, 2nd ed., 3 vols. (Rochester, NY: Charles Mann, 1889), 1:81.
55. Sarah Moore Grimké, *Letters on the Equality of the Sexes and the Condition of Woman. Addressed to Mary Parker, President of the Boston Female Anti-Slavery Society* (Boston: Isaac Knapp, 1838), accessed through *Google E-Books*, 4–5, 8, 11, 15–16. For the quotation see 16 and also 98 and 122.
56. Chapter 7 will discuss Grimké's impact on *Glances and Glimpses*.
57. Lerner, *Grimké Sisters from South Carolina*, 226.
58. Ibid., 170–222.
59. Lerner, *Feminist Thought of Sarah Grimké*, 92, does not believe that there was an "erotic" component to the relationship, yet she notes that Grimké was "uncharacteristically intimate and loving" when she addressed Hunt.
60. Sarah Moore Grimké to Harriot Kezia Hunt, December 16, 1847, Weld-Grimké Family Papers. Although Grimké did not note the year, it must have been 1847 because she wanted to know how Harvard Medical School would respond to Hunt's recent request to attend lectures there.
61. Grimké to Hunt, [1850?], ibid. Grimké's reference to the first of Hunt's lectures that she gave in the North End during the spring of 1850 suggests that her letter was written during this period.
62. Grimké to Hunt, October 19, [1851?], ibid. Once again Grimké did not write down the year. But her reference to the woman's rights convention that had just been held in Worcester, Massachusetts (October 15 and16), strongly argues for the year 1851.
63. Ibid.
64. Grimké to Hunt, December 16, 1847, ibid.
65. Grimké to Hunt, n.d., ibid.

Chapter 4: Battling Harvard Medical School, Becoming a Woman's Rights Activist

1. "She-Doctoring," *New York Daily Times*, June 3, 1854.
2. *1860 United States Federal Census*, Ward 5, Boston, Suffolk County, Massachusetts, p. 4, from ancestry.com.
3. Chapter 8 discusses Hunt's will in detail.
4. "Notice on Dr. Harriet K. Hunt," *Daily Ohio Statesman*, January 9, 1862.
5. Elizabeth Cady Stanton, Susan B. Anthony, and Matilda Joslyn Gage, eds., *History of Woman Suffrage*, 2nd ed., 3 vols. (Rochester, NY: Charles Mann, 1889), 1:259.
6. Bruce Kimball, *The "True Professional Ideal" in America: A History* (Cambridge, MA: Blackwell, 1992), 169; Lee Soltow, *Men and Wealth in the United States, 1850–1870* (New Haven, CT: Yale University Press, 1975), 22–23, 60–61.

7. Alice Kessler-Harris, *Out to Work: A History of Wage-Earning Women in the United States* (1982; repr., New York: Oxford University Press, 2003), 20–72. See p. 46 for the percentage of wage-earning women in 1860.
8. Ibid., 59, 37, 72.
9. Dianne Avery and Alfred S. Konefsky, "The Daughters of Job: Property Rights and Women's Lives in Mid-Nineteenth-Century Massachusetts," *Law and History Review* 10, no. 2 (Autumn 1992): 323–56; Norma Basch, *In the Eyes of the Law: Women, Marriage, and Property in Nineteenth-Century New York* (Ithaca, NY: Cornell University Press, 1982).
10. Sarah Moore Grimké, *Letters on the Equality of the Sexes and the Condition of Woman. Addressed to Mary Parker, President of the Boston Female Anti-Slavery Society* (Boston: Isaac Knapp, 1838), accessed through *Google E-Books*, 79.
11. Thomas H. O'Connor, *The Athens of America* (Amherst: University of Massachusetts Press, 2006).
12. For good introductions to these topics, see Anne M. Boylan, *The Origins of Women's Activism: New York and Boston, 1797–1840* (Chapel Hill: University of North Carolina Press, 2002), and Bruce Dorsey, *Reforming Men and Women: Gender in the Antebellum City* (Ithaca, NY: Cornell University Press, 2002).
13. Beth A. Salerno, *Sister Societies: Women's Antislavery Organizations in Antebellum America* (DeKalb: Northern Illinois University, 2005), 68–71; Gerda Lerner, *The Grimké Sisters from South Carolina: Pioneers for Women's Rights and Abolition*, 2nd rev. ed. (1967; repr., Chapel Hill: University of North Carolina Press, 2004), 131–34.
14. Marilyn Richardson, ed., *Maria W. Stewart, America's First Black Woman Political Writer: Essays and Speeches* (Bloomington: Indiana University Press, 1987).
15. Alise Portnoy, *Their Right to Speak: Women's Activism in the Indian and Slave Debates* (Cambridge, MA: Harvard University Press, 2005), esp. 78–86; Salerno, *Sister Societies*, 71–76; Susan Zaeske, *Signatures of Citizenship: Petitioning, Antislavery, and Women's Political Identity* (Chapel Hill: University of North Carolina Press, 2003).
16. My analysis builds on the scholarship of Jürgen Habermas in *The Structural Transformation of the Public Sphere: An Inquiry into a Category of Bourgeois Society*, trans. Thomas Burger with the assistance of Frederick Lawrence (1989; repr., Cambridge, MA: MIT Press, 1996).
17. See, for example, Ellen Carol DuBois, "Women's Rights and Abolition: The Nature of the Connection" (1979), reprinted in DuBois, *Woman Suffrage and Women's Rights* (New York: New York University Press, 1998), 54–67, and Blanche Glassman Hersh, *The Slavery of Sex: Feminist-Abolitionists in America* (Champaign: University of Illinois Press, 1978).
18. Jean V. Matthews, *Women's Struggle for Equality: The First Phase, 1828–1876* (Chicago: Ivan R. Dee, 1997), 84–115; Sylvia D. Hoffert, *When Hens Crow: The Women's Rights Movement in Antebellum America* (Bloomington: Indiana University Press, 1995), 32–52.
19. Nancy Isenberg, *Sex and Citizenship in Antebellum America* (Chapel Hill: University of North Carolina Press, 1998), esp. xiii, xviii, 37–39, 71–74, 195–96. See also Isenberg, "'Pillars in the Same Temple and Priests of the Same Worship': Woman's Rights and the Politics of Church and State in Antebellum America," *Journal of American History* 85, no.1 (June 1998): 98–128.
20. Isenberg, *Sex and Citizenship in Antebellum America*, 155–90; Françoise Basch, "Women's Rights and the Wrongs of Marriage in Mid-Nineteenth-Century America," *History Workshop*, no. 22, Special American Issue (Autumn 1986): 18–40. See also the works cited in n. 9.
21. For incisive discussions of these conventions, see Sally G. McMillen, *Lucy Stone: An Unapologetic Life* (New York: Oxford University Press, 2015), 89–98; Isenberg, *Sex and Citizenship in Antebellum America*, 15–39; Matthews, *Women's Struggle for Equality*, 65–69.
22. Bonnie S. Anderson, *Joyous Greetings: The First International Women's Movement, 1830–1860* (New York: Oxford University Press, 2000), 9; Jane Rendall, *The Origins of Modern Feminism: Women in Britain, France, and the United States, 1780–1860* (New York: Schocken Books, 1984), 311.
23. Jeanne Deroine Desroches, "Letter of Jeanne Deroine and Pauline Roland to the 1851 Women's Rights Convention, Assembled in Worcester, MA," in *Proceeding of the Woman's*

Rights Convention, Held at Worcester, October 15th and 16th, 1851 (New York: Fowler and Wells, 1852), 32–35, accessed from the website *Women and Social Movements in the United States, 1600-2000: Scholar's Edition*, ed. Kathryn Kish Sklar and Thomas Dublin, http://asp6new.alexanderstreet.com. See also Anderson, *Joyous Greetings*, 8, 180, and Rendall, *Origins of Modern Feminism*, 320.

24. *American National Biography Online*, s.v. "Flagg, Josiah Foster," http://www.amb.org/articles/12/12/00281.html.
25. "Woman's Rights Convention," *New York Herald*, October 28, 1850, reprinted in John McClymer, *How Do Contemporary Newspaper Accounts of the 1850 Worcester Woman's Rights Convention Enhance Our Understanding of the Issues Debated at That Meeting?* (Binghamton, NY: State University of New York at Binghamton, 2006), document 17, accessed from Sklar and Dublin, *Women and Social Movements in the United States*. Carol Faulkner also quotes the *New York Herald*'s comments in *Lucretia Mott's Heresy: Abolition and Women's Rights in Nineteenth-Century America* (Philadelphia: University of Pennsylvania Press, 2011), 151.
26. The quotations in this and the following paragraph are from Harriot K. Hunt, "An Address on the Medical Education of Women by Harriot K. Hunt (Excerpt)," *Proceedings of the Woman's Rights Convention, Held at Worcester, October 23rd and 24th, 1850* (Boston: Prentiss and Sawyer, 1851), 45–50, reprinted in John McClymer, *Contemporary Newspaper Accounts of the 1850 Worcester Woman's Rights Convention*, document 5B. Clymer noted in his introduction that the Convention Proceedings abridged Hunt's speech due to its length.
27. Carolyn Skinner, *Women Physicians and Professional Ethos in Nineteenth-Century America* (Carbondale: Southern Illinois University Press, 2014), 47–48.
28. Ibid., 30–31, 38, 70, 79. See also Nina Baym, *American Women of Letters and the Nineteenth-Century Sciences: Styles of Affiliation* (New Brunswick, NJ: Rutgers University Press, 2002), 174–84.
29. Skinner, *Women Physicians and Professional Ethos*, 41–68.
30. Ibid., 7–8, 13, 42, 49, 64–65, and Skinner, "Delicate Authority: Ethos in the Public Rhetoric of Nineteenth-Century American Women Physicians" (PhD diss., University of Louisville, 2006), 98–131, ProQuest (UMI 3228056), 98–131.
31. All quotations are from "An Address on the Medical Education of Women by Harriot K. Hunt (Excerpt)."
32. My interpretation differs from Carolyn Skinner's assertion that Hunt rarely invoked appeals to femininity in her public addresses. See Skinner, "Delicate Authority," 121.
33. Marie Zakrzewska echoed this view when she insisted that "science had no sex." Arlene Marcia Tuchman, *Science Has No Sex: The Life of Marie Zakrzewska, M.D.* (Chapel Hill: University of North Carolina Press, 2006), 7–8.
34. This section of Hunt's address does not appear in the truncated version of her talk published in the *Proceedings* of the Worcester Convention. Fortunately, a contemporary newspaper article discussed this part of Hunt's speech. See J. G. Forman, "Women's Rights Convention at Worcester, Mass.," *New York Daily Tribune*, October 26, 1850, reprinted in McClymer, *Contemporary Newspaper Accounts of the 1850 Worcester Woman's Rights Convention*, document 18.
35. "The Woman's Rights Convention," *Liberator*, November 1, 1850, document 22, ibid.
36. Forman, "Women's Rights Convention at Worcester, Mass.," *New York Daily Tribune*, October 26, 1850, document 18, ibid.
37. Matthews, *Woman's Struggle for Equality*, 70–71.
38. "Grand Demonstration of Petticoatdom at Worcester," *Boston Daily Mail*, October 24, 1850, and October 25, 1850, evening edition, documents 14 and 15 respectively in McClymer, *Contemporary Newspaper Accounts of the 1850 Worcester Woman's Rights Convention*.
39. "Grand Demonstration of Petticoatdom at Worcester," *Boston Daily Mail*, October 25, 1850, ibid.
40. "Woman's Rights Convention," *New York Herald*, October 28, 1850, document 20, ibid.
41. Ibid., October 26, 1850, document 19.
42. Hunt addressed her letter to the "Gentlemen of the Medical Faculty of Harvard College."

Harriot K. Hunt to O. W. Holmes, November 12, 1850, Harvard College Papers, 2nd ser., 17:373, HUA. Hunt's letter appeared in the *Boston Daily Evening Transcript*, January 7, 1851, and in *Glances and Glimpses*, 265–67. Nora N. Nercessian, *"Worthy of the Honor": A Brief History of Women at Harvard Medical School* (Boston: Prepared for the Committee on the Celebration of 50 Years of Women at Harvard Medical School, 1995), 15–20, discusses Hunt's second application to Harvard.

43. For detailed discussion of these cases and reprints of relevant primary documents, see Doris Y. Wilkinson, "The 1850 Harvard Medical School Dispute and the Admission of African American Students," *Harvard Library Bulletin*, Houghton Library, Harvard University Library, 13–27, http://pds.lib.harvard.edu. See also Ronald Takaki, "Aesculapius Was a White Man: Antebellum Racism and Male Chauvinism at Harvard Medical School," *Phylon* 39 (1978): 128–34.

44. Minutes for the Meeting of the President and Fellows of Harvard College, November 30, 1850, Records of the Harvard Medical Faculty. For the Countway Library's digitized copy of these minutes, see Harvard Medical School. Office of the Dean. Records, 1828–1904 (inclusive), 1869–1874 (bulk), RG M-DE01, ser. 00266, box C: Medical Education, 1828–1878, "Harvard Medical School Papers re admission of women," Oversized-box 7, folder 16, http://nrs.harvard.edu/urn-3:HMS.Count:med00110. These minutes are also found in the Harvard Corporation Records, 9:167, HUA.

45. O. W. Holmes to Jared Sparks, November 25, 1850, Harvard College Papers, 2nd ser., 17:378, HUA.

46. While no manuscript copy exists of the students' protests against Hunt's admission to the lectures, their resolutions were reprinted in "The Female Medical Pupil" by someone who was probably enrolled at the medical school, using the pseudonym "Scalpel." See the *Boston Daily Evening Transcript*, January 3, 1851. *Glances and Glimpses*, 269–70, also reprinted this article.

47. This student protest resolution, passed on December 10, 1850, and addressed to the Harvard Medical School faculty, is found in the Countway Library, "Petitions and correspondence, re admission of colored students," Oversized-box 7, folder 18.

48. In a December 10, 1850, letter to the medical faculty, the students noted that this resolution passed with "scarcely a dissenting vote"; see ibid. According to "Scalpel," "The Female Medical Pupil," the student resolution passed with only "*one* dissenting vote."

49. December 11, 1850, "Petitions . . . re admission of colored students," Oversized-box 7, folder 18, Countway Library.

50. Minutes for December 13, 1850, Records of the Harvard Medical Faculty, ibid.

51. In an undated draft of a letter to the American Colonization Society, the faculty noted it had made this decision at their December 26, 1850, meeting. "Petitions . . . re admission of colored students," box 4, folder 9, Countway Library. Unfortunately, the location of the original letter remains unknown.

52. "Petitions . . . re admission of colored students," January 3, 1851, ibid.

53. "Common Sense," "The Medical College," *Boston Daily Journal*, December 17, 1850.

54. April R. Haynes, *Riotous Flesh: Women, Physiology, and the Solitary Vice in Nineteenth-Century America* (Chicago: University of Chicago Press, 2016), esp. 56–62; Leonard L. Richards, *Gentlemen of Property and Standing: Anti-Abolition Mobs in Jacksonian America* (New York: Oxford University Press, 1970), 30–33, 40–46, 94–95, 114–15.

55. Ronald G. Walters, "The Erotic South: Civilization and Sexuality in American Abolitionism," *American Quarterly* 25, no. 2 (May 1973), esp. 181, 185, 192. For the quotation, see 185.

56. Carol Lasser, "Voyeuristic Abolitionism: Sex, Gender, and the Transformation of Antislavery Rhetoric," *Journal of the Early Republic* 28, no.1 (Spring 2008), 83–114.

57. "From the *Providence Morning Mirror*," *Liberator*, March 14, 1851.

58. "Fourth Annual Announcement of the Female Medical College of Philadelphia," 16, confirmed that Hunt received the honorary medical degree at the second annual commencement, January 27, 1853, Archives and Special Collections, Drexel University, College of Medicine, Philadelphia, PA.

59. Quotations from this paragraph and the next two paragraphs are from Harriot K. Hunt, "Speech of Harriot K. Hunt to the 1851 Woman's Rights Convention, Assembled in Worcester, MA," in *Proceedings of the Woman's Rights Convention, Held at Worcester, October 15th and*

16th, *1851* (New York: Fowler and Wells, 1852), 59–62, accessed from Sklar and Dublin, *Women and Social Movements in the United States*.
60. Isenberg, *Sex and Citizenship in Antebellum America*, 119–20.
61. Caroline Wells Dall, "Letter to Mrs. Paulina W. Davis," *Liberator*, November 8, 1850, reprinted in McClymer, *Contemporary Newspaper Accounts of the 1850 Worcester Woman's Rights Convention*, document 24.
62. See McClymer's introduction to the Dall letter in ibid.
63. *Proceedings of the Woman's Rights Convention, Held at Syracuse, September* 8th, 9th *& 10th, 1852* (Syracuse: Printed by J. E. Masters, 1852), 41, accessed from *Google*.
64. *Proceedings of the Woman's Rights Convention, Held at West Chester, Pa., June 2d and 3d, 1852* (Philadelphia: Merrihew and Thompson, 1852), 17, accessed from "Votes for Women: Selections from the National American Woman Suffrage Association Collection, 1848–1921" (Library of Congress), *American Memory*, http://memory.loc.gov.
65. *Proceedings of the Woman's Rights Convention, Held at Syracuse*, 76–77.
66. Ibid., 94.
67. Ibid., 13.
68. Stanton, Anthony, and Gage, *History of Woman Suffrage*, 1:852–53, reprints the comments from the *Syracuse Daily Star*, September 11, 1852.
69. "The Woman's Rights Convention—The Last Act of the Drama," *New York Herald*, September 12, 1852, reprinted in ibid., 1:853–54.

Chapter 5: Seeking Political Power, Gender Equality, and Female Friendship

1. See, for example, the obituaries in the *Boston Daily Advertiser*, January 5, 1875, and the *Boston Morning Journal*, January 5, 1875.
2. Hunt, *Glances and Glimpses*, 294–95, 308–9, 339–41, and 369–70, published her protests for the years 1852–55. They also appeared in various newspapers, especially in Boston and New York. The last year for which I found evidence of her protest appearing in print was "Miss Hunt's Protest," *Lowell (MA) Daily Citizen and News*, November 27, 1866. This chapter will analyze petitions which Hunt issued prior to the publication of her 1856 life narrative. Chapter 8 will discuss Hunt's petitions from 1856 to 1866.
3. Lori D. Ginzburg, *Elizabeth Cady Stanton: An American Life* (New York: Hill and Wang, 2009), 63–64; Nancy Isenberg, *Sex and Citizenship in Antebellum America* (Chapel Hill: University of North Carolina Press, 1998), 36–39; Ellen Carol DuBois, "The Radicalness of the Woman Suffrage Movement: Notes toward the Reconstruction of Nineteenth-Century Feminism" (1975), and "Outgrowing the Compact of the Fathers: Equal Rights, Woman Suffrage, and the United States Constitution, 1820–1878" (1987), reprinted in DuBois, *Woman Suffrage and Women's Rights* (New York: New York University Press, 1998), 30–42 and 81–113, respectively.
4. Barbara Young Welke, *Law and the Borders of Belonging in the Long Nineteenth Century United States* (New York: Cambridge University Press, 2010). See also Andreas Fahrmeir, *Citizenship: The Rise and Fall of a Modern Concept* (New Haven, CT: Yale University Press, 2007), esp. 7, 37, 53, 57–59; Evelyn Nakano Glenn, *Unequal Freedom: How Race and Gender Shaped American Citizenship and Labor* (Cambridge, MA: Harvard University Press, 2002), 1–55; Linda K. Kerber, *No Constitutional Right to be Ladies: Women and the Obligations of Citizenship* (New York: Hill and Wang, 1998), 3–123; Rogers M. Smith, *Civic Ideals: Conflicting Visions of Citizenship in U.S. History* (New Haven, CT: Yale University Press, 1997), esp. 165–242; and James H. Kettner, *The Development of American Citizenship, 1608–1870* (Chapel Hill: University of North Carolina Press, 1978), 287–333.
5. Glenn, *Unequal Freedom*, esp. 29–36. See also Manisha Sinha, *The Slave's Cause: A History of Abolition* (New Haven, CT: Yale University Press, 2016), esp. 199–200, 316–19; Stephen Kantrowitz, *More Than Freedom: Fighting for Black Citizenship in a White Republic, 1829–1889* (New York: Penguin Press, 2012), 24–25, and Alexander Keyssar, *The Right to Vote: The Contested History of Democracy in the United States*, rev. ed. (New York: Basic Books, 2009), 43–49.
6. Isenberg, *Sex and Citizenship in Antebellum America*, esp. 28–32, 153–54; Kerber, *No Constitutional Right*

to Be Ladies, 236–45; Rogers M. Smith, "'One United People': Second-Class Female Citizenship and the American Quest for Community," *Yale Journal of Law and the Humanities* 1 (1989): 229–93, esp. 243–44.
7. Rosemarie Zagarri, *Revolutionary Backlash: Women and Politics in the Early American Republic* (Philadelphia: University of Pennsylvania Press, 2007), esp. 115–80.
8. Lori D. Ginzburg, *Untidy Origins: A Story of Woman's Rights in Antebellum New York* (Chapel Hill: University of North Carolina Press, 2005), 3–4, reprints the petition.
9. Ginzburg, *Elizabeth Cady Stanton*, 60–62.
10. Isenberg, *Sex and Citizenship in Antebellum America*, 34–36.
11. For discussion of the history of the suffrage movement in Hunt's home state, see Harriet H. Robinson, *Massachusetts in the Woman Suffrage Movement: A General, Political, Legal and Legislative History from 1774 to 1881* (Boston: Roberts Brothers, 1881). For a good overview of this movement in the United States, see Suzanne M. Marilley, *Woman Suffrage and the Origins of Liberal Feminism in the United States, 1820–1920* (Cambridge, MA: Harvard University Press, 1996).
12. *Proceedings of the Woman's Rights Convention, Held at Syracuse, September 8th, 9th and 10th, 1852* (Syracuse: Printed by J. E. Masters, 1852), 34, accessed from *Google*.
13. Robinson, *Massachusetts in the Woman Suffrage Movement*, 22.
14. Margot Minardi, *Making Slavery History: Abolitionism and the Politics of Memory in Massachusetts* (New York: Oxford University Press, 2010), stresses this point.
15. Douglas Baynton, "Slaves, Immigrants, and Suffragists: The Uses of Disability in Citizenship Debates," *PMLA* 120, no. 2 (March 2005): 564; Isenberg, *Sex and Citizenship in Antebellum America*, esp. 32–39; Jean V. Matthews, *Women's Struggle for Equality: The First Phase, 1828–1876* (Chicago: Ivan R. Dee, 1997), 84–115, esp. 92–94, and "Race, Sex, and the Dimensions of Liberty in Antebellum America," *Journal of the Early Republic* 6, no. 3 (Fall 1986), 278–80.
16. Quoted in Welke, *Law and the Borders of Belonging*, 93. For the original source see Elizabeth Cady Stanton to Susan B. Anthony, December 23, 1859, in *Elizabeth Cady Stanton, Susan B. Anthony: Correspondence, Writings, Speeches*, ed. Ellen Carol DuBois (New York: Schocken Books, 1981), 69.
17. Elizabeth Cady Stanton, Susan B. Anthony, and Matilda Joslyn Gage, eds., *History of Woman Suffrage*, 3 vols. (1881; repr., New York: Arno and New York Times, 1969), 1:548.
18. *Proceedings of the Woman's Rights Convention Held at the Broadway Tabernacle, in the City of New York, on Tuesday and Wednesday, Sept. 6th and 7th, 1853* (New York: Fowlers and Wells, 1853), 60–63, accessed from "Votes for Women: Selections from the National American Woman Suffrage Association Collection, 1848–1921" (Library of Congress), *American Memory*, http://memory.loc.gov.
19. Ann D. Gordon, ed., *The Selected Papers of Elizabeth Cady Stanton and Susan B. Anthony*, 4 vols. (New Brunswick, NJ: Rutgers University Press, 1997–2006), 1:104–5. Ginzburg, *Elizabeth Cady Stanton*, 161–62, quotes from this address and notes that after the Civil War, Stanton ramped up her use of nativism to denounce women's continued disenfranchisement.
20. Stephen Puleo, *A City So Grand: The Rise of an American Metropolis, Boston, 1850–1900* (Boston: Beacon Press, 2010), 70–71.
21. Robinson, *Massachusetts in the Woman Suffrage Movement*, 91–95. Newspapers listed Hunt as one of the activists who were circulating their petition throughout Massachusetts in favor of "women's rights," including the right to vote. See, for example, "Female Legislators," *Boston Evening Transcript*, April 22, 1853.
22. *Official Report of the Debates and Proceedings in the State Convention, Assembled May 4, 1853, to Revise and Amend the Constitution of the Commonwealth of Massachusetts*, 3 vols. (Boston: White & Potter, Printers to the Convention, 1853), 1:159–60, notes the presentation of Hunt's May 17, 1853, petition to the Convention.
23. Robinson, *Massachusetts in the Woman Suffrage Movement*, 95.
24. "A Righteous Protest," *Liberator*, November 25, 1853.
25. "Political Rights of Women," *Liberator*, July 15, 1853.
26. "Woman's Rights," *New York Daily Times*, November 10, 1853.
27. "Taxation without Representation," *National Era*, November 4, 1852.

28. "Should Women Vote?" *Grand River Times*, November 23, 1853.
29. *New Hampshire Patriot and State Gazette*, November 22, 1854.
30. "XYZ," "Harriot K. Hunt and Her Protest," *Boston Daily Atlas*, November 27, 1854.
31. Stanton, *History of Woman Suffrage*, 1:555, 576.
32. "Dr. Harriot Hunt," *Plain Dealer*, November 10, 1852.
33. Isenberg, *Sex and Citizenship in Antebellum America*, esp. 15–39.
34. Sarah Moore Grimké, *Letters on the Equality of the Sexes and the Condition of Woman. Addressed to Mary Parker, President of the Boston Female Anti-Slavery Society* (Boston: Isaac Knapp, 1838), accessed through *Google E-Books*, 46, 47.
35. Mary Kelley, *Learning to Stand and Speak: Women, Education, and Public Life in America's Republic* (Chapel Hill: University of North Carolina, 2006), and Kelley, "Reading Women/Women Reading: The Making of Learned Women in Antebellum America," *Journal of American History* 83, no. 2 (September 1996): 401–24.
36. Thomas Woody, *A History of Women's Education in the United States*, 2 vols. (New York: Octagon Books, 1974), 1:519–21, 529–30; Charles K. Dillaway, "Education, Past and Present: The Rise of Free Education and Educational Institutions," and Edna Dow Cheney, "The Women of Boston," in *The Memorial History of Boston, Including Suffolk County, Massachusetts, 1630–1880*, ed. Justin Winsor, 4 vols. (Boston: James R. Osgood, 1881), 4:249–54; 343–45.
37. These activities were noted in "High School for Girls," *Liberator*, April 8, 1853.
38. Hunt echoed these comments at the September 1853 national woman's rights convention. See *Proceedings of the Woman's Rights Convention Held at the Broadway Tabernacle*, 60–63.
39. Elaine Frantz Parsons, *Manhood Lost: Fallen Drunkards and Redeeming Women in the Nineteenth-Century United States* (Baltimore, MD: John Hopkins University Press, 2003); Barbara Leslie Epstein, *The Politics of Domesticity: Women, Evangelism, and Temperance in Nineteenth-Century America* (Middletown, CT: Wesleyan University Press, 1981); Jed Dannenbaum, "The Origins of Temperance Activism and Militancy among American Women," *Journal of Social History* 15, no. 2 (Winter 1981): 235–52.
40. Stanton, *History of Woman Suffrage*, 1:499–506.
41. Beth A. Salerno, *Sister Societies: Women's Antislavery Organizations in Antebellum America* (DeKalb: Northern Illinois University Press, 2005), 100–103.
42. Stanton, Anthony, and Gage, *History of Woman Suffrage*, 1:52–53 and 501, stressed the opposition of clergy to women's participation in the antislavery and temperance conventions, respectively. See 1:501 for quotation.
43. Ibid., 1:506–12; see also "The Whole World's Temperance Convention, . . . Sept. 1st and 2d, 1853 . . . ," esp. 15, 65, accessed from "Votes for Women."
44. "The Whole World's Temperance Convention," 15, 65.
45. For an especially incisive discussion of these issues, see Bruce Dorsey, *Reforming Men and Women: Gender in the Antebellum City* (Ithaca, NY: Cornell University Press, 2002), esp. 2, 38–39, 83–85, 132–34.
46. Antebellum reformers who attacked drinking and prostitution especially proselytized an evangelical model of manhood. See ibid., 100–101, 113–31, and Parsons, *Manhood Lost*, esp. 53–74.
47. "A Convention without the Usual Distinctions," Worcester, MA, *National Aegis*, September 7, 1853.
48. Elizabeth Cazden, *Antoinette Brown Blackwell: A Biography* (Old Westbury, NY: Feminist Press, 1983), 82, notes Hunt's presence at the ordination.
49. *American National Biography Online*, s.v. "Smith, Gerrit," http://www .anb.org./articles/15/15-00627html. Isenberg, *Sex and Citizenship in Antebellum America*, 75–101; see 92–93 for quotation. See also Isenberg, "'Pillars in the Same Temple and Priests of the Same Worship': Woman's Rights and the Politics of Church and State in Antebellum America," *Journal of American History* 85, no. 1 (June 1998): 98–128.
50. Isenberg, *Sex and Citizenship in Antebellum America*, 94–95, 98–99, and "'Pillars in the Same Temple and Priests of the Same Worship,'" 113–14.
51. Hunt wrote that she delivered this talk during her 1852 lecture tour of Cape Cod, Provincetown,

and Harwich, Massachusetts (284–85). In June 1854, Hunt also lectured in New York City on this topic, which was noted by the *New York Daily Times*, June 3, 1854. The *Anti-Slavery Bugle*, January 27, 1855, indicated that Hunt was soon scheduled to deliver the talk in Salem and urged people to attend.
52. Unfortunately there is no record of what Hunt discussed at the mission.
53. *Records of the Meetings of the Ladies' Physiological Institute, January 1850 to January 1851. With the Meetings of the Board of Directors, from January 1850 to December 1860*. See October 30, 1850, p. 109, and November 2, 1850, p. 112, Schlesinger Library.
54. *Records of the Meetings of the Ladies' Physiological Institute of Boston and Vicinity, from January 1st, 1851 to May, 1854*; see January 29, 1851, 3:4, ibid.
55. Ibid., Third Annual Report, May 7, 1851, 41.
56. Hunt's paean to dancing appeared under slightly different titles in various newspapers and periodicals. See, for example, "Dancing," *Athens (TN) Post*, March 21, 1856; "A Physician on Dancing," *Ballou's Pictorial Drawing-Room Companion*, January 17, 1857; and "Physician's Evidence on Dancing," *Wellsboro (PA) Gazette*, March 26, 1857.
57. My analysis relies on Elizabeth McKinsey, *Niagara Falls: Icon of the American Sublime* (New York: Cambridge University Press, 1985), esp. 32–33, 38, 41–46, 86–98.
58. Joan Burbick, *Healing the Republic: The Language of Health and the Culture of Nationalism in Nineteenth-Century America* (New York: Cambridge University Press, 1994), 190.
59. Sarah Moore Grimké to Harriot Kezia Hunt, April 5, 1853, Weld-Grimké Family Papers.
60. Ibid., n.d. This letter was probably written shortly before the Massachusetts Constitutional Convention convened in early May 1853.
61. Ibid., ca. 1853.
62. Ibid., October 19, [1851]. Although Grimké did not note the year, her reference to the recently ended convention on October 15 and 16 indicates that it was 1851.
63. Ibid., January 3, 1852.
64. Gerda Lerner, *The Grimké Sisters from South Carolina: Pioneers for Women's Rights and Abolition*, 2nd rev. ed. (1967; repr., Chapel Hill: University of North Carolina Press, 2004), esp. 222–29. Katherine Du Pre Lumpkin, *The Emancipation of Angelina Grimké* (Chapel Hill: University of North Carolina Press, 1974), views Sarah as mostly to blame for troubles with her sister, but Lerner challenges this interpretation (*Grimké Sisters*, 335n15).
65. Grimké to Hunt, December 20, 1854, Weld-Grimké Family Papers.
66. Ibid., n.d.
67. Ibid., April 5, 1853.
68. Ibid., January 3, 1852.
69. Ibid., December 31, 1852.
70. Ibid., ca. 1853 and December 31, 1852.
71. Ann Lee Bressler, *The Universalist Movement in America, 1770–1880* (New York: Oxford University Press, 2001), 85–88.

Chapter 6: Forging New Connections in the Mid-1850s

1. Sarah Moore Grimké to Harriot Kezia Hunt, February 1854 [no day cited], Weld-Grimké Family Papers.
2. *American National Biography Online*, s.v. "Smith, Gerrit," http://www.anb.org./articles/15/15-00627html.
3. Ronald G. Walters, "The Erotic South: Civilization and Sexuality in American Abolitionism," *American Quarterly* 25, no. 2 (May 1973): esp. 181–85.
4. For a more recent discussion of this issue, see Ibram X. Kendi, *Stamped from the Beginning: The Definitive History of Racist Ideas in America* (New York: Nation Books, 2016), esp. 195.
5. April R. Haynes, *Riotous Flesh: Women, Physiology, and the Solitary Vice in Nineteenth-Century America* (Chicago: University of Chicago Press, 2016), esp. 56–80, discusses how antebellum black female reformers challenged this racialization of the concept of virtue.

6. Albert J. Von Frank, *The Trials of Anthony Burns: Freedom and Slavery in Emerson's Boston* (Cambridge, MA: Harvard University Press, 1998), esp. xii–xiii and 207.
7. Ibid., 208–11.
8. Ibid., 207.
9. "Woman's Right Convention," *Liberator*, June 16, 1854.
10. "New England Woman's Rights Convention," *New-Lisbon (OH) Anti-Slavery Bugle*, June 17, 1854.
11. "Woman's Right Convention," *Liberator*, June 16, 1854.
12. The resolutions and demands of this convention were reprinted in ibid.
13. Harriot Kezia Hunt to Anna Parsons, June 4, 1854, New England Hospital Records, box 23, folder 75, Sophia Smith Collection, Smith College Special Collections, Northampton, MA.
14. Quoted in Nancy Isenberg, *Sex and Citizenship in Antebellum America* (Chapel Hill: University of North Carolina Press, 1998), 110–11. Swift's comments originally appeared in the radical feminist newspaper *Lily*, August 1856, 105–6.
15. Nina Baym discusses Hale's public support for women doctors in *American Women of Letters and the Nineteenth-Century Sciences: Styles of Affiliation* (New Brunswick, NJ: Rutgers University Press, 2002), 36–53.
16. "Editor's Table," *Godey's Lady's Book*, August 1851. See also the August 1852, December 1853, and May 1854 issues.
17. Catharine E. Beecher, *Letters to the People on Health and Happiness* (New York: Harper & Brothers, 1855), 115–16, 119, 141–43. See also "Notes," 16 (at end of text).
18. Kathryn Kish Sklar, *Catharine Beecher: A Study in American Domesticity* (New York: W. W. Norton, 1973), 204–6.
19. Beecher, *Letters*, "Notes," 16.
20. Ibid., 119.
21. Sklar, *Catharine Beecher*, 209–10.
22. "Female Physicians," May 14, 1852, and "Mrs. Goulding, the Intelligent Agent of the College for Educating Female Physicians . . . ," July 10, 1852, both in *Bangor (ME) Daily Whig and Courier*.
23. "Female Physicians," *Cleveland (OH) Herald*, January 5, 1852.
24. "Female Medical College," *Western Reserve Chronicle*, July 11, 1855.
25. "Female Physicians," *Lowell (MA) Daily Citizen and News*, August 12, 1858.
26. "Female Physicians," *Herald of Freedom*, January 27, 1855.
27. "Female Physicians," *New York Daily Times*, July 27, 1853.
28. Mary Roth Walsh, *"Doctors Wanted: No Women Need Apply": Sexual Barriers in the Medical Profession, 1835–1975* (New Haven, CT: Yale University Press, 1977), 28, 90, 109, 133, 135, 142, 172–73, 198.
29. "Female Physicians," *Boston Medical and Surgical Journal*, February 16, 1853.
30. Ohio newspapers were reporting on Hunt's speeches through late February 1855. Carolyn Skinner, "Delicate Authority: Ethos in the Public Rhetoric of Nineteenth-Century American Women Physicians" (PhD diss., University of Louisville, 2006), ProQuest (UMI 3228056), 106–16, discusses Hunt's Ohio trip.
31. Virginia Elwood-Akers, *Caroline Severance* (Bloomington, NY: iUniverse, 2010).
32. Ibid., 48–49.
33. "Ladies as Physicians—The Movement in Ohio," *Columbus (OH) Daily Capital City Fact*, February 22, 1855, evening ed.
34. John White Chadwick, ed., *Sallie Holley, a Life for Liberty: Anti-Slavery and Other Letters of Sallie Holley* (1899; repr., New York: Negro Universities Press, 1969), 147.
35. John S. Haller Jr., *Medical Protestants: The Eclectics in American Medicine, 1825–1939* (Carbondale: Southern Illinois Press, 1994), 94–124.
36. "Special Notices," *Cleveland Daily Plain Dealer*, February 3, 1855, evening ed.; "The Annual Meeting," *Cleveland Morning Leader*, February 5, 1855, morning ed.; "Female Physicians," *Columbus Daily Ohio State Journal*, February 17, 1855, evening ed.; "Ladies as Physicians—The Movement in Ohio," *Columbus Daily Capital Fact*, February 22, 1855, evening ed.

37. "Ladies as Physicians—The Movement in Ohio," *Daily Capital City Fact*, February 22, 1855, evening ed.
38. "The Annual Meeting," *Cleveland Morning Leader*, February 5, 1855, morning ed.
39. "Female Physicians," *Daily Ohio State Journal*, February 17, 1855, evening ed.
40. "Human Rights," *Cincinnati Daily Times*, February 24, 1855, evening ed.
41. "Ladies as Physicians—The Movement in Ohio," *Daily Capital City Fact*, February 22, 1855, evening ed.
42. "Woman's Rights Convention," *Liberator*, September 28, 1855, offered an extensive account of the convention and printed Hunt's resolutions.
43. Walsh, *"Doctors Wanted,"* 46–48.
44. Ibid., 150–51, 104.
45. Elizabeth Blackwell, *An Appeal in Behalf of the Medical Education of Women* (New York: n.p., 1856), 13. See also Walsh, *"Doctors Wanted,"* 81–83, 33n73.
46. Arleen Marcia Tuchman, *Science Has No Sex: The Life of Marie Zakrzewska, M.D.* (Chapel Hill: University of North Carolina Press, 2006), 62–69; Agnes C. Vietor, ed., *A Woman's Quest: The Life of Marie E. Zakrzewska, M.D.* (1924; repr., New York: Arno Press, 1972), esp. 134–35; see also Walsh, *"Doctors Wanted,"* 76–105.
47. Vietor, *A Woman's Quest*, 137, 134–35.
48. Tuchman, *Science Has No Sex*, 171–72; Vietor, *A Woman's Quest*, 149–50, 336; Walsh, *"Doctors Wanted,"* 81–82, 88–89.
49. Various historians have stressed this point. See, for example, Tuchman, *Science Has No Sex*, 12, 60–62, 93–95; Regina Markell Morantz-Sanchez, *Sympathy and Science: Women Physicians in American Medicine* (1985; repr., Chapel Hill: University of North Carolina Press, 2000), 73–75.
50. Besides the sources cited above, see Walsh, *"Doctors Wanted,"* 84.
51. Quoted in Tuchman, *Science Has No Sex*, 134. For the original source, see *A Practical Illustration of "Woman's Right to Labor"; or, A Letter from Marie E. Zakrzewska, M.D. Late of Berlin, Prussia*, ed. Caroline H. Dall (1860; repr., n.p.: Dodo Press, n.d.), 34.
52. Carla Bittel, *Mary Putnam Jacobi and the Politics of Medicine in Nineteenth-Century America* (Chapel Hill: University of North Carolina Press, 2009), 97–98, 117.
53. Mary Putnam Jacobi, "Woman in Medicine," in *Woman's Work in America*, ed. Annie Nathan Meyer (New York: Henry Holt, 1891), 139–205. For the quotation, see 157.
54. Sarah Moore Grimké to Harriot Kezia Hunt, May 23, 1855, Weld-Grimké Family Papers.
55. The following works have shaped my understanding of spiritualism in antebellum America: Robert S. Cox, *Body and Soul: A Sympathetic History of American Spiritualism* (Charlottesville: University of Virginia Press, 2003); Ann Taves, *Fits, Trances, and Visions: Experiencing Religion and Explaining Experience from Wesley to James* (Princeton, NJ: Princeton University Press, 1999), 166–206; Bret E. Carroll, *Spiritualism in Antebellum America* (Bloomington: Indiana University Press, 1997); Ann Braude, *Radical Spirits: Spiritualism and Women's Rights in Nineteenth-Century America* (Boston: Beacon Press, 1989); and R. Laurence Moore, *In Search of White Crows: Spiritualism, Parapsychology, and American Culture* (New York: Oxford University Press, 1977), 1–69.
56. Grimké to Hunt, December 16, 1847, Weld-Grimké Family Papers.
57. Carroll, *Spiritualism in Antebellum America*, 22–23, 30.
58. Emma Hardinge Britten, *Modern American Spiritualism: A Twenty Years' Record of the Communion between Earth and the World of Spirits* (New York: Published by the Author, 1870), reprints the scientists' report. See also Moore, *In Search of White Crows*, 33–34, and Cox, *Body and Soul*, 124.

Chapter 7: *Glances and Glimpses*—Harriot Hunt's "Heart History," Jeremiad, and Reform Manifesto

1. Sarah Moore Grimké to Harriot Kezia Hunt, December 20, 1854, Weld-Grimké Family Papers. Although Grimké did not note the year, internal evidence dates her letter as 1854.
2. Marie Zakrzewska noted this fact when she recalled meeting Grimké and Angelina and

Theodore Weld at Hunt's house. See Agnes C. Vietor, *A Woman's Quest: The Life of Marie E. Zakrzewska, M.D.* (New York: D. Appleton, 1924), 149–50.
3. The title page states the publication date as 1856.
4. *Boston Daily Atlas*, December 12, 1855.
5. See, for example, *Liberator*, November 30, 1855; *Boston Recorder*, December 6, 1855; *Inventor*, January 1, 1856; and *California Farmer and Journal of Useful Sciences* (Sacramento, CA) 5, no. 14 (April 11, 1856): 2.
6. *New York Daily Tribune*, January 28 and 30, 1856; *Liberator*, February 8, 15, and 29 and March 14, 1856.
7. *Boston Daily Atlas*, April 24, 1856; *New-York Daily Tribune*, April 28, 1856; *Liberator*, June 27, 1856.
8. Major theoreticians who have shaped the study of autobiographical writing include Sidonie Smith and Julia Watson, *Reading Autobiography: A Guide for Interpreting Life Narratives* (Minneapolis: University of Minnesota Press, 2001); Philippe Lejeune, *On Autobiography*, ed. and introduction by Paul John Eakin (Minneapolis: University of Minnesota Press, 1989); see also Eakin's own works, esp. *Living Autobiography: How We Create Identity in Narrative* (Ithaca, NY: Cornell University Press, 2008), and two of his other books published by Princeton University Press: *Touching the World: Reference in Autobiography* (1992), and *Fictions in Autobiography: Studies in the Art of Self Invention* (1985), and James Olney, ed., *Autobiography: Essays Theoretical and Critical*, and *Metaphors of Self: The Meaning of Autobiography*, both published by Princeton University Press in 1980 and 1972, respectively. Major scholarship on women's life narratives include Martine Watson Brownley and Allison B. Kimmich, eds., *Women and Autobiography* (Wilmington, DE: Scholarly Resources, 1999); Martha Watson, *Lives of Their Own: Rhetorical Dimensions in Autobiographies of Women Activists* (Colombia: University of South Carolina Press, 1999); Sidonie Smith and Julia Watson, eds., *Women, Autobiography, Theory: A Reader* (Madison: University of Wisconsin Press, 1998); Mary Jean Corbett, *Representing Femininity: Middle-Class Subjectivity in Victorian and Edwardian Women's Autobiographies* (New York: Oxford University Press, 1992); Personal Narratives Group, ed., *Interpreting Women's Lives: Feminist Theory and Personal Narratives* (Bloomington: Indiana University Press,1989); Carolyn G. Heilbrun, *Writing a Woman's Life* (New York: W.W. Norton,1988); Shari Benstock, ed., *The Private Self: Theory and Practice of Women's Autobiographical Writings* (Chapel Hill: University of North Carolina Press,1988); Sidonie Smith, *A Poetics of Women's Autobiography: Marginality and the Fictions of Self-Representation* (Bloomington: Indiana University Press, 1987); Estelle C. Jelinek, ed., *Women's Autobiography: Essays in Criticism* (Bloomington: Indiana University Press, 1980).
9. Louis Kaplan, comp., *A Bibliography of American Autobiographies* (Madison: University of Wisconsin Press, 1962).
10. Estelle Jelinek, *The Tradition of Women's Autobiography: From Antiquity to the Present* (Boston: Twayne Press, 1986), xiii; Jelinek, *Women's Autobiography*, 17, 19.
11. Although Jelinek asserts that women's autobiographies were generally briefer than men's, a review of the antebellum female narratives cited in Kaplan, *A Bibliography of American Autobiographies*, shows that in the 1850s these texts did become noticeably longer.
12. See, for example, Abigail Bailey, *Memoirs*. . . . (Boston: Samuel T. Armstrong, 1815).
13. Anna Matlack Richards, *Memories of a Grandmother, by a Lady of Massachusetts* (Boston: Gould & Lincoln, 1854).
14. *Notable American Women, 1607–1950: A Biographical Dictionary*, 1:598–600, s.v. "Farnham, Eliza Wood Burhans."
15. Eliza W. Farnham, *Life in Prairie Land* (1846; repr., Champaign: University of Illinois Press, 1988), and *California, In-doors and Out; or, How We Farm, Mine, and Live Generally in the Golden State* (New York: Dix, Edwards, 1856).
16. Lucy Richards, *Memoirs*. . . . (New York: G. Lane & P. P. Sandford, 1842); Harriet Livermore, *A Narration of Religious Experience: In Twelve Letters* (Concord, NH: Printed by Jacob B. Moore, for the author, 1826).
17. Jarena Lee, *The Life and Religious Experience of Jarena Lee, a Coloured Lady*. . . . (Philadelphia:

Published for the author, 1836), and Zilpha Elaw, *Memoirs*. . . . (London: Published by the author, 1846). William L. Andrews has edited and introduced these works in *Sisters of the Spirit: Three Black Women's Autobiographies of the Nineteenth Century* (Bloomington: Indiana University Press, 1986), 25–160. For more recent analyses of these and other autobiographies by female preachers in the nineteenth century, see Rosetta Renae Haynes, *Radical Spiritual Motherhood: Autobiography and Empowerment in Nineteenth-Century African American Women* (Baton Rouge: Louisiana State University Press, 2010), and Elizabeth Elkin Grammer, *Some Wild Visions: Autobiographies by Itinerant Female Preachers in Nineteenth-Century America* (New York: Oxford University Press, 2003). On Jacobs, see Jennifer Fleischner, ed., *Incidents in the Life of a Slave Girl Written by Herself, by Harriet Jacobs, with Related Documents* (Boston: Bedford/St. Martin's Press, 2010). See also Jean Fagan Yellin, *Harriet Jacobs: A Life* (New York: Basic Civitas Books, 2004).

18. George Gusdorf, "Conditions and Limits of Autobiography," reprinted in Olney, *Autobiography*, 28–48.
19. Carol Gilligan, *In a Different Voice: Psychological Theory and Women's Development* (1982; repr., Cambridge, MA: Harvard University Press, 1993), and Nancy Chodorow, *Psychoanalysis and the Sociology of Gender* (Berkeley: University of California Press, 1978), esp. 167–69, 176–78, are seminal texts on this issue.
20. Smith, *A Poetics of Women's Autobiography*, esp. 3–19, 44–62; Shari Benstock, "The Female Self Engendered: Autobiographical Writing and Theories of Selfhood," in Brownley and Kimmich, *Women and Autobiography*, 3–13; Benstock, "Authorizing the Autobiographical," esp. 19–20, and Susan Stanford Friedman, "Women's Autobiographical Selves: Theory and Practice," esp. 34–44, both in Benstock, *Private Self*.
21. Heilbrun, *Writing a Woman's Life*, 12–13.
22. Ann Fabian, *The Unvarnished Truth: Personal Narratives in Nineteenth-Century America* (Berkeley: University of California Press, 2000), esp.7, 171–73, discusses how the narratives of antebellum marginal people, such as beggars, convicts, and slaves, did this.
23. Patricia Spacks, "Selves in Hiding," in Jelinek, *Women's Autobiography*, 112–32. See also Heilbrun, *Writing a Woman's Life*, esp. 12–26, and Heilbrun, "Woman's Autobiographical Writings: New Forms," 15–32, and Sidonie Smith, "Construing Truth in Lying Mouths: Truthtelling in Women's Autobiography, esp. 46–47, both in Brownley and Kimmich, *Women and Autobiography*.
24. *Notable American Women, 1607–1950*, 2:596–98, s.v. "Mowatt, Anna Cora Ogden."
25. Anna Cora Mowatt, *Autobiography of an Actress; or, Eight Years on the Stage* (Boston: Ticknor, Reed, and Fields, 1854).
26. Grimké to Harriot Kezia Hunt, December 20, 1854, Weld-Grimké Family Papers. On the Hunt-Mowatt relationship, see *Glances and Glimpses*, 168, 321–22, 332–34.
27. Mowatt, *Autobiography of an Actress*, 3, 371.
28. Ibid., 139.
29. Elizabeth Blackwell, *Pioneer Work in Opening the Medical Profession to Women: Autobiographical Sketches* (1895; repr., New York: Source Book Press, 1970). More recent scholarly analyses of Blackwell's autobiography also stress these points: Mary Daniels Brown, "Personal and Social Identity in the Life Stories of Five Nineteenth-Century Women Physicians" (PhD diss., Saybrook University, 2011), ProQuest (UMI 3464640), 53–78; Carolyn Skinner, "Delicate Authority: Ethos in the Public Rhetoric of Nineteenth-Century American Women Physicians" (PhD diss., University of Louisville, 2006), ProQuest (UMI 3228056), 168–88; Nina Baym, *American Women of Letters and the Nineteenth-Century Sciences: Styles of Affiliation* (New Brunswick, NJ: Rutgers University Press, 2002), 180–83.
30. Blackwell, *Pioneer Work in Opening the Medical Profession to Women*, 154–57, 198.
31. Ibid., 197.
32. Ibid., 178–79.
33. Elizabeth Cady Stanton, *Eighty Years and More: Reminiscences, 1815–1897* (1898; repr., New York: Schocken Books, 1971), preface.

34. Lori D. Ginzberg, *Elizabeth Cady Stanton: An American Life* (New York: Hill and Wang, 2009), 181.
35. Ibid.; Watson, *Lives of Their Own*, 63–81, esp. 75–76; Jelinek, *Tradition of Women's Autobiography*, 107-27.
36. Patricia Spacks, "Stages of Life: Notes on Autobiography and the Life Cycle," *Boston University Journal* 25, no. 2 (1977):14–15.
37. Heilbrun, *Writing a Woman's Life*, 15.
38. Spacks, "Stages of Life," 9–10.
39. Cynthia Davis, *Bodily and Narrative Forms: The Influence of Medicine on American Literature, 1845–1915* (Stanford, CA: Stanford University Press, 2000), 70.
40. Ibid., 63–72.
41. Fred Somkin, *Unquiet Eagle: Memory and Desire in the Idea of American Freedom, 1815–1860* (Ithaca, NY: Cornell University Press, 1967), explores this theme.
42. See esp. 82–90; 122; 151–55; 172–73; 216; 271.
43. April R. Haynes, *Riotous Flesh: Women, Physiology, and the Solitary Vice in Nineteenth-Century America* (Chicago: University of Chicago Press, 2015), esp. 58, 60, 76–77, 79; Mary P. Ryan, "The Power of Women's Networks: A Case Study of Female Moral Reform in Antebellum America," *Feminist Studies* 5, no. 1 (Spring 1979): 66–85.
44. Sarah Moore Grimké, *Letters on the Equality of the Sexes and the Condition of Woman. Addressed to Mary Parker, President of the Boston Female Anti-Slavery Society* (Boston: Isaac Knapp, 1838), esp. 74-97, accessed through *Google E-Books*. For quotations see 86 and 74.
45. *The Proceedings of the Woman's Rights Convention, Held at Worcester, October 15th and 16th, 1851*. . . . (New York: Fowlers and Wells, 1852), 29 and 37, accessed from *Women and Social Movements in the United States, 1600-2000: Scholar's Edition*, ed. Kathryn Kish Sklar and Thomas Dublin, http://asp6new.alexanderstreet.com.
46. Ann Russo and Cheris Kramarae, eds., *The Radical Women's Press of the 1850s* (New York: Routledge, 1991), 69–94. For quotations see 74–75, 86, and 79–80.
47. Quotations are from Elizabeth Oakes Smith, *Woman and Her Needs* (New York: Fowlers and Wells, 1851). For a more recent discussion of Smith's life and work, see Adam Tuchinsky, "'Woman and Her Needs': Elizabeth Oakes Smith and the Divorce Question," *Journal of Woman's History* 28, no. 1 (Spring 2016): 38–59.
48. Patricia Cline Cohen, "The 'Anti-Marriage Theory' of Thomas and Mary Gove Nichols: A Radical Critique of Monogamy in the 1850s," *Journal of the Early Republic* 34, no.1 (Spring 2014): 2.
49. T. L. Nichols and Mary S. Gove Nichols, *Marriage: Its History, Character, and Results: Its Sanctities and Its Profanities; Its Science and Its Facts*. . . . (New York: T. L. Nichols, 1854). For more recent discussions of this work, see Cohen, "'Anti-Marriage Theory' of Thomas and Mary Gove Nichols," esp. 1, 6, and Jean Silver-Isenstadt, *Shameless: The Visionary Life of Mary Gove Nichols* (Baltimore, MD: Johns Hopkins University Press, 2002), 178–85.
50. Cohen, "'Anti-Marriage Theory' of Thomas and Mary Gove Nichols," 1.
51. [Mary S. Gove Nichols], *Mary Lyndon: Revelations of a Life* (New York: Stringer and Townsend, 1855).
52. Margaret Fuller, *Woman in the Nineteenth Century: An Authoritative Text, Backgrounds, Criticism*, ed. Larry J. Reynolds, Norton Critical Edition (New York: W. W Norton, 1998), 68–69.
53. Ibid., 20.
54. Anthony's speech "Homes for Single Women," first delivered in October 1877, appears in Ellen Carol DuBois, ed., *Elizabeth Cady Stanton, Susan B. Anthony: Correspondence, Writings, Speeches* (New York: Schocken Books, 1981), 146–51.
55. "New Publications," *Boston Daily Atlas*, December 27, 1855.
56. "New Publications," *Salem (MA) Register*, December 31, 1855.
57. Frank Luther Mott, *A History of American Magazines, 1850–1865* (Cambridge, MA: Belknap Press of Harvard University Press, 1957), surveys the political/religious affiliations of different mid-nineteenth-century American journals.
58. "Book Notices," *Happy Home and Parlor Magazine*, February 1, 1856.

59. *New Englander* 14, no. 54 (May 1856): 321.
60. "Literary Notices," *Country Gentleman* 7, no. 2 (January 10, 1856): 35.
61. *Evening Star*, January 3, 1856.
62. "A Hint for Political Leaders," *Cape Ann Light and Gloucester Telegraph*, January 19, 1856.
63. *New Englander* 14, no. 54 (May 1856): 321.
64. "New Books," *New Hampshire Patriot and State Gazette*, February 20, 1856.
65. "New Publications," *New York Daily Times*, March 27, 1856.
66. "J. C. B.," "Glances and Glimpses," *Ohio Cultivator* 12, no. 6 (March 15, 1856): 91.
67. *Christian Examiner and Religious Miscellany* 60, no. 2 (March 1856): 314.
68. "New Publications," *New York Daily Times*, March 27, 1856.
69. "A Grandmother," "Glances and Glimpses," *Boston Evening Transcript*, February 2, 1856.
70. "C," "Glances and Glimpses," ibid., February 7, 1856.
71. "New Books," *New Hampshire Patriot and State Gazette*, February 20, 1856.
72. *California Farmer and Journal of Useful Sciences* (Sacramento, CA) 5, no. 5 (February 8, 1856): 38.
73. *North American Review* 82, no. 171 (April 1856): 577–78.
74. "H. B.," "A Live Book," *Liberator*, July 25, 1856.
75. *Universalist Quarterly and General Review* 13 (April 1856): 218.
76. "New Publications," *Boston Daily Atlas*, December 27, 1855; "New Publications," *Salem (MA) Register*, December 31, 1855.
77. Angelina Grimké Weld to Harriot Kezia Hunt, April 24, 1856, Weld-Grimké Family Papers.
78. Sarah Moore Grimké to Harriot Kezia Hunt, March 8, [1856?], ibid. Haynes, *Riotous Flesh*, 73, 74, 132–62, discusses Douglass and her friendship with Grimké.
79. Ronald J. Zboray and Mary Saracino Zboray, "Reading and Everyday Life in Antebellum Boston: The Diary of Daniel F. and Mary D. Child," *Libraries and Culture* 32, no. 3 (Summer 1997): 285–323.
80. Neither the newspaper obituaries on Hunt nor published remembrances of her mentioned that she had authored an autobiography. According to WorldCat, *Glances and Glimpses* was not reprinted until 1970 (Source Book Press, New York), a time when the renewed interest in women's history led to the publication of various long-out-of-print works by nineteenth-century women.

Chapter 8: Confronting War, Old Age, and Other Challenges

1. "Silver Wedding," *Liberator*, July 13, 1860. See also "A Celebration among Our Strong-Minded Women," *American Traveller*, July 9 and 14, 1860; Ednah Dow Cheney, *Reminiscences of Ednah Dow Cheney* (Boston: Lee & Shepard, 1902), 52–53; Elizabeth Cady Stanton, Susan B. Anthony, and Matilda Joslyn Gage, eds., *History of Woman Suffrage*, 3 vols. (Rochester, NY: Charles Mann Printing, 1889), 1:260. Mary Safford Blake, "A Visit to Dr. Harriet [sic] K. Hunt," *Woman's Journal* 3, no. 47 (November 23, 1872): 376, noted that fifteen hundred people, including three generations of patients, came to congratulate Hunt during her anniversary celebration.
2. Stanton, Anthony, and Gage, *History of Woman Suffrage*, 1:260.
3. *Notable American Women, 1607–1950: A Biographical Dictionary*, 1:325–27, s.v. "Cheney, Ednah Dow Littlehale"; Cheney, *Reminiscences*, 52.
4. Martha Coffin Wright to Elizabeth Cady Stanton, July 5, 1860, William Lloyd Garrison Family Papers, box 266, folder 2, Sophia Smith Collection, Smith College Special Collections, Northampton, MA.
5. Harriot K. Hunt to Anna Parsons, May 30, 1860, New England Hospital Records, box 23, folder 75, ibid.
6. *Notable American Women: 1607–1950*, s.v. "Safford [Blake], Mary Jane," http://www.credoreference.com.
7. Blake, "A Visit to Dr. Harriet K. Hunt."
8. Records of the Meetings of the Ladies' Physiological Institute of Boston and Vicinity from

May 1854 to May 1857, vol. 4, Eighth Annual Report, May 7 and October 31, 1856, Schlesinger Library; Martha H. Verbrugge, *Able-Bodied Womanhood: Personal Health and Social Change in Nineteenth-Century Boston* (New York: Oxford University Press, 1988), 65.

9. Records of the Meetings of the Ladies' Physiological Institute, vol. 4, Eighth Annual Report, October 15, 1856, December 10 and 24,1856, Schlesinger Library; Verbrugge, *Able-Bodied Womanhood*, 78.

10. Records of the Meetings of the Ladies' Physiological Institute, vol. 4, Ninth Annual Report, May 6, 1857, Schlesinger Library.

11. Ibid., May 14, 1857.

12. Sarah Moore Grimké to Harriot Kezia Hunt, June 28, 1857, Weld-Grimké Family Papers.

13. Hunt's protest is reprinted in "Taxation without Representation," *Liberator*, December 31, 1859.

14. Sally G. McMillen, *Lucy Stone: An Unapologetic Life* (New York: Oxford University Press, 2015), 139–40; Andrea Moore Kerr, *Lucy Stone: Speaking Out for Equality* (New Brunswick, NJ: Rutgers University Press, 1992), 103.

15. "Protest of Sarah E. Wall. To the Treasurer and Assessors of the City of Worcester" is reprinted in the *Liberator*, October 15, 1858. See also Harriet H. Robinson, *Massachusetts in the Woman Suffrage Movement: A General, Political, Legal and Legislative History from 1774 to 1881* (1881; repr., Forgotten Books, 2012), 241–42.

16. Linda K. Kerber, *No Constitutional Right to Be Ladies: Women and the Obligations of Citizenship* (New York: Hill and Wang, 1998), 97, 334n43.

17. Ann Russo and Cheris Kramarae, eds., *The Radical Women's Press of the 1850s* (New York: Routledge, 1991), 244–45, reprinted Hasbrouck's untitled February 1862 essay in the *Sibyl*.

18. Diane Avery and Alfred S. Konefsky, "The Daughters of Job: Property Rights and Women's Lives in Mid-Nineteenth-Century Massachusetts," *Law and History Review* 10, no. 2 (Autumn 1992): esp. 326–27n18.

19. Several sources reprinted these speeches. See, for example, "The Political Rights of Women," *New-Bedford-Mercury* (MA), March 13, 1857; Stanton, Anthony, and Gage, *History of Woman Suffrage*, 1:258–59; Robinson, *Massachusetts in the Woman Suffrage Movement*, 232–33.

20. Hunt's remarks appeared in the *Boston Evening Transcript*, February 4, 1858.

21. "From Our Own Correspondent," *New York Tribune*, February 10, 1858.

22. Their comments are discussed and/or excerpted in ibid. See also Robinson, *Massachusetts in the Woman Suffrage Movement*, 233–35.

23. Nina Moore Tiffany, ed., *Samuel E. Sewall: A Memoir* (Boston: Houghton, Mifflin, 1898), offers a useful introduction to his work.

24. "Right of Suffrage for Women. Remarks of Hon. Sam'l E. Sewall," *Liberator*, February 19, 1858. See also "The Rights of Women to Vote," *Massachusetts Spy* (Worcester, MA), February 10, 1858.

25. *Boston Evening Transcript*, February 4, 1858, noted this exchange.

26. Harriot Kezia Hunt to Samuel E. Sewall, October 18, 1857, Robie-Sewall Family Papers, Massachusetts Historical Society, Boston, MA.

27. "Abolishing Women," *New York Times*, February 15, 1858.

28. "Taxation without Representation," *Boston Investigator*, December 29, 1858.

29. "Woman's Rights Meeting," *Liberator*, June 10, 1859.

30. Report of the Woman's Rights Meeting, at Mercantile Hall, May 27, 1859. . . . p. 11, http://memory.loc.gov.

31. "The Women in Council," *Boston Post*, May 30, 1859.

32. Grimké to Hunt, June 28, 1857, Weld-Grimké Family Papers.

33. On Severance see Virginia Elwood-Akers, *Caroline Severance* (Bloomington, NY: iUniverse, 2010). On Dall see Helen R. Deese, ed., *Daughter of Boston: The Extraordinary Diary of a Nineteenth-Century Woman, Caroline Healey Dall* (Boston: Beacon Press, 2005); Deese, "Caroline Healey Dall and the American Women's Movement, 1848–75," *American Nineteenth Century History* 3, no. 3 (Fall 2002): 1–28; Nancy Bowman, "Caroline Healey Dall: Her Creation

and Reform Career," in *Women of the Commonwealth: Work, Family, and Social Change in Nineteenth-Century Massachusetts*, ed. Susan L. Porter (Amherst: University of Massachusetts Press,1996), 121–46.
34. Deese, *Daughter of Boston*, 139, Dall's diary entry for February 3, 1851.
35. See Dall's diary entries for September 19 and September 29, 1855, in ibid., 233–34, 237.
36. Dall recounted this incident in her September 20, 1855, diary entry in ibid., 234.
37. Records of the Meetings of the Ladies' Physiological Institute, vol. 4, Ninth Annual Report, May 6, 1857.
38. Mary Roth Walsh, *"Doctors Wanted: No Women Need Apply": Sexual Barriers in the Medical Profession, 1835–1975* (New Haven, CT: Yale University Press, 1977), 79–80, 82.
39. Her lectures, which advocated for women in medicine and other professions, appeared in Caroline H. Dall, *The College, the Market, and the Court; or, Woman's Relation to Education, Labor, and Law* (1867; repr., New York: Arno Press, 1972).
40. *A Practical Illustration of "Woman's Right to Labor"; or, A Letter from Marie E. Zakrzewska, M.D. Late of Berlin, Prussia*, ed. Caroline H. Dall (1860; repr., Dodo Press). See also Arleen Marcia Tuchman, *Science Has No Sex: The Life of Marie Zakrzewska, M.D.* (Chapel Hill: University of North Carolina Press, 2006), 121–36, 285n4.
41. "The Women in Council," *Boston Post*, May 30, 1859.
42. Report of the Woman's Rights Meeting, at Mercantile Hall, 7, 15–23. Dall's address was reprinted in the *Liberator*, March 5, 1858.
43. Dall, *The College, the Market, and the Court*, esp. 26–27, 202–4, 358–61.
44. "Mrs. Dall's 'Fraternity' Lecture," *Liberator*, October 26, 1860.
45. Quotes from this paragraph and the next are from Dall, *The College, the Market, and the Court*, 364.
46. Lee V. Chambers, *The Weston Sisters: An Abolitionist Family* (Chapel Hill: University of North Carolina Press, 2014), 139–47.
47. Sallie Holley, *A Life for Liberty: Anti-Slavery and Other Letters of Sallie Holley*, edited with introductory chapters by John White Chadwick (1899; repr. New York: Negro Universities Press, 1969), 147–50; Dall's diary entry for September 19, 1855, found in Deese, *Daughter of Boston*, 233.
48. Cheney, *Reminiscences*, 60.
49. Marie E. Zakrzewska to Harriot K. Hunt, May 14, 1857, Caroline Wells Healey Dall Papers, Massachusetts Historical Society, Boston, MA.
50. Unpublished journal of Edmund Wentworth Wright, 1856–1863, private family collection of Gary Wentworth Wright and Justin Frank DeFreitas. The passages quoted in paragraphs below are from the following diary entries: April 5, 1857; June 2, 1858; August 5, 1858; December 2, 1859; May 6 and 7, 1857; June 27, 1860; April 10 and 23, 1862; July 15, 1862; and October 10, 1862.
51. Grimké to Hunt, April 13, 1859, Weld-Grimké Family Papers.
52. Grimké to Hunt, June 28, 1857, ibid.
53. *New York Times*, April 14, 1859; *Boston Traveler*, September 23, 1859. See also "A Woman Preacher," *St. Albans (VT) Messenger*, October 13, 1859; *Highland Weekly News* (Hillsboro, IL), May 12, 1859; *Cincinnati (OH) Daily Press*, April 21, 1859; "Woman," *Boston Evening Transcript*, April 11, 1859, and September 9, 1859.
54. *Boston Evening Transcript*, September 9, 1859. For similar comments see the *Boston Traveler*, September 23, 1859.
55. "A. B.," "Dr. Harriot K. Hunt," *Liberator*, September 30, 1859.
56. See the following entries in the Wright journal: April 7, 1861; August 18 and 25, 1861; and September 20, 1861.
57. Catherine A. Brekus, *Strangers and Pilgrims: Female Preaching in America, 1740–1845* (Chapel Hill: University of North Carolina Press, 1998), esp. 1–264; on "biblical feminists," see 6–7, 221–27. See also Brekus, "Harriet Livermore, the Pilgrim Stranger: Female Preaching and Biblical Feminism in Early-Nineteenth-Century America," *Church History* 65, no. 3 (September 1996): 389–404.

58. See chapter 1 for a fuller discussion of this issue.
59. Dall, *The College, the Market, and the Court*, 443.
60. Brekus, *Strangers and Pilgrims*, 267–306.
61. Ibid., 307–35.
62. Ibid., 337–39; see also Nancy Isenberg, "'Pillars in the Same Temple and Priests of the Same Worship': Woman's Rights and the Politics of Church and State in Antebellum America," *Journal of American History* 85, no. 1 (June 1998): 105–14, and Beverly A. Zink-Sawyer, "From Preachers to Suffragists: Enlisting the Pulpit in the Early Movement for Woman's Rights," *American Transcendental Quarterly* 14, no. 3 (September 2000): 193–209.
63. Sarah Allaback, "'Better Than Silver and Gold': Design Schools for Women in America, 1848–1860," *Journal of Women's History* 10, no. 1 (Spring 1998): 88–107.
64. Ibid., 91–92. See also Cheney, *Reminiscences*, 72.
65. Hunt to Parsons, January 4, 1854, New England Hospital Records, box 23, folder 75, Sophia Smith Collection.
66. Allaback, "'Better Than Silver and Gold,'" 99.
67. Hunt to Parsons, n.d. [probably 1860], New England Hospital Records, box 23, folder 75, Sophia Smith Collection.
68. Jeanie Attie, *Patriotic Toil: Northern Women and the American Civil War* (Ithaca, NY: Cornell University Press, 1998); Wendy Hamand Venet, *Neither Ballots nor Bullets: Women Abolitionists and the Civil War* (Charlottesville: University of Virginia Press, 1991), 94–122; Stanton, Anthony, and Gage, *History of Woman Suffrage*, 2:50–89.
69. Lori D. Ginzburg, *Elizabeth Cady Stanton: An American Life* (New York: Hill and Wang, 2009), 103.
70. Ibid., 108.
71. *Proceedings of the Meeting of the Loyal Women of the Republic, Held in New York, May 14, 1863* (New York: Phair, Steam Printers, 1863). The "Loyal Women of the Republic" was one of the many variations of the name the Women's National Loyal League used.
72. Venet, *Neither Ballots nor Bullets*, 12.
73. Hunt to Grimké, January 1, 1860, Weld-Grimké Family Papers. It was not unusual for Hunt to refer to herself as "HKH" in her personal correspondence.
74. Grimké to Hunt, June 28, 1857, ibid.
75. *1860 United States Federal Census*, Ward 5, Boston, Suffolk County, Massachusetts, p. 4, from ancestry.com.
76. Ibid.
77. *Daily Ohio Statesman*, January 9, 1862; *Providence (RI) Evening Press*, January 6, 1862.
78. "Incomes in the Fourth District. Internal Revenue Returns from Wards One, Two, Three, and Five," *Boston Evening Transcript*, July 14, 1865.
79. *Historical Statistics of the United States Millennial Edition Online*, Table Ba 4280–4282, https://hsus.cambridge.org/HSUSWeb/HSUSEntryServlet.
80. The quotes from this paragraph and the next are from Hunt's 1861 annual protest, printed in "Taxation without Representation," *Liberator*, January 3, 1862. Other newspapers also noted her protest. See, for example, *Cincinnati (OH) Daily Press*, January 8, 1862.
81. "The War Record of Massachusetts," *Boston Daily Advertiser*, November 16, 1866. See also "A Patriotic Record," *Boston Traveler*, November 8, 1866.
82. "The Woman Movement," *Ladies' Repository; A Monthly Periodical, Devoted to Literature, Art...*, May 1870, 383.
83. The quotes from this paragraph and the next are from "Taxation without Representation," *Liberator*, December 23, 1864.
84. For more recent discussions of the postwar woman's rights movement and how it intersected with that for African American rights, see Laura E. Free, *Suffrage Reconstructed: Gender, Race, and Voting Rights in the Civil War Era* (Ithaca, NY: Cornell University Press, 2015), and Faye E. Dudden, *Fighting Chance: The Struggle over Woman Suffrage and Black Suffrage in Reconstruction America* (New York: Oxford University Press, 2011).

85. Several newspapers reprinted "Miss Hunt's Protest," including the *Lowell (MA) Daily Citizen and News*, November 27, 1866, and the *Manchester (NH) Mirror and Farmer*, December 8, 1866.
86. Untitled, *Springfield (MA) Republican*, November 23, 1863.
87. These comments were reprinted in the *Liberator*, January 13, 1865.
88. Ibid.
89. "Dr. Holland's Lecture," *Liberator*, February 3, 1865.
90. Elizabeth Blackwell to Kitty Brown Blackwell, November 18, 1865, Blackwell Family Papers, box 74 (corresponds to reel 57), Manuscript Division, Library of Congress, Washington, DC.
91. I have been unable to find newspaper accounts of any such tours or other public activities of Hunt's of the type that were regularly reported in earlier years.
92. Blake, "A Visit to Dr. Harriet K. Hunt," noted this fact.
93. "Woman's Rights. The Convention in Horticultural Hall," *Boston Traveler*, November 20, 1868.
94. Karen J. Blair, *The Clubwoman as Feminist: True Womanhood Redefined, 1868–1914* (New York: Holmes & Meier Publishers, 1980), esp. 31–38.
95. Julia A. Sprague, *History of the New England Women's Club from 1868 to 1893* (Boston: Lee and Shepard Publishers, 1894), 3, 7.
96. Ibid. discusses these activities. See also the New England Women's Club Records, Minutes and Annual Reports from February 18, 1868, to May 3, 1873, and May 31, 1873, to May 7, 1881, vols. 22 and 23; Record Book of the "Weekly Social Meetings," November 6, 1868–February 27, 1871, vol. 39, both in Schlesinger Library. On Zakrzewska's involvement with the club, see also Tuchman, *Science Has No Sex*, 121, 247.
97. The Schlesinger Library has a copy of Hunt's death certificate. The original is in MJA, death records, vol. 276, no. 59, p. 3. Bright's disease is also listed as the cause of Hunt's death in *Massachusetts, Death Records, 1841–1915*, from ancestry.com.
98. See, for example, the *Boston Daily Advertiser*, January 5, 1875, and *Salem (MA) Register*, January 7, 1875.
99. *Massachusetts, Death Records, 1841–1915*, from ancestry.com.
100. Gerda Lerner, *The Grimké Sisters from South Carolina: Pioneers for Women's Rights and Abolition*, 2nd rev. ed. (1967; repr., Chapel Hill: University of North Carolina Press, 2004), 262.
101. Will of Harriot Kezia Hunt, Suffolk Probate File Papers, Docket no. 56530, MJA. The Schlesinger Library also has a copy of this document titled "Last will & testament of Harriot K. Hunt, dated October 4, 1871. Filed January 6, 1875." All future quotes from Hunt's will are from this source.
102. "The Will of Dr. Harriot Keziah [sic] Hunt," *Boston Journal*, January 7, 1875, and "Will, of the Late Dr. Harriot K. Hunt," *Boston Daily Advertiser*, January 8, 1875.
103. There is no reason given as to why one nephew, Theodore Francis Wright, did not receive a $300 bequest.
104. In her will Hunt stipulated that Lewis was to receive the remaining half of her commission once she delivered the completed statue of Hygeia. On Lewis and her career, see *Notable American Women: 1607–1950*, s.v. "Edmonia Lewis," http:search.credoreference.com.
105. Cheney, *Reminiscences*, 51–53. For other reminiscences stressing Hunt's laugh and her buoyant spirits, see Blake, "A Visit to Dr. Harriet K. Hunt," and Emily Faithful, *Three Visits to America* (Edinburgh: David Douglas, 1884), 105.
106. Cheney, *Reminiscences*, 52.

Index

"Abolishing Women" (*New York Times* editorial), 170
abolitionists and abolitionist movement: American Revolution legacy and, 93; in Boston, 118; churches and, 105, 177–78; democratization of antebellum America and, 27; feminists and, 119–20, 180; Harvard Medical School and, 82; Hunt's involvement in, 111–13; male physicians supporting, 29; racial amalgamation fears and, 84; Universalists and, 13; Woman's National Loyal League and, 179–80; woman's rights movement and, 73, 75; women's participation in, 72, 102–3, 207n42. *See also* antislavery; Grimké, Angelina; Grimké, Sarah; slavery; Weld, Theodore Dwight
"Address on the Medical Education of Women, An," 76
affluence, 39–40
African Americans: female authors, 139; female preachers, 177; medical school applicants, 82–84; men, 183; school for girls, 114
Agassiz, Louis, 134–35
alcohol abuse, 101–2, 207n46
Alcott, Bronson, 56, 172, 175
Alcott, William, 60
alternative health care movement, 26–28, 38–42, 126, 132, 134
alternative medicine, spiritualizing of, 38–39
American and Foreign Anti-Slavery Society, 103

American Antislavery Society, 72, 102–3
American Colonization Society, 82
American Medical Society, 28
American Revolution, 92–94, 149–50, 169, 171
Animal Kingdom (Swedenborg), 51–52
Anthony, Susan B., 93, 102–3, 129, 159, 180, 183
anti-Catholicism, 47, 95
Antimasonic Party and movement, 20–21
antislavery, 64, 66, 72, 105, 111–19, 124. *See also* abolitionists and abolitionist movement
Anti-Slavery Bugle, 118–19
Antislavery Conventions of American Women, 72
Associated Housewrights, 9
autobiographies in antebellum America, 136–42, 211n11. *See also Glances and Glimpses*
Autobiography of an Actress (Mowatt), 140–41

Babcock, Rachael, 180
Ballou, Hosea, 13, 23, 50
Baltimore, Maryland, 116
Bangor Daily Whig and Courier, 122
Beecher, Catharine, 121–22
Beecher, Thomas, 122
Belleville, New Jersey, 67–68
Bennett, James Gordon, 80
Bennett, Judith, 66
Bethel (church for sailors), 108–9
Bibliography of American Autobiographies, A, 138–39

Blackwell, Antoinette Brown. *See* Brown, Antoinette
Blackwell, Elizabeth: Beecher's praise of, 122; distancing self from Hunt, 132; femininity rhetoric and, 141; Hale's praise of, 121; heart histories and, 42; Hunt's advocacy for, 2, 130; Hunt's twenty-fifth anniversary in medicine and, 165; medical degree earned by, 1, 28, 55, 82, 121; New York Infirmary for Women and Children and, 2, 130; on visit to Hunt after Civil War, 184
Blackwell, Emily, 28, 126, 165
Blake, Mary Safford, 166
blistering, 25, 27
bloodletting, 27
Boston, Massachusetts: American Revolution legacy in, 93; in early nineteenth century, 8–13, 17, 22, 219 n 52; female physicians marginalized in, 129–30; Fugitive Slave Act and, 118–20; Harriot's medical practice established in, 35–37; medical establishment in, 26–31, 37, 54, 124, 129–30; reform activism in, 72, 111–12, 178; slavery and racial discrimination in, 72; Swedenborgianism in, 50
Boston Courier, 134–35
Boston Daily Advertiser, 1
Boston Daily Atlas, 159
Boston Daily Journal, 84
Boston Daily Mail, 79–80
Boston Evening Transcript, 161, 176
Boston Female Medical College. *See* New England Female Medical College
Boston Medical and Surgical Journal, 123
Boston Music Hall, 177
Boston Post, 171, 173
Boston Traveler, 33–34, 176
Bowditch, Henry Ingersoll, 29–30, 132
Bremer, Fredrika, 63–65, 109, 131, 137, 146
Brown, Antoinette, 75, 103–6, 125, 132, 160
Brown, John, 93, 167, 175
Brown, Olympia, 15, 177–78
Buchanan, Joseph, 27–28, 126, 129
Buckingham, Joseph T., 11–12
Buffalo, New York, 106
Bunker Hill Monument, 149
Burbick, Joan, 108

Burns, Anthony, 118–20
Bush, George, 50–51

California Farmer and Journal of Useful Sciences, 162
calomel, 25, 27
Calvinism, 13, 50
Canton trade, 17, 195n52
capital punishment, 19
celibacy, 55, 57
Central Medical College, 28
Chambers, John, 103
Channing, William Henry, 75, 86
Chapin, Augusta, 15
Cheney, Ednah Dow, 166, 174, 179, 185, 188
Child, Daniel, 164
Child, Lydia Maria, 108
Child, Mary, 164
childbirth, 57–58, 60
childhood, nostalgia for, 7–8, 43, 50–51, 62, 108–9, 144–45
childrearing, gender-neutral, 158
Christian anarchism, 75
Christian Examiner and Religious Miscellany, 161
Christianity, 7, 9, 16, 75–76, 105, 115, 158. *See also* ministry; Quakers; Shakers; Unitarians and Unitarianism; Universalists and Universalism
Christian missionaries, 139
Christian Science Church, 39
Christian socialism, 63
Church of New Jerusalem. *See* New Church
Cincinnati, Ohio, 129
Cincinnati Daily Times, 128
citizenship, limitation of rights of, 91–92, 98
Civil War, 166–67, 179–82
Claremont, New Hampshire, 168
Clarke, James Freeman, 168–69
Clarke, Nancy, 130, 132
class prejudice, 94–95, 99–100, 183
Cleveland, Ohio, 124–27, 129–31
Cleveland Herald, 122
Cleveland Medical College. *See* Western Reserve Medical College
Cleveland Medical Loan Fund Association, 130
Cleveland Morning Leader, 128
Coates, Sarah, 60
Columbus, Ohio, 126, 128–29
Combe, George, 37–38, 52

"Common Sense," 84–85
Congregational Church, 11–12
Constitution of Man (Combe), 38
Cooper, James Fenimore, 56
corporal punishment, 18–19
Corson, Hiram, 29
Country Gentleman, 160

Daily Capital City Fact, 128
Daily Ohio State Journal, 128
Dall, Caroline Wells Healey, 86–87, 172–74, 178
Dana, Richard Henry, 182
dancing, 107
Darlington, William, 60
Davis, Andrew Jackson, 39
Davis, Cynthia, 148
Davis, Paulina Wright: at Hunt's home, 64, 174; as public lecturer, 60, 64; Shakers and, 57; woman's rights conventions and, 75, 86, 88, 129
Declaration of Independence, 97, 168–69, 181–82
Declaration of Sentiments and Resolutions, 92
Delany, Martin R., 82
Democratic Party, 114
Deroine, Jeanne, 73–74
Dickens, Charles, 56
disabled people, discrimination against, 91
divorce, 58, 124–25, 155
Dolley, Sarah Adamson, 28
domesticity. *See* femininity and domesticity
Douglass, Frederick, 183
Douglass, Sarah Mapps, 163

East of United States, 124, 128
Eclectic Medical Institute, 126, 129
eclectic medical schools, 28–29
economic discrimination, 151–52, 173
Eddy, Mary Baker. *See* Patterson, Mary
education, sexualizing, 100–101
education of women: avoidance of oppression in marriage and, 157; as controversial idea, 14; Hunt's advocacy for, 2, 70, 76, 79–80, 90, 98–101; in medicine, 76, 79, 99; New England Women's Club and, 185. *See also under* medical schools
Elaw, Zilpha, 139
Emancipation Proclamation, 182
Embargo Act (1807), 10

Emerson, George B., 182
Emerson, Ralph Waldo, 23–24, 56, 118
"Enfranchisement of Women" (H. T. Mill), 73
Erie Canal, 11
Everett, Edward, 182

Faneuil Hall, 149
Farnham, Eliza Wood Burhans, 139
fashion, 99, 107, 156, 158, 163
Federalists, 10
female friendships, 63–68, 109–11, 131, 146, 172, 174–75
Female Medical College of Pennsylvania, 29–30, 81, 85, 122–23, 130, 204n58
female physicians. *See* physicians, female
femininity and domesticity: in autobiographies, 140–41, 143–44, 147; in Hunt's public addresses, 203n32; Hunt's views on, 104; marketing of *Glances and Glimpses* and, 137–38; oppression of women and, 156–57; practice of medicine and, 122–23, 133; preventive medicine and, 86
feminism and feminists: abolitionist movement and, 119–20, 180; American Revolution legacy and, 93; autobiographies and, 136, 140–42; divisions after Civil War, 182–83; educated women and, 99; founding mothers of, 1, 75, 142; hostility toward, 88; Hunt's friendships and, 109, 113, 124–25, 131, 144, 147–48, 172; male predatory sexuality and, 152; ministry and churches and, 105; prostitution and, 86–87; religious unorthodoxy and, 159–60; Universalism and, 14–15. *See also* Bremer, Fredrika; gender equality; Grimké, Sarah; suffrage, female; woman's rights advocacy; woman's rights conventions
Fifteenth Amendment, 183
Finch, Marianne, 56, 59, 199n27
Finney, Charles Grandison, 125
Five Points Mission, 106
Flagg, Josiah Foster, 75, 179
Fleet Street home, 8, 22, 26, 31–32, 43–44, 186–87
Fourier, Charles, 64
Fourteenth Amendment, 183
Fowler, Lorenzo, 57
Fowler, Lydia Folger, 28, 57

Fox sisters, 133
France, 10
franchise, demands for. *See* suffrage, black man's; suffrage, female
Franklin, Benjamin, 138
Franklin Institute School, 179
free churches, 105
free-love doctrine, 60, 154–55, 167
Freemasons. *See* Masons
friendships, female. *See* female friendships
Fugitive Slave Act (1850), 114–15, 118
Fuller, Margaret, 1, 108, 158, 172, 174
Fuller, Robert, 38
Fussell, Bartholomew, 29

Gage, Frances D., 103, 109, 165, 175
Garrison, William Lloyd, 75, 96, 129, 168, 171–72, 184
gender equality: in citizenship, 73; female physicians and, 77; heart histories and, 148; Hunt's advocacy for, 90, 158; North American Phalanx and, 64; Quakers and, 29; Sarah Grimké and, 66–67; Shakers and, 55–58, 64; Universalism and, 14–15. *See also* feminism and feminists; woman's rights advocacy
gender fluidity, 158
General Association of Massachusetts Congregational Churches, 66
Geneva Medical College, 1, 28, 55, 130
Girls' High and Normal School, 100
Girls' Latin School in Boston, 185
Glances and Glimpses (Hunt), 136–64; on amalgamation fears, 84–85; childhood home portrait in, 7–8, 144–45, 161–62; conflictedness of, 146–47; disillusionment with conventional medicine, 25–26; on economic discrimination, 151–52; Edmund Wright and, 45; on education of women, 157–58; femininity and domesticity rhetoric in, 143–44, 161–63; friendship with Bremer and, 65; on gender equality, 158–59, 161; on home, desire for, 159; Kezia Hunt's love of politics, 94; Ladies' Physiological Institute and, 48, 167; loneliness and depression themes in, 145; as major achievement, 2–4; male physicians criticized in, 43, 150–51; on marriage, oppression in, 120, 153–57; medical career beginning, 35, 37; on ministry, women's exclusion from, 150; on moral decline in United States, 148–49; Motts, controversy surrounding, 31; Motts, Hunts' relationship with, 34; obituaries, lack of mention in, 214n80; Ohio tour, 128–29; patients described in, 36; patriarchy denounced in, 147–48; plates of, 187–88; on politics, women's exclusion from, 149–50; pride in achievements, 145; privacy protected in, 145–46; publication of, 70, 135–38; public lecturing, 60–61, 70; reviews of, 159–64; on seduction of young women, 152–53, 157; self-deprecation in, 142–43; on slavery and sexual exploitation of women, 152; on spiritual approach to medicine, 39; teaching career described in, 19; U.S. Congress visit, 114–15; woman's rights advocacy and, 61–62, 70; woman's rights conventions and, 81
"Gleaner" essays (J. Sargent Murray), 14
Gleason, Rachel, 28, 42
Gleason, Silas, 28
Gleason water cure, 122
Godey's Lady's Book, 121
Graham, Sylvester, 60
Great Britain, 10
Greeley, Horace, 79–80
Green Street home, 43–44, 186–87
Gregory, Samuel, 28–29
Grimké, Angelina: as abolitionist, 72, 105; Hunt's autobiography and, 163; Hunt's reform network and, 174; Hunt's will and, 186–87; ministry and, 105; Quakers and, 66; sister Sarah and, 67–68, 110–11, 208n64; Whole World's Temperance Convention and, 103; Woman's National Loyal League and, 180; Zakrzewska and, 132
Grimké, Sarah: as abolitionist, 72, 105; death of, 185–86; Hunt's autobiography and, 136, 141, 144, 163; Hunt's friendship with, 66–68, 90, 109–11, 146, 172, 176, 180, 201nn59–62; Hunt's protests and, 170; Hunt's reform network and, 174; *Letters on the Equality of the Sexes*, 66–67, 99, 110, 153; on licensed female physicians, 133;

on marriage, 71; ministry and, 105, 150, 177; Mowatt's autobiography and, 140–41; Quakers and, 66–67; sister Angelina and, 67–68, 110–11, 208n64; spiritualism and, 134; Zakrzewska and, 132
Grosvenor, Roxalana L., 57–58, 186
Gunn's Domestic Medicine, 27
Gusdorf, George, 139

Hale, Sarah, 121
Half a Century (Swisshelm), 136
Hamilton, Gail, 18
Hamlet, 24
Hanaford, Phebe, 15
Happy Home and Parlor Magazine, 160
Harper's Ferry, Virginia, 167
Hartford Convention (1814), 10
Harvard, Massachusetts, Shaker community in, 56–57, 59, 64, 175
Harvard Medical School: Hunt rejected by, 52, 54–55, 61, 74, 78–79; Hunt's criticism of, 78–79, 87, 151, 158–59; Hunt's first application to, 2, 54–55, 68, 199n19; Hunt's reapplication to, 2, 69, 81–85; inexpedient, use of term, 55, 79, 87, 96; refusal to admit women, 129
Harvard University, 134–35
Hasbrouck, Lydia Sayer, 168
health, women's, 48, 54, 59–61, 64, 106–7
health reform: alternative health care movement, 26–28, 38–42, 126, 132, 134; Hunt as champion of, 2–4; lecturing on, 60, 86–87, 106. *See also* heart histories; physicians, female; preventive medicine
heart histories: gender discrimination and, 74; gendered approach to medicine and, 78; gender equality and, 148; *Glances and Glimpses* as, 145; Hunt as priestly confessor and, 47–48; Hunt's, told to Bremer, 65; Hunt's need to move beyond, 70; Hunt's reputation for, 1–2; partnerships with patients and, 41–42; Shaker women and, 58, 61; spiritualism and, 39; Swedenborgianism and, 133; unhappy relationships with men and, 40–41, 61; wealthy women and, 39–40, 61; of women in abusive marriages, 61, 101, 148; women's anguish and, 39–40, 61–62;

working-class women and, 39, 61–62, 151–52. *See also* mind-cure approach to medicine
Heilbrun, Carolyn, 140, 144
heroic therapies, 27, 47, 61
Hertha (Bremer), 64
Higginson, Thomas Wentworth, 103
History of Woman Suffrage (vol. 1), 1, 166
Holley, Sallie, 125, 174
Holmes, Oliver Wendell, 54–55, 79, 82, 199n19
home instinct, 159
homeopathy and homepaths, 27, 48, 51, 75, 122, 132
Homes of the New World, The (Bremer), 63
homosexuality, suggestions of, 65–67, 146, 201n59
Hopkinton Springs, 63
Horsford, Eben Norton, 134–35
Hosmer, Harriet, 165
human rights: feminism and, 131; Hunt's activism and, 143; Lucretia Mott, and, 75; slavery as violation of, 27, 111–12, 119; Stanton and, 94; woman's rights as, 62, 70, 110, 119, 173
Hunt, Harriot Kezia: death of, 1, 90, 185; early years of, 7–24; family tragedy and, 49–54, 187; financial independence of, 70–72, 92, 180–81; illnesses of, 22, 62–64, 82, 164, 166, 170, 185; loneliness of, 53, 60–61, 109, 135, 145; obituaries on, 214n80; professional rejection of, 36–37, 69, 130, 158–59; will of, 186–88, 218nn103–4
Hunt, Joab: birth of, 190n1; career of, 7–9; charitable activities of, 9, 12; death of, 20–23, 31, 49, 52; education of daughters, 15–16; Harriot's childhood and, 7–8; Harriot Wright's resemblance to, 49; marriage of, 192n1; as Mason, 9–10, 12; praise for, 20, 195n63; Universalism and, 12–13
Hunt, Kezia Wentworth: birth of, 190n1; death of, 44, 52–53, 61; education of daughters, 15–16; Harriot's childhood and, 7, 51, 62–63; Harriot's support of, 47; Joab Hunt's death and, 20, 22, 45; marriage of, 190n1; Motts and, 26, 33; support from, 20, 37, 43, 53; Universalism and, 12–13, 15, 49–50

Hunt, Sarah: birth of, 192n2; birth of first child, 49; childhood of, 7–8, 16; death of, 185–86, 192n2; family life of, 52–53, 59; Harriot's medical practice with, 33–37, 39, 43–46; Harriot's relationship with, 53–54, 59, 62–63, 109, 165; illness and recovery of, 24–26, 31–32; marriage of, 44–46, 144–45; as teacher, 22
Hunt family: death of Harriot Wright and, 49–51; death of Kezia Hunt and, 53–54; education valued by, 16; financial difficulties of, 17, 22–24, 31; Universalism and, 12–13; War of 1812 ending and, 10
Hutchinson, Thomas, 8
hydropathy, 27–28, 34, 48, 132
Hygeia, marble statue of, 188

immigration and immigrants, 11–12, 94–95, 99–100, 102, 170
Incidents in the Life of a Slave Girl (Jacobs), 139
industrial design, 179
Industrial School for impoverished girls, 15
inexpedient, use of term, 55, 79, 87, 96
intromission, 50
Irish immigrants, 12, 94–95, 99–100, 102, 170

Jacobi, Mary Putnam, 3–4, 132–33
Jacobs, Harriet, 139
John P. Jewett and Company, 136–38
Joint Special Committee on the Qualifications of Voters, 169

Kansas, 114–15, 122
Kansas-Nebraska Act, 114–16, 118–19
Kelley, Mary, 15, 99
Kentucky, 126
Kessler-Harris, Alice, 71

labor movement, antebellum, 13
Ladies Medical Oracle, The (E. Mott), 30–31
Ladies' Physiological Institute, 2, 48–49, 106–7, 166–67, 172, 175
Ladies Repository, 182
Lawrence, Amos, 118
Lawrence, Kansas, 122
Laws of Life, The (Elizabeth Blackwell), 122
Le Berceau (French corvette), 8–9
Lee, Ann, 56–57

Lee, Jarena, 139
leeches, 25–26
Lerner, Gerda, 67, 110, 201n59, 208n64
lesbian-like friendships, 66. *See also* homosexuality, suggestions of
Letters on the Equality of the Sexes (S. Grimké), 66–67, 99, 110, 153
Letters to the People on Health and Happiness (C. Beecher), 121–22
Lewis, Edmonia, 188, 218n104
Liberator: Garrison as editor of, 75; on *Glances and Glimpses*, 162–63; on Harvard's medical class, 85; on Hunt's Maine tour, 176; Hunt's twenty-fifth anniversary and, 165; rebuttal of *Springfield Republican*, 184; woman's rights conventions and, 79, 119, 171
"Life Elixir" of Elizabeth Mott, 30, 34
Life in Prairie Land (Farnham), 139
Lily, 154
Lincoln, Abraham, 180, 182
Livermore, Harriet, 139, 177
Livermore, Mary L., 168
Longfellow, Henry Wadsworth, 182
Longshore, Joseph, 29
Lowell, James Russell, 182
Lowell Daily Citizen and News, 122
Lynn, Massachusetts, 154
Lyon, Mary, 14

Maine, 176
manhood, evangelical model of, 104, 207n46
manufacturing, rise of, 11
market revolution in United States, 11
marriage: abusive, 58, 61, 101, 120, 139, 148, 154–55; egalitarian, support for, 133–34; oppression in, 120, 153–57; patriarchal power within, 153–55; property rights in, 168; status of women and, 71, 73, 75; unhappy, 40–41, 58, 116–18, 139, 151, 154–56
Marriage (M. G. and T. L. Nichols), 154–55
Mary Lyndon (M. G. Nichols), 155
Masons, 9–10, 12–14, 20–22. *See also* St. Andrew's Lodge (Masons)
Massachusetts: Constitution of, 168; economy of, 10–12, 96; female medical education and, 127, 129; New England Women's Club and, 185; representative recruits in Civil War, 181–82; school

teaching in, 18, 195n55; Shaker communities in, 56–57, 59, 64; taxation without representation protests, 92; Universalism in, 12–13; woman's rights conventions in, 73–81, 85–86, 110. *See also* Boston, Massachusetts
Massachusetts Charitable Mechanic Association, 9, 12
Massachusetts Constitutional Convention (1853), 90, 95–96, 98, 109
Massachusetts Judiciary Committee, 168–70, 173
Massachusetts Medical Society, 130
Massachusetts State Legislature, 17, 26, 110, 168–70, 173
May, Samuel J., 109
medical career, 25–44; in 1860, 180; autobiography and, 136–37; Combe's influence on, 37–38; decision to pursue, 23–24; gendered nature of, 78; medical establishment in Boston and, 26, 30–31; medical practice with Sarah Hunt, 33–37, 39, 43–44; relationship with Motts, 31–34; Sarah Hunt's illness and establishment of, 24–26; spiritualizing of alternative medicine and, 38–39; successful medical practice established, 1–2; twenty-fifth anniversary of, 165–66, 175, 214n1. *See also* heart histories
medical establishment in antebellum era, 26–31, 37, 54, 86, 124, 150–51
medical parishes, 106
medical schools: admission of women into, 4, 78–79, 88–89, 127, 173; African American applicants to, 82–84; all-female, 28–30, 81, 121; denounced by health reformers, 27–28; eclectic, 28–29; female graduates of, 42, 121; immorality and, 87; monopoly over practice of medicine and, 26–27; refusals to admit women, 54–55, 83, 87, 129. *See also specific medical school names*
medicine, professionalization of, 29
medicine, women in. *See* physicians, female
mercury, 25, 27
mesmerists and mesmerism, 38–39, 51, 126
Mexican-American War, 114
Middling Interest movement, 11–12

Midwest of United States, 2
Mill, Harriet Taylor, 73
Mill, John Stuart, 73
Millerites, 178
mind-cure approach to medicine, 39, 51–52, 78, 126, 132. *See also* heart histories
ministry: abolitionist and temperance movements and, 103–5, 207n42; Hunt's criticism of men in, 150; Hunt's experience in, 176–79; ordination of women into, 15, 58, 90, 104–6, 150, 177–78
miscegenation, 116
Missouri Compromise (1820), 114–15
Morgan, William, 20–21
Morison, Samuel Eliot, 10
Mott, Elizabeth, 26, 30–34, 42, 77
Mott, Lucretia: *History of Woman Suffrage* and, 1; Hunt linked to, 160; Hunt's admiration for, 75–76, 105–6; Hunt's protests and, 170; Hunt's socializing with, 109, 145; Hunt's twenty-fifth anniversary in medicine and, 165–66; tribute to Tyndale, 87
Mott, Richard, 26, 30–33
Mount Auburn Cemetery, 188
Mount Holyoke Seminar, 14
Mowatt, Anna Cora, 140–41
Murray, John, 13–17, 45, 165
Murray, Judith Sargent, 14–15

Napoleonic Wars, 10
National American Woman's Suffrage Association, 53
National Era, 97
Native Americans, 40, 108
nativism, 94–95, 99–100, 102, 183, 206n19
Nebraska, 114
New Church, 50, 52–53, 61, 134–35
New England: economy of, 10–11, 17; religion in, 12–13; support for female physicians, 122
New Englander, 160
New England Female Medical College (formerly Boston Female Medical College), 28–29, 81–82, 122
New England Galaxy and Freemason's Weekly, 12
New England Hospital for Women and Children, 2, 30, 131–32, 165, 185
New England School of Design, 179

New England Woman's Rights Convention (1854), 118–20
New England Woman's Rights Convention (1855), 129
New England Women's Auxiliary Association, 179–80
New England Women's Club, 2, 184–85, 187
New Guide to Health (Thomson), 27
New Hampshire Patriot and State Gazette, 160–61
New Lebanon, New York, Shaker community in, 59
New York, 10–11, 17, 21, 92, 106, 195n52
New York City: Bremer's meeting of Hunt in, 63; Elizabeth Blackwell's practice in, 130; Elizabeth Mott's practice in, 34; Five Point Mission in, Hunt's lecture at, 106; Hunt's lectures in, reactions to, 69; Joab Hunt's death and, 21; prostitution in, 87; Water Cure College in, 28; Whole World's Temperance Convention in, 102–3; Woman's National Loyal League first meeting in, 180; woman's rights convention in (1853), 94, 97
New York Daily Times, 69, 96–97, 123, 160–61
New York Daily Tribune, 79, 97
New York Herald, 80, 88
New York Infirmary for Women and Children, 2, 130–31, 167, 174
New York State Legislature, 26–27
New York Times, 168, 170, 176
New York Tribune, 110, 154
Niagara Falls, New York, 106–8
Nichols, Clarina Howard, 75
Nichols, Mary Gove, 28, 60, 154–55, 167
Nichols, Thomas Low, 154–55
Nineteenth Amendment, 91, 169
non-resistance, 75
North American Phalanx, 64
North American Review, 162
Northeast of United States, 2, 139
North End of Boston, 8–12, 22, 44, 68, 108–9, 193n15

Oberlin College, 125–26
Ohio: Coates's tour of, 60; Hunt's travels to, 113, 116, 124–29, 172, 209n30; woman's rights conventions in, 73, 106, 111

Ohio Female Medical Education Society, 128
Ohio Female Medical Loan Fund Association, 127–28
Ohio Woman's Rights Association, 124
"On the Equality of the Sexes" (J. Sargent Murray), 14

Panic of 1819, 11
pantheism, 107
Parker, Theodore, 124
Parsons, Anna, 119, 166, 179
patriarchy: erosion of, and elder sisters, 46; feminist attacks on, 73; *Hertha,* and challenge to, 64; Hunt's anger at power of, 138, 147–48, 152–53; mainline churches and, 105; role in behavior of women, 163; spiritualism and, 133–34; Universalism and, 14; women preachers and, 178
Patterson, Mary (later Mary Baker Eddy), 39
Peirce, Benjamin, 134–35
penitentiaries, 19
Pennsylvania, 73
people churches, 105
petitions, 90, 92–94, 96, 98, 100
Philadelphia, Pennsylvania, 179
Philadelphia County Medical Society, 30
Phillips, Wendell, 75, 168–69
phrenology and phrenologists, 37, 57, 126
physicians, female: Bowditch's advocacy for, 29–30; Dall's advocacy for, 172–73; female ministers and, 106; femininity and, 76–78, 122–23, 203n33; girls' higher education and, 99; Hunt's advocacy for, 2, 69–70, 88–89, 106, 120–21, 207–8n51; Hunt's support for, 130–32; licensed, and distancing from Hunt, 132–33; loans for female students and, 127; male physicians' hostility toward, 29, 47, 123, 128; marginalization of, in Massachusetts, 129–30; newspaper debates about, 122–24; next generation of, 113; press hostility toward, 80, 88; promotion of, for female patients and children, 77–78, 82, 87, 121–22, 129, 173; prostitution and, 86–87; public resistance and hostility toward, 36–37, 69, 76; spiritualism and, 133–34; support for, in Ohio, 126–29. *See also* medical schools

physicians, male: criticism of, 42–43, 77–78, 87, 121, 129; Elizabeth Blackwell's reluctance to criticize, 141; hostility toward female physicians, 29, 47, 123, 128; supporters of abolitionist movement, 29; supporters of female physicians, 29–30, 122–24
Physiological Institutes of Woburn and Charlestown, 165
Physiological Society of Cleveland, 130
political interest, 15–16, 149
poverty, 39–40, 151
Practical Illustration of "Woman's Right to Labor," A (Zakrzewska), 172
preventive medicine: Combe's regimen and, 38; Elizabeth Blackwell and Catharine Beecher on, 122; failure of male physicians to practice, 150–51; as feminine, 86; Ladies' Physiological Institute and, 48; medicated champoo baths as, 33; public lecturing on, 127; Swedenborg and, 51
Price, Abby, 86
professional witnessing, 76
prohibition of alcohol, 101
property rights in marriage, 168
prostitutes and prostitution, 72, 77, 86–87, 152, 157, 207n46
prussic acid, 25
public lecturing: gender equality promotion and, 76–77; Grimkés and, 68; at Ladies' Physiological Institute, 106–7; by Mary Gove Nichols, 154; in Massachusetts, 207–8n51; as new endeavor for Hunt, 59–61; in New York City, 69, 106, 207–8n51; in North End of Boston, 68; in Ohio, 113, 127–29; press coverage of, 69–70, 79–81, 128; on preventive medicine, 127; prostitution and, 86–87; in upstate New York, 106; at woman's rights conventions, 76–81, 85–90, 153; women in medicine and, 76–79, 86–87, 127–28, 207–8n51; on women's health, 59–60, 106–7, 109
Punch, 69

quackery, 78, 86, 129, 150–52
Quakers, 29, 66–67, 75–76, 105–6, 115, 125, 177
Quimby, Phineas, 39

racial amalgamation, fears of, 84–85, 116–17
racism, 82–84, 91, 95
Reconstruction, 166–67
reform activism: in Boston, 72, 111–12, 178; Bremer and, 64–65; female physicians and, 77; *Glances and Glimpses* and, 145; Grimkés and, 66–68, 72, 90; Hunt's network for, 90, 174; late in Hunt's life, 166–67; news coverage of, 69–70, 88; women's participation in, 72–74. *See also* abolitionists and abolitionist movement; health reform; temperance movement; woman's rights advocacy; woman's rights movement
religious revivals, 27
republican motherhood, 14
Republican Party, 114, 183
Revere, Paul, 9
Richards, Lucy, 139
Richmond, Virginia, 116
Roland, Pauline, 73–74
Rose, Ernestine, 75, 80, 88, 153–54, 180
Royal Charité hospital (Berlin), 130

Sawin, Martha A., 130
school teaching: discipline and, 17–19, 22, 24, 195n55; pay for, 100–101, 151
Scott, Walter, 69
séances, 133–35
Second Universalist Church in Boston, 13, 23
self-reliance, 24, 27, 53, 141, 157
"Self-Reliance" (R. W. Emerson), 23–24
Seneca Falls, New York, 92, 109
Severance, Caroline, 113, 124–25, 129–32, 165, 172–75, 185, 187
Severance, Theodoric Cordenio, 124–25
Sewall, Samuel E., 169–70, 187
sex, science and mind as separate from, 77–78, 82, 86, 100–101, 123, 126, 132
Shakers: Bremer and, 64; Finch and, 56, 199n27; gender equality and, 55–58, 64; Hunt's relationship with, 54–59, 61, 105, 109, 201nn27–28, 200n31; sanctuary for abused women and, 200n34; women preachers and, 177; Wright family and, 175
ship-news, 8, 16
Shirley, Massachusetts, Shaker community in, 56, 59
Sibyl, 168

sisterhood, 46, 198n3
Skinner, Carolyn, 76, 203n32
slavery: Hunt's revulsion at, 116–18, 167, 181; Kansas-Nebraska Act and, 114–16; marriage compared to, 120; sectional controversy over, 113–14, 119, 167, 171; sexual exploitation by slaveholders, 152. *See also* abolitionists and abolitionist movement; antislavery
Smith, Elizabeth Oakes, 154, 172
Smith, Gerrit, 105, 109, 113, 115–17, 145, 163
socialism, 63–64
"Solitude of Self" (Stanton), 53
South Butler, New York, 104
South of United States, 11, 84, 114, 117
Southwark, Philadelphia, 13
Spacks, Patricia, 143
Sparks, Jared, 82
spinsterhood, 54
spiritualists and spiritualism, 39, 51, 126, 133–35
Springfield Republican, 183–84
Stack, David, 37
St. Andrew's Lodge (Masons), 9–10, 12, 20–22, 193n15
Stanton, Elizabeth Cady: on churches, 105; Civil War and, 180–81; *Declaration of Sentiments and Resolutions* and, 92; *Eighty Years and More*, 136, 142; femininity rhetoric and, 141–42, 144; Hunt's autobiography and, 145; Hunt's twenty-fifth anniversary in medicine and, 166; memories of Hunt, 1, 71; nativism, class prejudice, and gender grievances expressed by, 94–95, 206n19; Sarah Grimké's criticism of, 111; self-reliance and, 53; socializing with Hunt, 109; suffrage after Civil War and, 183; on wish to be a man, 93–94
Starling Medical College, 126, 129
Stewart, Maria, 72
Stone, Lucy: "Abolishing Women" editorial and, 170; biography of, 3–4; graduation from Oberlin, 125; Hunt linked to, 160; Judiciary Committee addressed by, 168–69; on oppression in marriage, 153; suffrage movement and, 168–69; taxation without representation and, 92, 168, 173; Woman's National Loyal League and,

180; at woman's rights conventions, 75, 88, 92, 103, 119
Stowe, Harriet Beecher, 116, 143
suffrage, black man's, 183
suffrage, female: abolitionist movement and, 119; female physicians and, 77, 125, 131; Hunt's advocacy for, 1, 68, 89–99, 167–73, 182–84, 187; New England Women's Club and, 2, 185; temperance movement and, 101; Universalism and, 15
Swedenborg, Emanuel, and Swedenborgianism: *Glances and Glimpses* reviews and, 160; Hunt's embrace of, 50–53, 86, 105, 114, 125, 198n40; spiritual approach to healing and, 51–52, 86, 133, 198n40; spiritualism and, 133–34
Swift, Adeline, 120
Swisshelm, Jane, 136
Syracuse, New York, woman's rights convention at, 85–88, 92, 109, 172
Syracuse Daily Star, 88

talking cure, 42
taxation without representation: Hunt's petition to constitutional convention and, 96; Hunt's protests against, 1, 70, 90, 92–93, 96–98, 137, 167, 170–73, 181–84, 187; Lucy Stone and, 92, 168, 173; Massachusetts State Legislature and, 168–69; refusals to pay taxes and, 167–68; woman's rights conventions and, 92
tax on sales by auction, 17
teachers. *See* school teaching
temperance movement: female physicians and, 77; Hunt's participation in, 4, 60, 90, 101–4; Universalists' involvement in, 13; women's involvement in, 72, 207n42
Thomson, Samuel, 27
Thoreau, Henry David, 118
Tiffin, Ohio, 127–28
traveling for pleasure, 107
Troy Female Seminary, 14
Truth, Sojourner, 177
Tyndale, Sarah, 87

Una, 154
Uncle Tom's Cabin (Stowe), 116, 143
Unitarians and Unitarianism: Channing and, 75; Daniel and Mary Childs and,

164; Higginson and, 103; R. W. Emerson and, 23; Swedenborg and, 50; woman's rights and, 75, 103, 109, 168–69; women preachers and, 177–78
United Society of Believers in Christ's Second Appearing. *See* Shakers
United States Congress, 114–16, 119
United States Constitution, 168
United States Sanitary Commission, 179–80
Universalist Church, 13, 16–17, 176
Universalist Quarterly and General Review, 162–63
Universalists and Universalism: abolition movement and, 13, 112; education of women and, 14–16; *Glances and Glimpses* reviews and, 160; growing numbers of, 194n35; Hunt family and, 12–13, 15–17, 105; Hunt's waning commitment to, 49–50; Masons and, 13–14; May and, 109; ordination of women into ministry and, 177–78; spiritualism and, 133–34; Swedenborg and, 50; Unitarian views and, 23; woman's rights and, 14–15, 168–69, 178; Wrights and, 45

Verbrugge, Martha, 48
Virginia, 118–19
virtue, racialized and gendered, 117, 208n5

wages in antebellum America, 71, 100–101, 151, 173
Wall, Sarah, 168–69
Wall Street, 151
War of 1812, 10
Warren, Ohio, 122
Washington, D.C., 113–16
water, health benefits of, 34, 47
Water Cure College, 28
water cures, 28, 36, 60, 63, 121–22
Weld, Angelina Grimké. *See* Grimké, Angelina
Weld, Theodore Dwight, 67–68, 132, 136, 174
Wells, Susan, 42
Wesley, John, 34
Wesleyan Chapel, Seneca Falls, 109
West Chester, Pennsylvania, woman's rights convention at, 85, 87, 109
Western Reserve Medical College, 2, 126, 130–31
Westminster Review, 73

West of United States, 11, 114, 122, 124, 127–29
Whig Party, 114, 118
Whole World's Temperance Convention, 102–4
Willard, Emma, 14
Wollstonecraft, Mary, 1
Woman and Her Needs (E. O. Smith), 154
"Woman as Physician," 106, 207–8n51
Woman's Christian Temperance Union, 101
Woman's Medical College of Pennsylvania. *See* Female Medical College of Pennsylvania
"Woman's Movement, Educationally Considered, The," 100
Woman's National Loyal League, 179
woman's rights advocacy: black rights linked to, 182; Bremer and, 64–65; criticism of, 160–61; economic discrimination, 151–52; Grimkés and, 66–68, 109–11; health reform, 2, 60, 69–70, 86–87; heart histories and, 61–62; by women preachers, 178. *See also* education of women; feminism and feminists; gender equality; physicians, female; suffrage, female; taxation without representation
woman's rights conventions: Antoinette Brown and, 106; in Boston (1859), 171, 173; in *Glances and Glimpses,* 81; Hunt's lecturing and involvement in, 85–88, 94, 97, 100, 109–11, 207n38; Hunt's support for, 184; Lucretia Mott and, 105; Lucy Stone and, 75, 88, 92, 103, 119; New England Woman's Rights Convention (1854), 118–20; New England Woman's Rights Convention (1855), 129; in New York City, 94, 97, 207n38; in Ohio, 73, 106, 111; patriarchal power in marriage and, 153–54; press coverage of, 79–81, 97, 119, 171; in Seneca Falls, New York, 109; Severance and Dall and, 172–73; Severance's attendance at, 124; in Syracuse, New York, 85–88, 92, 109, 172; taxation without representation and, 92; in West Chester, Pennsylvania, 85, 87, 109; in Worcester, Massachusetts, 73–81, 85–86, 100, 110, 141
woman's rights movement, 73–81, 85–89, 180, 182–83. *See also* feminism and feminists; woman's rights advocacy; woman's rights conventions

women's health. *See* health, women's
Woody, Thomas, 17, 195n55
Worcester, Massachusetts: Wall's protest in, 168; woman's rights conventions in, 73–81, 85–86, 100, 110, 141
Wright, Edmund, 45, 49, 59
Wright, Edmund Wentworth, 175–77
Wright, Harriot Augusta, 49–52, 187
Wright, Lucy, 56
Wright, Martha C., 166
Wright, Sarah Hunt. *See* Hunt, Sarah
Wright, Theodore Francis, 218n103
Wright family, 53–54, 62, 109, 167, 175–76, 186–87

Yearly Meeting of Friends (1851), 106, 115

Zagarri, Rosemarie, 91
Zakrzewska, Marie: biography of, 3–4; Bowditch and, 30; Hunt's autobiography and, 210n2; Hunt's friendship with, 174–75; Hunt's reform network and, 174; Hunt's support for, 2, 130–32; Hunt's twenty-fifth anniversary and, 165; New England Hospital for Women and Children and, 2, 30, 131–32, 185; New England Women's Club and, 185; New York Infirmary for Women and Children and, 2, 131, 167, 174; "science has no sex" and, 132, 203n33; Severance and Dall and, 172; Severance's support for, 130–32

MYRA C. GLENN, professor of American history at Elmira College, earned her PhD in history from the State University of New York at Buffalo. She has authored numerous articles in nineteenth-century American cultural and intellectual history and also published three books—*Jack Tar's Story: The Autobiographies and Memoirs of Sailors in Antebellum America* (2010), *Thomas K. Beecher: Minister to a Changing America, 1824–1900* (1996), and *Campaigns Against Corporal Punishment: Prisoners, Sailors, Women, and Children in Antebellum America* (1984). An indefatigable traveler, Glenn has studied in India and taught in Brazil. She also taught as a Fulbright lecturer at the University of Lleida in Spain and the National University of Córdoba in Argentina.

www.ingramcontent.com/pod-product-compliance
Lightning Source LLC
Chambersburg PA
CBHW030540230426
43665CB00010B/968